The Midwife's Labour
and Birth

DATE DUE

The Midwife's Labour and Birth Handbook

Second Edition

Edited by

Vicky Chapman
RGN, RM(Dip), MA

and

Cathy Charles
RGN, RM, BA(Hons), BSc(Hons)

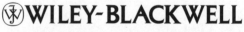

WILEY-BLACKWELL

A John Wiley & Sons, Ltd., Publication

This edition first published 2009
© 2009 by Blackwell Publishing Ltd

Blackwell Publishing was acquired by John Wiley & Sons in February 2007. Blackwell's publishing programme has been merged with Wiley's global Scientific, Technical, and Medical business to form Wiley-Blackwell.

Registered office
John Wiley & Sons Ltd, The Atrium, Southern Gate, Chichester, West Sussex, PO19 8SQ, United Kingdom

Editorial offices
9600 Garsington Road, Oxford, OX4 2DQ, United Kingdom
350 Main Street, Malden, MA 02148-5020, USA

For details of our global editorial offices, for customer services and for information about how to apply for permission to reuse the copyright material in this book please see our website at www.wiley.com/wiley-blackwell.

A catalogue record for this book is available from the British Library.

Library of Congress Cataloging-in-Publication Data

The midwife's labour and birth handbook / edited by Vicky Chapman and Cathy Charles. – 2nd ed.
     p. ; cm.
   Includes bibliographical references and index.
   ISBN: 978-1-4051-6105-3 (pbk. : alk. paper)
1. Midwifery – Handbooks, manuals, etc.
2. Childbirth – Handbooks, manuals, etc.   I. Chapman, Vicky.   II. Charles, Cathy.
   [DNLM: 1. Midwifery – Handbooks. 2. Labor, Obstetric – Handbooks. 3. Parturition – Handbooks.
4. Prenatal Care – Handbooks. WQ 165 M6295 2008]

   RG950.M526 2008
   618.2–dc22

                                                                                    2008006194

Set in 9.5/12 pt Palatino by Aptara Inc., New Delhi, India
Printed in Singapore by C. O. S. Printers Pte Ltd

3   2010

Contents

Preface

If midwifery is both art and science then this book aims to maintain that balance.

The aim of the book is to provide students and practicing midwives with a good working knowledge of midwifery care in the real world, with a special emphasis on support for the mother. It has been written predominantly by practicing midwives combining the latest evidence, knowledge, skills and ideas, aiming to describe best practice rather than just current practice.

Most chapters follow a consistent format for ease of use; the introduction is followed by 'incidence and facts', and then describes the role of the midwife in giving evidence-based, women-centred care. Some chapters use illustrations as visual prompts, for example interpreting fetal head position from vaginal examinations, current suturing techniques and knot tying. Most chapters finish with a summary of the main points and a list of useful organisation and website links.

A pharmacopoeia and blood reference ranges are also included as useful reference material.

This second edition has expanded to include more illustrations and a number of new chapters including twins, induction of labour and caesarean section as well as new chapters on bullying and risk management/litigation.

The latest national guidelines are included where appropriate, but not always accepted uncritically. Guidelines may at times be really helpful in assisting midwives to improve labour care for women; however, they are not without their limitations and obstetric bias. While in many settings it is hard for midwives to 'go against' national or local guidelines, providing midwifery care that is individualised, safe and flexible to the woman's wishes remains paramount. Should a midwife wake a woman in early labour who has dozed off at last to perform a VE because NICE recommends 4-hourly VEs in the first stage of labour? A midwife should assess the total picture and use sensible clinical judgement.

Whilst quantitative research can help determine what constitutes good care, women's stories ('anecdotal accounts') can also provide real insight into what women want and what works for them. How women feel about their labour care may directly influence their progress: the effect of stress hormones on labour has been proved so conclusively that it is amazing that there are still obstetricians and midwives who practise as if it is not so. There is simply no excuse for creating a harsh birthing environment with bright fluorescent overhead lights and loud noise, where people can wander into a room without permission, fail to smile or communicate with the woman, or deny her the support of a second birthing partner even though these are non-clinical issues and do not compromise on 'safety'. It is so sad when a woman is told that she cannot have a water birth because 'no-one here knows how to do them'.

Midwives have a difficult job to do. We work in many different settings including homes, birthing centres and acute obstetric units. Sometimes the needs of the organisation can make us feel that the needs of the women we care for are coming second: witness the lone midwife trying to offer skin-to-skin contact for a 32-week baby whilst a sceptical room looks on.

This book recognises the problems many midwives face working within the hospital system. Providing woman-centred care can be a real challenge, especially if it means that a midwife supports a woman who wants something that appears out of step with the care usually provided in that setting. A solid knowledge base helps to give the midwife confidence to provide care that is safe and supportive, and in accordance with the woman's wishes.

Good midwives never forget that at the centre of the birth drama there is a real person, bringing another real person into the world.

Acknowledgements

I would like to extend my appreciation and thanks to Cathy Charles who has done the majority of the work producing this book (amazingly she has retained her great sense of humour and clear midwifery perspective throughout).

I would also like to thank my very good friend Ulrike who has supported me in so many ways, and generously given up her time to help me with my younger children when trying to write.

My thanks must also go to my husband, Kelvin, for his all round support; also to my wonderful grandmother, Grace Page, for her ongoing interest and encouragement and lastly my sister Sue.

Vicky Chapman

I would like to extend similar thanks to Vicky Chapman for her endless support and wise guidance. I thank the writers for their hard work and patience, and my wonderful husband, Nigel, for his tolerance of me tapping on the laptop in bed at 3 a.m.

Cathy Charles

Contributors

The Editors

Vicky Chapman, *RGN, RM(Dip), MA*
As a midwife Vicky has worked in a variety of hospital settings and as a caseload midwife. She has a particular interest in normal birth, as well as an interest the politics of childbirth and their impact on women's birth experiences. She is presently a full-time mother of four, including twins.

Cathy Charles, *RGN, RM, BA(Hons), BSc(Hons)*
Cathy is a midwife and ventouse practitioner, practising in acute and community settings within the Wiltshire Health Care Trust. In this trust, 1500 out of 5000 births take place in one of five stand-alone midwife-led community units or at home. Cathy has acted as a visiting lecturer, and written articles on practising as a midwife ventouse practitioner in a community unit. Like Vicky, Cathy has an interest in water and home births. She teaches aquanatal classes. She also gained experience of investigating adverse events in a former post as clinical audit/risk management co-ordinator and has been a supervisor of midwives.

Contributors

Annette Briley, *SRN, RM, MSc*
Annette is a clinical trials midwifery manager and consultant midwife within the Maternal and Fetal Research Unit at St Thomas' Hospital, London. She was a clinical midwife for many years, working in all areas of maternity provision, including obstetric ultrasound. Annette joined the St Thomas' research team in 1997 and was involved in a major study on vitamins in pre-eclampsia. She has since worked on numerous pregnancy-related research projects. Annette has worked with Tommy's, the baby charity, and Parentalk, a charity that aims to inspire and aid parents, and has written a book with Tim Mungeam, Parentalk's CEO, about the first six weeks of parenthood.

Nick Castle, *DipIMC, RCS(Ed), RGN, ENB 100, SRParamedic, MSc(Dist)*
Nick is a nurse consultant in resuscitation and emergency care in a large district general hospital and undertakes a wide range of training, research, audit and clinical duties. Nick is married with twin girls.

Jo Coggins, *DipHE (Midwifery) (Dist), BSc(Hons)*
Jo is a team midwife in Wiltshire where she lives with her partner Mark. She previously practised in both acute and community settings in Bath. Following recent closure of the local birthing unit, Jo and her colleague have adopted a 'team midwifery' model to

ensure women in the area continue to receive a quality service, in which their needs and choices are foremost. A steep rise in the homebirth rate has been a particular success. In addition to her clinical role, Jo enjoys writing and has published articles in various midwifery journals. She is currently undertaking an MSc in Advanced Practice at the University of the West of England, Bristol.

Julie Davis, *RGN, RM*
Julie Davis qualified as a midwife in 1994. She is a mother of two children and works part-time at Frimley Park Hospital in Surrey.

Mary-Lou Elliott, *RM, BA(Hons)*
Mary-Lou qualified as a midwife in 1998 and is a midwife at the Royal United Hospital in Bath. Her experience is varied, having worked with the risk management team, a community birthing centre and on the community teams in the city. She is currently also employed by the University of the West of England as a student support mid-wife/visiting clinical educator.

Hilary Field, *RGN, RSCN, RM, DHyp, PDCHyp, MBSCH*
Hilary has been a midwife since 1983 and is currently working part-time at a midwife-led maternity unit in Witshire. Having a keen interest in complementary therapy, she qualified as a reflexologist in 1995 and clinical hypnotherapist in 2005. Hilary now lectures on clinical hypnosis in pregnancy, childbirth and postnatally at the University of the West of England and the London College of Clinical Hypnosis, having presented a masterclass for hypnotherapists. She also works in a voluntary capacity for the Birth Trauma Association using Eye Movement Desensitisation and Reprocessing for resolving birth trauma. More details on her website www.sojustrelax.co.uk.

Janet Gwillim, *RGN, RM, ADM*
Janet trained as a general nurse in 1968 and a midwife in 1969. After suspending her career to have two children, she returned to midwifery and completed the Advanced Diploma in Midwifery and the Supervisor of Midwives course. Janet attended the first woman to have a water birth in East Kent, and she has been an enthusiastic teacher and resource on water and home births. Following the Changing Childbirth Report in 1993, Janet helped to change the way midwives work in southeast Kent by gaining funding for a pilot scheme for a midwifery group practice called JACANES, which provided choice and continuity for midwives and women. Janet retired from midwifery in February 2002 and is now thoroughly enjoying being a grandparent.

Sheila Miskelly, *RGN, RM, Dip HE*
Sheila is a practice development midwife, teaching skills drills and other clinical skills who until recently worked in a stand-alone midwifery-led unit for 8 years, enjoying all the pleasures of woman-centred care and homebirths.

Bryony Read, *RM, BA(Hons)*
Bryony completed her midwifery degree from Oxford Brookes in 2001 and worked at the John Radcliffe in Oxford until 2003. Since then she has worked at the Princess Royal University Hospital in Kent, working mainly on delivery suite with rotations to the

maternity ward and community. In 2005, after completing a course on aromatherapy in childbirth, Bryony was part of a team that implemented aromatherapy for use on the delivery suite and postnatal ward.

Caroline Rutter, *Cert Ed, RM Dip(HEM), BSc(Hons)*
Caroline was an NCT teacher prior to becoming a midwife in 1993. She now works as a midwife in a stand-alone midwife-led maternity unit in Wiltshire. Caroline is also a visiting lecturer at University of the West of England.

Lesley Shuttler, *RN(Dip), RM, BSc(Hons)*
Lesley is married with two daughters. She is an antenatal teacher and tutor with the National Childbirth Trust and has been a midwife since 1995. Lesley strongly believes in women's innate ability to birth their babies and the need to promote and support informed choice at all times.

List of abbreviations

AFE   Amniotic fluid embolism
AFI   Amniotic fluid index
AIDS   Acquired immunodeficiency syndrome
ALT   Alanine transaminase
APTT   Activated partial thromboplastin time
ARM   Artificial rupture of the membranes
AST   Aspartate transaminase
BLS   Basic life support
BNF   British National Formulary (of drugs)
BP   Blood pressure
bpm   Beats per minute
BVM   Bag-valve-mask (device)
CPD   Cephalopelvic disproportion
CS   Caesarean section
CTG   Cardiotocograph/cardiotocography
CVP   Central venous pressure
DIC   Disseminated intravascular coagulation
ECV   External cephalic version
EDTA   Ethylenediamine tetra acetic acid
EFM   Electronic fetal monitoring
ETT   Endotracheal tube
FBC   Full blood count
FBS   Fetal blood sampling
FHR   Fetal heart rate
FSE   Fetal scalp electrode
Hb   Haemoglobin
HELLP   Haemolysis, elevated liver enzymes, low platelets
HDN   Haemorrhagic disease of the newborn
HIV   Human immunodeficiency virus
IA   Intermittent auscultation
IM   Intramuscular
IOL   Induction of labour
IUGR   Intrauterine growth restriction/retardation
ICU   Intensive care unit
ITU   Intensive therapy unit
IV   Intravenous
MAP   Mean arterial pressure
MCV   Mean corpuscular volume
MROP   Manual removal of the placenta

NHS	National Health Service
NICE	National Institute for Health and Clinical Excellence
NICU	Neonatal intensive care unit
OA	Occipitoanterior
OP	Occipitoposterior
PCV	Packed cell volume
PPH	Postpartum haemorrhage
PPROM	Preterm prelabour rupture of the membranes
PROM	Prelabour rupture of the membranes
PT	Prothrombin time
RBC	Red blood cell
RCM	Royal College of Midwives
RCT	Randomised controlled trial
RCOG	Royal College of Obstetricians and Gynaecologists
RDS	Respiratory distress syndrome
SCBU	Special care baby unit
SOM	Supervisor of midwives
TENS	Transcutaneous electrical nerve stimulation
VBAC	Vaginal birth after caesarean
VKDB	Vitamin K deficiency bleeding
VE	Vaginal examination
VF	Ventricular fibrillation
VT	Ventricular tachycardia
WBC	White blood cells

1 Labour and normal birth

Cathy Charles

Introduction

'Undisturbed birth . . . is the balance and involvement of an exquisitely complex and finely tuned orchestra of hormones' (Buckley, 2004a).

The most exciting activity of a midwife is assisting a woman in labour. The care and support of a midwife may well have a direct result on a woman's ability to labour and birth her baby. Every woman and each birthing experience is unique.

Many midwives manage excessive workloads and, particularly in hospitals, may be pressured by colleagues and policies into offering medicalised care. Yet the midwifery philosophy of helping women to work with their amazing bodies enables many women to have a safe pleasurable birth. Most good midwives find ways to provide good care, whatever the environment, and their example will be passed on to the colleagues and students with whom they work.

Some labours are inherently harder than others, despite all the best efforts of woman and midwife, and the midwife should be flexible and adaptable, accepting that it may be neither the midwife's nor the mother's fault if things do not go to plan. The aim is a healthy happy outcome, whatever the means.

This chapter aims to give an overview of the process of labour, but it is recognised that labour does not simplistically divide into distinct stages. It is a complex phenomenon of interdependent physical, hormonal and emotional changes, which can vary enormously between individual women. The limitation of the medical model undermines the importance of the midwife's observation and interpretation of a woman's behaviour.

Facts

- The National Service Framework recommends that women should have as normal a labour and birth as possible, and medical intervention should be used only when beneficial to mother and/or baby (Department of Health (DoH), 2004).
- Women should be offered the choice of birth at home, in a midwife-led unit or in an obstetric unit (National Institute for Health and Clinical Excellence (NICE), 2007). An obstetric unit may be advised for women with certain problems, but it remains their choice.
- Women should be offered one-to-one care in labour (NICE, 2007). The presence of a caring and supportive caregiver has been proved to shorten labour, reduce intervention and improve neonatal outcomes (Green *et al.*, 2000; Hodnett *et al.*, 2004).
- Women tend to rate midwifery support as positive, although a few midwives are regarded as 'off-hand', 'bossy' or 'unhelpful' (Redshaw *et al.*, 2007).
- A pleasurable labour can bring great joy but 5–6% mothers develop birth-related post-traumatic stress disorder (Kitzinger & Kitzinger, 2007).
- The attitude of the caregiver seems to be the most powerful influence on women's satisfaction in labour (NICE, 2007).

Signs that precede labour

Women often describe feeling restless and strange prior to going into labour, sometimes experiencing spurts of energy or undertaking 'nesting' activities (Burvill, 2002). Physical symptoms of prelabour may include:

- low backache and deep pelvic discomfort as the baby descends into the pelvis;
- upset stomach/diarrhoea;
- intermittent episodes of regular tightening for days or weeks prior to birth;
- loss of operculum ('show') usually clear or lightly bloodstained;
- increased vaginal leaking or 'cervical weep'; and
- spontaneous rupture of membranes (ROM) – usually unmistakeable, but sometimes less so, particularly if the head is well engaged (see Boxes 1.1 and 1.2 for diagnosis and management of ROM).

Box 1.1   Diagnosis of PROM.

Woman's history
- This is usually conclusive in itself (Walsh, 2001a).
- Clarify the time of loss and the appearance and approximate amount of fluid.

Observe the liquor
- The pad is usually soaked: if no liquor evident, ask the woman to walk around for an hour and check again.
- Liquor may be:
  - Clear, straw-coloured or pink: it should smell fresh.
  - Bloodstained: if mucoid contamination, this is probably a show – but perform CTG if you doubt this (NICE, 2007).
  - Offensive smelling: this may indicate infection.
  - Meconium-stained (green): a term baby may simply have passed meconium naturally, but always pay close attention to meconium. Light staining is less of a concern,

Box 1.1   (*Continued*)

but dark green or black colouring and/or thick and tenacious meconium means it is fresh, and this could be more serious. NICE (2007) advises continuous EFM for significant meconium and 'consider' continuous EFM for light staining, depending on the stage of labour, any other risks, volume of liquor and FHR.

Speculum examination
- If the history is unmistakable or the woman is in labour, there is no need for a speculum examination.
- Never perform a vaginal examination unless the woman is having regular strong contractions and there is a good reason to do so: it risks ascending infection.
- To perform:
  - Suggest that the woman lies down for a while to allow liquor to pool.
  - Lubricate the speculum and gently insert it: the mother may find that raising her bottom (on her fists or a pillow) allows easier and more comfortable access.
  - If no liquor visible, ask her to cough: liquor may then trickle through the cervix and collect in the speculum bill.
  - Amnisticks (nitrazine test) are no longer recommended due to high false positive rates.

Box 1.2   Management of PROM at term.

Await labour
The woman can await the onset of labour in the comfort of her home, away from potential infection and unnecessary interventions. There is no need to perform vaginal swabs (NICE, 2007).

Check temperature
Ask her to do this 4-hourly during waking hours (NICE, 2007).

Observe liquor
Observe liquor and report any change in colour or smell.

Listen to the fetal heart
Intermittent auscultation is fine: there is no need for a CTG unless meconium-stained liquor observed. Observe fetal activity.

General advice
- Suggest that the woman avoids sexual intercourse or putting anything into her vagina.
- Suggest that she wipes from front to back after having her bowels opened.
- Inform her that bathing or showering is not associated with any increase in infection.
- Advise her to report any reduced fetal movements, uterine tenderness, pyrexia or feverish symptoms.
- Ask her to come back after 24 hours if labour has not started.
- Tell her that 60% women go into labour within 24 hours.
  If no labour within 24 h (NICE, 2007)
- NICE advises induction of labour after 24 hours of PROM (see Chapter 18). The woman will then be advised to remain in hospital for 12 hours afterwards so that the baby can be observed.
- **If a woman chooses to wait longer**, continue as above and review every 24 hours.
- After birth observe asymptomatic babies (PROM > 24 hours) for 12 hours: at 1 hour, 2 hours and then 2-hourly for 10 hours: observe general well-being, chest movements and nasal flare, colour, tone, feeding temperature, heart rate and respiration. Ask the mother to report any concerns.

Not all women seek advice at this stage. For those who do, the midwife should act as a listener and reassure the woman that these prelabour signs are normal. Avoid using negative terms such as 'false labour'.

First stage of labour

Latent stage

Characteristics of latent stage

NICE (2007) describes this as:

> '...a period of time, not necessarily continuous, when:
> - there are painful contractions, and
> - there is some cervical change, including cervical effacement and dilatation up to 4 cm'

Midwifery care in latent phase

Women may be excited and/or anxious. They will need a warm response and explicit information about what is happening to them. In very early labour they may need just verbal reassurance; they may make several phone calls.

While not offered everywhere, home assessment is preferable to hospital; it reduces analgesia use, labour augmentation and caesarean section (CS) and is therefore probably also cost-effective. Women report greater feelings of control and an improved birth experience (McNiven *et al.*, 1998; Walsh, 2000a; Lauzon & Hodnett, 2002).

Some women experience a prolonged latent phase, which may be tiring and demoralising, requiring more support (see section 'Prolonged latent phase', Chapter 8). These women may undergo repeated visits/assessments and feel that something is going wrong. Most women however cope well.

- Always greet a woman warmly and make her feel special.
- Observe, listen and acknowledge her excitement. Her first contact with a midwife is important as it will establish trust.
- Be positive but realistic: many women, especially primigravidae, are overoptimistic about progress.
- Women whose first language is not English may need extra reassurance, careful explanations and sensitivity to personal and cultural preferences. A translator that the woman is comfortable with should have been arranged prior to labour, but this is sometimes not the case.
- If labour is not established, gently explain that she is not in strong labour yet and, if it is night time, suggest she attempts to go back to sleep, or at least tries to rest. During the day she should try to relax, try warm baths or distractions such as shopping, walking or watching a film.
- If the woman has sougth direct contact, then if all is well she should be left at home, or discharged home if in hospital, to establish in labour.
- Encourage her to eat and drink at not to focus on labour and coping techniques too early; instead she should try to get on with everyday life (Simkin & Ancheta, 2005).

Table 1.1   Baseline observations in labour.

Observation	Frequency	Significance
Blood pressure Normal range: Systolic: 100–140 mm Hg Diastolic: 60–90 mm Hg (Baston, 2001)	Tested at labour onset and then hourly (NICE, 2007)	Hypertension can be caused by: • Anxiety and pain • General anaesthesia • Pre-eclampsia Pre-eclampsia is defined as: • Diastolic BP ≥ 90 mm Hg on two or more occasions at least 4 hours apart • Diastolic BP ≥ 110 mm Hg on one occasion • Systolic >160 mm Hg or diastolic ≥ 110 mm Hg or a mean arterial pressure >125 mm Hg • BP ≥ 140/90 mm Hg with proteinuria (≥2+) (see Chapter 19) Hypotension can be caused by: • An epidural/top-up • Aortocaval occlusion secondary to lying supine • Haemorrhage and hypovolaemic shock (see Chapter 15)
Pulse rate Normal range: 55–90 beats/min	Tested at labour onset and then hourly when checking the fetal heart (NICE, 2007)	Tachycardia ≥100 bpm can be caused by (Baston, 2001): • Anxiety, pain, hyperventilation • Dehydration, pyrexia • Exertion • Obstructed labour • Haemorrhage, anaemia and shock Bradycardia ≤55 bpm can be caused by: • Rest and relaxation • Injury and shock • Myocardial infarction
Temperature Normally 36–37°C	Tested at labour onset and then 4-hourly (NICE, 2007) or hourly if in birthing pool	Pyrexia >37°C can be caused by: • Infection • Epidural – usually low-grade pyrexia but rises with time • Dehydration • Overheated birth pool (see Chapter 7)

- The physical check includes the following:
  - **Baseline observations.** Blood pressure (BP), pulse and temperature (see Table 1.1).
  - **Urinalysis.** Testing a sample at labour onset is recommended by NICE (2007), although its helpfulness in a normotensive woman is debatable since vaginal secretions, e.g. liquor, often contaminate the sample and abnormal findings are often ignored.
  - **Abdominal palpation.** Ascertain fundal height, lie, presentation, position and engagement (see Fig. 1.1). Ask about fetal movements.
  - **Fetal heart (FH) auscultation.** Low-risk women should be offered intermittent auscultation. There is no place for a 'routine admission trace' for low-risk women (NICE, 2007) (see Chapter 3 for more detail).

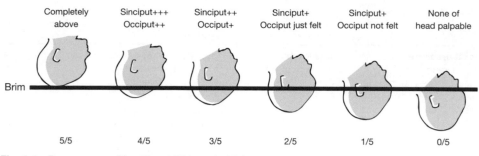

Fig. 1.1 Engagement of fetal head (fifths palpable).

- **Vaginal examination** (VE) is not usually warranted if contractions are <5 min apart and lasting >60 seconds unless the woman really wants one.
- **Ruptured membranes** (see Box 1.1 for diagnosis) are usually obvious. If the woman is contracting, there is no need to do anything other than note the history and observe the liquor. Do not perform a VE unless the woman really wants one and she is contracting strongly and regularly, due to risk of infection.

Prelabour rupture of the membranes at term

Some women experience prelabour rupture of the membranes (PROM) at term. There are some risks, including infection, cord prolapse and sometimes the iatrogenic consequences of intervention. However, most women with PROM will go into labour spontaneously and have a good outcome. For management see Box 1.2. Refer to Chapter 18 for more information.

Established first stage of labour

Characteristics of the established first stage

In early labour:
- The woman may eat, laugh and talk between contractions.
- Contractions become stronger and increasingly painful, 2–5 minutes apart lasting ≤60 seconds.
- The cervix is mid to anterior, soft, effaced (not always fully effaced in multiparous women) and >4 cm dilated.

As labour advances:
- The woman usually becomes quieter, behaves more instinctively, withdrawing as the primitive parts of the brain take over (Ockenden, 2001).
- During contractions she may become less mobile, holding someone/something during a contraction or stand legs astride and rock her hips. She may close her eyes and breathe heavily and rhythmically (Burvill, 2002), moaning or calling out during the most painful contractions.
- Talking may be brief, e.g. 'water' or 'back'. This is not the time for others to chat. Lemay (2000) echoes Dr Michel Odent's constant advice in advising midwives: 'the most important thing is *do not disturb the birthing woman*'. Midwives are usually adept

at reading cues. Others unfamiliar with labour behaviour, including her partner and students, may need guidance to avoid disturbing her, particularly during a contraction. Before auscultating the FH, first speak in a quiet voice or touch the woman's arm; do not always expect an answer.

Midwifery care in established first stage

The *Royal College of Midwives (RCM) Campaign for Normal Birth* (available at: www. rcmnormalbirth.org.uk) has produced eight top tips to enhance women's birth experience. These are listed over the page in Box 1.3.

- **Make sure your manner is warm.** Involve her partner. Clarify how they prefer to be addressed. Ideally, the woman will have already met her midwife antenatally. However this is not always possible. A good midwife, familiar or not, will quickly establish a good rapport. Kind words, a constant presence and appropriate touch are proven powerful analgesics.
- **Take a clear history.** Discuss previous pregnancies, labours and births: how does the woman feel about these? Ask about vaginal loss, 'show', time of onset of tightenings. Look for relevant risk factors.
- **Review the notes.** Check any ultrasound scans for placental location and dating or size estimation. Ensure you have a blood group and recent haemoglobin result. Check any allergies.
- **Offer continuous support.** Cochrane review (Hodnett *et al.*, 2004) found that continuous support in labour:
  - reduces use of pharmacological analgesia including epidural;
  - makes a spontaneous birth more likely, with fewer instrumental deliveries and caesarean sections;
  - shortens labour; and
  - increases women's satisfaction with labour.

Supporting a woman and her partner in labour is an intense relationship, hour after hour, and can be physically and mentally demanding. Providing emotional support, monitoring labour and documenting care may mean that the midwife can hardly leave the woman's side. Involving the birth partner(s) or a doula can both support the midwife and enhance the quality of support the woman receives. There should be no restriction on the number of birth partners present, although be very sure that they are the people the mother really wants. Sometimes women accede to the desires of sisters or friends to be at the birth. Birth however is not a spectator sport: if they are chatting amongst themselves and not supporting the woman then the midwife may need to offer them some direction or tactfully suggest they leave the room.

- **"Listen to her" (RCM, 2005).** Talk through any birth plans early, while the woman is still able to concentrate. As labour progresses, observe her verbal and body language and tell her how well she is coping, offering simple clear information. Try not to leave her alone unless she wishes this.
- **"Build her a nest" (RCM, 2005).** In order to make the birth environment welcoming prepare the room before she arrives.
  - Mammals like warm dark places to nest, so keep it relaxed with low lighting.

- ○ Remove unnecessary monitors/equipment.
- ○ Noise, particularly other women giving birth, can be distressing; low music may help cut out such noise. Avoid placing a woman arriving in labour adjoining someone who is noisy.
- ○ Keep interruptions to a minimum; always knock before entering a room and do not accept anyone else failing to do this.
- ○ If there is a bed in the room, consider pushing it to the side so that it is not the centrepiece (National Childbirth Trust (NCT), 2003).

Box 1.3   Eight top tips for normal birth.

---

(1) Wait and see

The single practice most likely to help a woman have a normal birth is patience. In order to be able to let natural physiology take its own time, we have to be very confident of our own knowledge and experience.

(2) Build her a nest

Mammals try to find warm, secure, dark places to give birth – and human beings are no exception.

(3) Get her off the bed

Gravity is our greatest aid in giving birth, but for historical and cultural reasons (now obsolete) in this society we make women give birth on their backs. We need to help women understand and practise alternative positions antenatally, feel free to be mobile and try different positions during labour and birth.

(4) Justify intervention

Technology is wonderful, except where it gets in the way. We need to ask ourselves 'Is it really necessary?' And not to do it unless it is indicated.

(5) Listen to her

Women themselves are the best source of information about what they need. What we need to do is to get to know her, listen to her, understand her, talk to her and think about how we are contributing to her sense of achievement.

(6) Keep a diary

One of the best sources for learning is our own observations. Especially when we can look back at them and realise what we have learned and discovered since then. Write down what happened today: how you felt and what you learned.

(7) Trust your intuition

Intuition is the knowledge that comes from the multitude of perceptions that we make, which are too subtle to be noticed. With experience and reflection we can understand what these patterns are telling us – picking up and anticipating a woman's progress, needs and feelings.

(8) Be a role model

Our behaviour influences others – for better or worse. Midwifery really does need exemplars who can model the practices, behaviour and attitudes that facilitate normal birth. Start being a role model today.

RCM (2005).

- • **Eating and drinking.** Women often want to eat in early (rarely later) labour. Offer her what she feels like, e.g. high-calorie snacks, fruit juice, tea, toast, cereal and biscuits (Johnson *et al.*, 2000). Drinking well will prevent dehydration, and a light diet is appropriate unless the woman has recently had opioids or is at higher risk of a general anaesthetic (NICE, 2007). Ensure her birth attendants eat too.

- **Basic observations (see Table 1.1).** There is a lack of evidence supporting many routine labour observations (Crowther *et al.*, 2000; NICE, 2007), but NICE (2007) recommends hourly pulse (checked simultaneously with the fetal heart rate (FHR)) and BP, 4-hourly temperature. Consider hourly temperature if water birth (see Chapter 7).
- **Frequent micturition.** It should be encouraged, but urinalysis in labour is probably pointless. NICE (2007) recommends testing one sample at the onset of labour but the benefit is unclear as vaginal secretions and liquor commonly contaminate the sample and 'abnormal findings' are often, in practice, ignored.
- **Observe vaginal loss discreetly**, e.g. liquor, meconium, blood and offensive smell.
- **FH auscultation:** NICE (2007) recommends every 15 min for 1 min following a contraction. Midwives may disagree with this guidance that is based on consensus opinion rather than clear evidence of benefit and may choose to monitor less than every 15 min early in labour or, more frequently, at other times, e.g. following spontaneous rupture of the membranes or a VE. For more information see Chapter 3.

Assessing progress in labour

'... Justify intervention' (RCM, 2005).

Unless birth is imminent, most midwives undertake *abdominal palpation* when taking on a woman's care and, periodically thereafter, to ascertain the lie, position and presentation of the baby. Engagement is particularly helpful to monitor descent of the presenting part and thus labour progress (see Fig. 1.1). However some women may find this examination painful, particularly in advanced labour.

The assessment of progress can also be judged *observationally*: by the woman's contractions and her verbal and non-verbal response to them (Stuart, 2000; Burvill, 2002; see Table 1.2). Some midwives also observe the 'purple line', which may gradually extend from the anal margin up to the nape of the buttocks by full dilatation (Hobbs, 1998).

Vaginal examination and artificial rupture of the membranes

VEs in labour are an invasive, subjective intervention of unproven benefit (Crowther *et al.*, 2000). However, they do remain the accepted method for assessing the progress of labour (see Chapter 2).

It can be difficult for woman to decline a VE or for the midwife to choose to perform one more selectively (i.e. when she/he feels one is best indicated). Even in low-risk births, midwives often feel pressured to adhere to guidelines which lack good evidence and have a medical bias.

NICE (2007) recommends the following:

- Four-hourly VEs in the first stage of labour.
- Cervical dilatation of 0.5 cm/hour as reasonable progress (Crowther *et al.*, 2000; NICE, 2007).

Table 1.2   Contractions and women's typical behaviour.

Criteria	Cervical dilatation (cm)				
	0–3	3–4	4–7	7–9	9–10
Frequency of contractions	May be irregular and may sometimes stop; gradually increasing in frequency	2:10 min Increasingly regular, lasting 20–40 seconds	3:10 min Regular, lasting ≥60 seconds	3–4:10 min Regular, lasting ≥60 seconds	4–5:10 min Sometimes almost continuous, although can 'fade away' for a while in transition
Pain of contractions	Varying from painless/mild/ stronger	Becoming more painful but usually bearable		Increasingly painful	Often almost (sometimes completely) unbearable pain, although if in transitional stage may have some respite
Behaviour	Chatty, nervous, excited, able to make jokes and laugh; often able to talk through contractions; may use learned breathing techniques too early and need reminding to pace herself		Withdrawing more; deeper 'sighing' breathing; sense of humour fading	Becoming vocal: crying out with some contractions; may express irritation when touched	Appears withdrawn, in another world; may not reply or answer sharply; concentrating on breathing, which slows and deepens with a contraction; throaty grunting noises, crying out with expiration: may panic and express desperate ideas: 'I *can't do this!*'
Movement and posture	Mobile during contractions		Needing to stop and concentrate during contractions	Grasps abdomen and leans forward; may rock, curl toes	Less mobile, holding on to something during a contraction; often eyes closed, but may open wide in surprise with pushing urge

N.B. This is only a broad guide, intended to stimulate awareness of external signs. There is in reality no such thing as a 'typical labour' and women's behaviour will of course vary. Most women exhibit the above to some degree.

- A 4-hour rather than 2-hour action line on the partogram. This appears to reduce intervention for primigravidae with no adverse maternal or neonatal outcomes (Lavender *et al.*, 2006; NICE, 2007).
- In normally progressing labour, amniotomy should not be performed routinely (NICE, 2007). The decision should only be made in consultation with the woman,

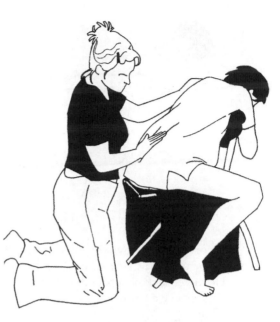

Fig. 1.2 Hands on comfort: massage and touch.

when the evidence is discussed and the intervention justified and not minimised (RCM, 2005) (see also Chapter 2 for more on ARM).

(For more on partograms and assessing progress see Chapter 8.)

- *Document* all care on the partogram and in the notes, including any problems, interventions or referrals (for more on record keeping see Chapter 22).

Analgesia

Most midwives encourage natural and non-interventionist methods first, with pharmacological methods only if these methods are deemed insufficient. Pain is a complex phenomenon and a pain-free labour will not necessarily be more satisfying; working with women's pain rather than alleviating it underpins many midwives' practice (Downe, 2004).

The following is a brief overview.

Non-pharmacological analgesia

- **Massage and touch.** These can be powerful analgesics (Fig. 1.2), e.g. back rubbing, breathing and relaxation, massage and touch. These encourage pain-relieving endorphin release. Never underestimate the effect of being 'with woman'.

    Be sensitive. Labour can induce flashbacks for sexual abuse victims (see Chapter 2) and some women come from cultures where touching by strangers can feel invasive.
- **Distraction**, e.g. breathing patterns, music and television.
- **Position changes with aids.** These include beanbags, wedges, stools and birthing balls (e.g. Figs. 1.3 and 1.4).
- **Transcutaneous electrical nerve stimulation (TENS).** Despite conflicting opinions on effectiveness of TENS, including possible placebo effect, many women

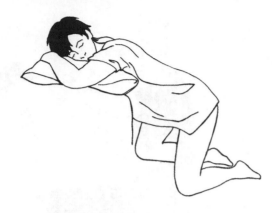

Fig. 1.3   Kneeling forwards onto a pillow.

report that it provides good pain relief, especially in the first stage of labour (Johnson, 1997). There is no adverse effect on the mother or baby (Mainstone, 2004). However lack of substantial non-anecdotal evidence has led NICE (2007) to conclude, very controversially, that TENS should not be recommended in established labour.

- **Aromatherapy.** Only oils known to be safe in pregnancy should be used: some are contraindicated in pregnancy (Tiran, 2000). Continuous vaporisation may impede concentration and have adverse maternal effects (Tiran, 2006). Oils should be diluted, preferably to half the usual dilution in pregnancy. For a bath, adding the drops to milk prior to putting them in water helps them disperse.
- **Other methods, e.g. acupuncture/pressure, reflexology, shiatsu, yoga, hypnosis (including self-hypnosis), homeopathic and herbal remedies.** Normally only midwives trained in these specialist areas or qualified practitioners offer these therapies. Non-pharmacological methods are notoriously difficult to evaluate by standard research methods. Acupuncture and hypnosis are the only complementary therapies that have been clinically proved to work (Smith *et al.*, 2006; NICE, 2007).
- **Water.** Deep-water immersion has unique benefits (see Chapter 7). The opportunity to labour in water should be more widely adopted as part of routine care and is recommended by NICE (2007).

Pharmacological analgesia

- **Entonox (nitrous oxide).** This is possibly the most commonly used labour analgesic in the UK. There is little evidence on the effects of entonox on a mother or baby,

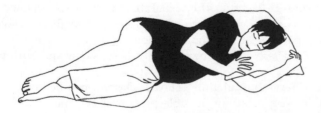

Fig. 1.4   Side lying.

and it is usually assumed that it is fairly safe. There are minor side effects, e.g. dry mouth or nausea, but entonox is quickly excreted from the woman's system and so the effects wear off rapidly if the woman stops using it. Long-term exposure risks are well documented, including the risk to pregnant staff with high labour ward workloads (Robertson, 2006).

- **Opioids, e.g. pethidine.** It is usually given intramuscularly but occasionally by patient-controlled analgesia. Antiemetics should be given prophylactically (NICE, 2007). Opioids can 'take the edge off' the pain for some women, inducing a feeling of well-being and allowing some rest. Many midwives will recount stories of anxious, scared women who on receiving pethidine fall into a doze and wake up fully dilated. Arguably, this 'emotional dystocia' (Simkin & Ancheta, 2005) can be addressed in other ways, e.g. good caring support. There are considerable doubts about effectiveness of opioid and concern about potential maternal, fetal and neonatal side effects. Opioids can cause maternal nausea, vomiting and hypotension (Elbourne & Wiseman, 2004). Some women feel disorientated and out of control.

  Neonatal side effects include respiratory depression (which may require injection of the antagonist **naloxone**), subdued behaviour patterns, including a lack of responsiveness to sights and sounds, drowsiness and impaired early breastfeeding (Elbourne & Wiseman, 2004; NICE, 2007). Babies of mothers receiving opiates in labour appear more likely to become addicted to opiates/amphetamines in later life (Jacobsen *et al.*, 1988, 1990; Nyberg *et al.*, 2000).

- **Regional anaesthesia** is used by around a third of UK women for birth (NHS Maternity Statistics, 2007) and aims to remove pain from the lower half of the body. It can take the form of an epidural, a spinal or a combination of both.
  ○ *Epidural anaesthesia* involves administration of local anaesthetic and/or opiates into the epidural space around the spinal column.
  ○ *Spinal anaesthesia* involves an opiate, and sometimes anaesthetic drug injected through the covering of the spinal cord, and is usually short acting.
  ○ *Combined epidural–spinal anaesthesia* appears no better than epidural alone (Simmons *et al.*, 2007), but it is rapid (NICE, 2007).

  Women should be informed about the implications for their labour before choosing regional anaesthesia (NICE, 2007). Whilst for many women regional anaesthesia may provide welcome relief from pain, regional anaesthetic drugs can cause pyrexia, leg weakness, poor mobility, longer labour, increased malposition, increased oxytocin augmentation and significant perineal trauma due to increased instrumental delivery (Leighton & Halpern, 2002; Lieberman & O'Donaghue, 2002; Howell, 2004). Opiates cross the placenta and can sedate the fetus: some studies have reported decreased mother–baby interaction and poorer breastfeeding rates following epidural anaesthesia (Buckley, 2004b).

  Care for a woman with regional anaesthesia includes:
  ○ intravenous (IV) access, hourly sensory block check and continual pain assessment;
  ○ BP monitoring every 5 min for 15 min, particularly following establishment of block and following bolus administration (top-up) (NICE, 2007);
  ○ continuous cardiotocography (CTG) for 30 min following establishment of block and following bolus administration (top up) (NICE, 2007);

○ regular position changes and non-supine (NICE, 2007), side lying or all four position (this will depend on the block) (Downe, 2004) with attention to pressure areas;

○ bladder care: regular (in and out catheter) or continuous bladder drainage; and

○ avoidance of aortocaval compression.

See pharmacopoeia (Chapter 24) for more information.

Mobility and positions

'Get her off the bed' (RCM, 2005).

Midwives are the major influence on whether a woman is free to mobilise or not. Actively encouraging women to mobilise during childbirth is a fundamental component of good midwifery practice and is a safe, cost-effective way of reducing complications caused by restricted mobility and semi-recumbent postures (Gupta *et al.*, 2004), as well as enriching the woman's birth experience.

Women's expectations of how to behave in labour, unfamiliar surroundings, the bed in the labour room, lack of privacy and the medical model of care, all inhibit mobility in labour. Many women spend their labour lying on their backs propped up by pillows or wedges. Most women labouring upright say they would do the same again, and those who remained supine would prefer to be upright for any subsequent labour and birth (MIDIRS, 2007). Evidence supports this choice.

However, one in five women still report that they were not enabled to choose the most comfortable position in labour (Redshaw *et al.*, 2007).

'Think about how you can help the woman to adopt other positions in labour – observe what works and what doesn't, and review when and why these positions were most successful. Your knowledge of anatomy can also help you to understand how different positions aid the physiological processes (e.g., the curve of Carus)' (RCM, 2005).

Try to witness other midwives during deliveries or ask a colleague for support when the mother is giving birth in a non-supine position.

● Have you discussed with the woman in labour why it is important to mobilise in labour? By pointing out that labour is more likely to be shorter and less painful, you will give her 'permission' to move around freely and do what she feels is best for her.

● Women often get stuck on the bed following an examination or during electronic fetal monitoring (EFM). Suggest that she changes position or walks out to the toilet.

● Mind your back. A birth on a bed involves twisting, which is not the optimal position for your back. Any position where you face directly to the woman is better. You may need to kneel down or temporarily squat (Fig. 1.5) as the baby is born, depending on your own preference and on the mother's position (see second stage).

Transition

Towards the end of the first stage contractions may become almost continuous or, conversely, space out a little. Many women may have a sensation to bear down during the peak of the contraction as the cervix approaches full dilatation. This stage may be the most painful and distressing. Labour stress hormones peak; this has a positive physiological effect in producing the surge of energy shortly needed to push (Odent, 1999; Buckley, 2004a). It can last a few contractions, but for some women it lasts much longer.

> 'The diagnosis of the transitional stage . . . is a far more women-centred and subjective skill . . . essentially a midwifery observation and as such is dependent on knowing the woman . . . and recognising any changes in her behaviour. Progress can thus be diagnosed without the need to resort to a VE' (Mander, 2002).

The woman experiencing the 'extreme pain' of transition has a decreased ability to listen or concentrate on anything but giving birth (Leap, 2000). She becomes honest in vocalising her needs and dislikes, 'unfettered by politeness'! This should not be misinterpreted as rejection or rudeness by the midwife or birth partner (Robertson, 1996).

Typical behaviour may include:

- distressed or panicky statements: 'I want to go home now', 'Get me a caesarean/ epidural . . . ', 'I've changed my mind';
- non-verbal sounds: groaning or shouting, involuntary pushing sounds;
- body language: agitated, restless, toes curling, closed eyes due to intense concentration and pain (Leap, 2000);
- withdrawing from the activities and conversation of people around (Leap, 2000; Burvill, 2002);

Midwifery care in transition

Support birth partners. They can become tired, be stressed and want something done to help the woman. This common reaction sometimes leads to inappropriate analgesia, e.g. epidural (Mander, 2002), and then subsequent discovery of a fully dilated cervix. It can be a difficult situation for the midwife to judge.

Keep it calm. Change the dynamics if the women panics; e.g. suggest a walk to the toilet, a position change or focus on her breathing.

Avoid the temptation of VE. Unless the woman really wants it, VE is likely to yield disappointment: at this stage it is painful and the cervix is often 8–9 cm dilated (Lemay, 2000).

To push or not to push? Telling women that they must not push when they cannot stop themselves at the end of the first stage is unnecessary and distressing for the woman (Sleep *et al.*, 2000). The belief that pushing on an undilated cervix will cause an oedematous cervix is based on very limited old evidence (Perez-Botella & Downe, 2006). Remember however that a strong urge to push in earlier labour should alert the midwife to a possible problem e.g. fetal malposition (see Chapter 8).

Second stage of labour

This has traditionally been defined as the stage from full cervical dilation until the baby has been born. Usually, the actual time of onset of the second stage is uncertain

(Walsh, 2000b). There is much debate about the limitations of the medical definitions of labour as separate 'stages' which determine set care and rigid time frames, rather than care aimed at what the woman's body is doing. Long (2006) suggests that 'I would encourage others...to consider redefining the second stage, so that the emphasis is placed on descent and station of the presenting part instead of cervical dilatation'.

Lemay (2000) describes the majority of a primigravida's pushing phase as 'shaping of the head' rather than 'descent of the head':

> 'Each expulsive sensation shapes the head of the baby to conform to the contours of the mother's pelvis. This can take time and...often...is erroneously interpreted as "lack of descent", "arrest" or "failure to progress". I tell mothers at this time, "It's normal to feel like the baby is stuck. The baby's head is elongating and getting shaped a little more with each sensation. It will suddenly feel like it has come down". This is exactly what happens.'

Characteristics of second stage

The woman may experience/exhibit the following:

- **Vomiting** often accompanied by involuntary pushing.
- **Show** or bright red vaginal loss.
- **Spontaneous rupture of the membranes** can occur at any time but often at full dilatation.
- **Slowing of the FH** (early deceleration) at the peak of a contraction; usually due to head compression (see Chapter 3).
- **'Purple line'.** Hobbs (1998) describes a line which gradually extends from the anus to the nape of the buttocks (just below the sacrococcygeal joint where the coccyx starts to curve inwards) relative to cervical dilatation. The line starts just above the anal margin at 0–2 cm dilatation. It does not rise in strict proportion: there is a longer gap between 4 and 7 cm than there is before and after. Hobbs suggests that when it reaches the nape of the buttocks, the woman is fully dilated. Checking the purple line can be quite invasive and is not appropriate for everyone.
- **Urge to push.** Powerful, expulsive contractions every 2–3 minute, lasting <60 seconds. Most women make a distinctive throaty expulsive sound at the peak of a contraction. Others may groan: 'I'm *push*ing!' This urge can precede full dilatation or occur some time afterwards.
- **Rectal pressure.** As the presenting part descends it exerts great pressure on the bowel. The woman often feels she needs to have her bowels opened and may do so.
- **External signs**, e.g. anal dilatation, bulging perineum, gaping vagina.

Midwifery care in second stage

Duration of second stage

The NICE (2007) guidelines are more flexible than previous national guidelines, although some challenge any second-stage time limit if there is progress and no fetal or maternal concern, claiming that there is no link between time per se and poor neonatal outcome (Sleep *et al.*, 2000; Walsh, 2000b). There is some evidence that maternal morbidity increases after 3 hours in second stage (Cheung *et al.*, 2004) but there is known maternal morbidity with instrumental delivery (Sleep *et al.*, 2000; Dupuis *et al.*, 2004).

It is disappointing that some hospitals still appear to have a 1-hour second-stage 'limit'. Rightly or wrongly, midwives have been known to 'fudge' VE results in the face of such restrictive policies, claiming that a woman has an anterior lip, to allow her more time without medical intervention.

NICE (2007) suggests the following:

- Perform a VE after an hour of 'active second stage' for nulliparous women, then artificial rupture of the membranes (ARM) if membranes intact and consider further analgesia.
- If no birth after 2 active hours (or after 1 hour for multiparous women), then obstetric review every 15 min as long as there are no concerns about fetal well-being and not to start oxytocin.
- Instrumental delivery after 3 hour of active pushing for a nulliparous woman and 2 hours for a multiparous woman (in the absence of fetal well-being concerns).

Vaginal examination. It has become the norm for full dilatation to be confirmed by VE. While it can be helpful, it is not always necessary, particularly if the external signs are evident or in multiparous women.

Monitoring the FH. As the baby descends with pushing, the FH can be difficult to locate and monitoring may feel invasive and uncomfortable. Early decelerations are more common in the second stage, sometimes becoming late decelerations or even an end-stage bradycardia (see Chapter 3).

In the second stage of labour, NICE (2007) recommends FHR auscultation every 5 minutes following a contraction.

Pushing

Bergstrom *et al.* (1997) ask, 'Why does the clinician's definition of second stage take precedent, regardless of what the woman's body is instinctively doing?'

Bergstrom *et al.* describe how midwives expend great energy, discouraging a woman from pushing prior to confirmation of full dilatation, and then coerce her into exaggerated active pushing once full dilatation is confirmed. As stated earlier, there is no evidence that cervical swelling occurs with premature pushing (Walsh, 2000b) and active pushing is thought to do more harm than good (see also Chapter 2, 'Anterior lip', p. 36).

Enable spontaneous involuntary pushing. Women simply push as they wish, most women take a short breath, hold their breath for ≤6 seconds as they bear down and then give an expiratory grunt (Thomson, 1995). They may give multiple short pushes with a contraction.

Push only when ready. Women naturally push as the contraction builds up and the urge is present. The earliest part of the contraction pulls the vagina taut, preventing it from being pushed down in front of the descending presenting part (Gee & Glynn, 1997).

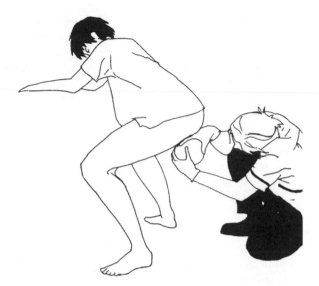

Fig. 1.5   Standing/hanging from a bed (second stage).

Forced pushing (valsalva). This is inadvisable in a normal birth as it involves directed, prolonged breath-holding and prolonged bearing down (Sleep *et al.*, 2000), which can result in FH abnormalities, lower Apgars, perineal trauma, episiotomy and instrumental birth (Thomson, 1995; Sleep *et al.*, 2000). Pelvic dysfunction and urinary incontinence can also result from forced pushing (Schaffer *et al.*, 2005).

Try stopping pushing or even trying to 'suck the baby back in' for a few contractions if pushing feels ineffective: paradoxically (perhaps it is psychological), some women find that this increases their pushing urge (Lemay, 2000).

Pushing with an epidural. Many women do not experience a pushing urge and may need more direction. Delaying pushing for an hour or two (Roberts *et al.*, 2004), allowing 3–4-hour second stage (NICE, 2007), may help achieve a normal delivery and avoid other complications (Simpson & James, 2005). Discontinuing the epidural can be distressing for the woman and does not increase the spontaneous birth rate (Torvaldsen *et al.*, 2004). See Chapter 8 for ideas to improve the spontaneous birth rate in epidural.

Slow progress may be normal for that woman or the sign of problems (see Chapter 8).

Birthing positions. Squatting, kneeling or side lying, as opposed to lying semi-recumbent, increases the maximum pelvic outlet significantly. Gravity-enhancing upright positions (Figs. 1.1, 1.3, 1.5 and 1.6) appear to be less painful and may shorten the second stage compared with supine or lithotomy positions which increase fetal heart anomalies, dystocia, episiotomy and instrumental delivery (Gupta *et al.*, 2004; RCM, 2005). Side lying appears to reduce perineal trauma the most, while squatting may increase it (Shorten *et al.*, 2002; Bedwell, 2006). Blood loss appears higher following upright birth (Gupta *et al.*, 2004), but this may be due to the ease of measuring blood loss when upright. Upright positions may also benefit the perineum in making episiotomies difficult to perform (Albers *et al.*, 2005): as a result there are more second-degree tears instead (Gupta *et al.*, 2004). Many women instinctively take up the position that feels right for them; encourage them to do so.

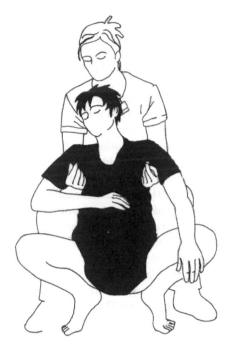

Fig. 1.6 Supported squat (second stage).

Verbal support. Speak soothingly, give simple explanations and praise the woman for doing so well. Insincere and overeffusive praise can sound false. Most midwives tend to instinctively know the right things to say and when to say them.

The birth

As the birth approaches the perineum bulges, the vagina gapes and the anus flattens. Often the woman opens her bowels when pushing. The presenting part becomes visible and advances with contractions. A surge of birth hormones, including oxytocin and catecholamines, known as the 'fetal ejection reflex' increases the energy needed to expel the baby (Odent, 2000). The woman may cry out as she feels the stretching, burning sensation of the stretching perineum. She may be immensely focused or, conversely, may panic, and writhe around maybe even resisting pushing because of the pain.

Low lighting and privacy. There is no justification for putting on bright fluorescent lights. They are harsh and institutional and may cause a stress reaction, inhibiting natural oxytocin production. Birthing mammals tend to prefer darker environments and need nests where they feel safe (Johnston, 2004). A light source near the perineum may reassure some midwives who wish to view the perineum, but continual staring and focusing on the perineum and/or the woman's face may put her under pressure and make her feel exposed. This can feel particularly voyeuristic for sexual abuse victims (Kitzinger, 1992). Also think of the baby: the transition from womb to outside world is likely to be quite a shock as it is, without a bright light shining into its eyes.

Neither method appears to have any ill effects on the baby (Prendiville & Elbourne, 2000). Delayed cord clamping (occurring naturally with physiological management, but still achievable with active management) allows 20–50% increased blood flow to the baby (Prendiville & Elbourne, 2000), increasing neonatal haemoglobin and haematocrit without significantly increasing symptomatic polycythaemia or jaundice (Mercer, 2001; Hutton & Hassan, 2007). It may reduce fetomaternal transfusion, benefiting rhesus-negative women with rhesus-positive babies (Prendiville & Elbourne, 2000).

All midwives should be knowledgeable about both methods of third stage management. Some midwives lack experience and confidence of physiological third stage management, having assisted only a very few physiological third stages and never really learned what to do – and what, more importantly, not to do.

Physiological third stage (expectant management)

If the woman has had a positive birth followed by unhurried, quality contact with her newborn, this will facilitate oxytocin release (Odent, 1999), the hormone that stimulates uterine muscle contraction. Breastfeeding and/or nipple stimulation will also increase natural oxytocin. The woman may use her contractions, upright postures and maternal pushing efforts to aid placenta delivery, or it may just suddenly emerge.

Midwifery care for a physiological third stage

'Watchful waiting' – resist the urge to intervene.

Do not

- Administer an oxytocic.
- Palpate the uterus (fundal fiddling).
- Apply cord traction.
- Routinely clamp and cut the cord. Levy (1990) suggests clamping the baby's end of the cord and then cutting, leaving the maternal end of the cord free to bleed *only if* mother and baby have to be separated (e.g. the baby requires resuscitation or the mother wishes to move from a pool to a bed to deliver the placenta and the cord is short). If possible, wait until the cord has stopped pulsating so that the baby receives plenty of maternal blood, unless the situation is urgent.

Do

- Encourage skin-to-skin contact.
- Encourage breastfeeding to increase oxytocin levels. (Nipple self-stimulation can also help.)
- Wait a while (typically >20–30 min).

Watch blood loss and **observe for signs of separation**, e.g.:

- Cord lengthening
- Trickle of blood/passage of small clots
- The woman may groan, have a period-type ache or urge to push
- The placenta may be visible at the vagina

Assist the mother to an upright posture, e.g. kneeling, squatting or sitting: gravity will help her birth the placenta.

Push with a contraction as expulsive efforts are usually more effective then.

If the placenta does not emerge after several attempts, relax and wait a while before trying again. A quiet darkened room may reduce the woman's stress hormones and increase oxytocin production.

If the woman has tried pushing, utilising gravity, changing position, breastfeeding and passing urine, you may wish to check that the placenta has actually separated: a gentle VE may reveal the partially/totally separated placenta in the os or vagina.

If the placenta is slow, but there is no heavy bleeding, then encourage the baby to nuzzle and feed at the breast. Encourage the woman to relax . . . and try to do the same.

Most women (95%) deliver the placenta within 1 hour of physiological third stage (NICE, 2007), with multiparous women averaging 20 minutes (Begley, 1990). There is little good evidence to guide midwives in the safe time to wait for a placenta to deliver, as most PPH studies look only at active management. NICE (2007) recommends proceeding to active management (oxytocic+cord traction) after 1 hour, citing one study suggesting that PPH risk rises after 30 minutes and peaks at 75 minutes with both active and physiological management (Combs & Laros, 1991), but this old US data (i.e. 1976–1985) may not be applicable to current UK physiological management.

Active management of the third stage of labour

Active management usually achieves delivery of the placenta within around 10 minutes of birth. Initial blood loss is reduced (Prendiville *et al.*, 2000).

- **Give a prophylactic oxytocic** with the delivery of the anterior shoulder or following birth. Oxytocic agents are listed in Chapter 24. Syntometrine is commonly used, although NICE (2007) recommends oxytocin (syntocinon) 10 IU IM as this appears to be as effective as syntometrine at preventing haemorrhage and reduces the likelihood of retained placenta.
- **Clamp and cut the cord.** This is often in practice done immediately, and NICE (2007) recommends this in the absence of substantive Western trials; however, delayed cord clamping for several minutes is shown to benefit the babies with anaemia in developing countries (NICE, 2007), with only a small rise in hyperbilirubinaemia. Further research is needed. If syntocinon has been given as NICE suggests, which may take >2 minutes to take effect through an intramuscular route, the benefits of early cord clamping are debatable. Surely until an oxytocic has started to take effect the cord should not be clamped: this would be mixing physiological and active management. NICE do not address this contradiction however, and midwives must make their own judgement on this issue.
- Cochrane review suggests **unclamping the maternal end** and allowing it to drain into a bowl may reduce the length of the third stage and possibly reduce the incidence of retained placenta (Soltani *et al.*, 2005).
- **Deliver the placenta by controlled cord traction.** Press the lower uterine area ('guard the uterus') with one hand while gently but firmly pulling the placenta with the other, typically several minutes after the administration of the oxytocic. Some midwives wait for placental separation first, i.e. a small gush of blood indicating that the placenta has sheared off the uterine wall.
- **Retained placenta.** NICE (2007) defines a 'prolonged third stage' as an undelivered placenta after 30 minutes of active management since PPH risk is increased after this time (see Chapter 15 for PPH management).

Possible third-stage problems (physiological or active management)

The placenta is delivered, but the membranes remain stuck:

- Suggest that the mother gives a few hearty coughs: this usually releases the membranes and they slide out.
- It is also possible to gently twist the placenta round and move it up and down, to coax them out (Davis, 1997).

Bleeding is heavy, gushing or continuous:

- Rub up a contraction.
- Administer oxytocic: local policy may apply. Syntocinon may be preferable to syntometrine/ergometrine if the placenta is still in situ as the latter cause the cervical os to close (Crafter, 2002) but ergometrine is faster acting; consider IV administration if giving syntocinon.
- Refer to Chapter 15 for PPH management.

Following delivery of the placenta

Check that the woman's uterus is well contracted and the blood loss normal. Examine the placenta (Fig. 1.7): some women are fascinated by their placenta and wish to watch this.

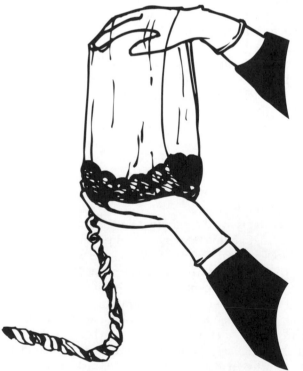

Fig. 1.7 The midwife should check that there are three vessels (two arteries and a vein): a chorion and an amnion. Observe for completeness and record any abnormalities.

After the birth

Immediately after the birth. Women's reactions vary enormously. Some may enjoy being congratulated: others are in their own new world at this point and simply do not know the midwife exists. Stand back: let her or her birth partner explore the baby to discover the sex; resist the urge to talk loudly or take control unless it is clear that guidance is wanted.

The baby. Babies are individuals too and may have had a hard birth. Some gaze calmly around: others cry pitifully and need lots of comfort. Mothers are known to use a particular high soothing voice to their newborn.

Babies are vulnerable to heat loss. Keep the baby snuggled up with its mother and/or birth partner for skin-to-skin contact for as long as they want. A warm hat and blanket over the outside of the mother and baby will keep them both warm. The World Health Organization (WHO) (1997) has suggested a list of actions to reduce neonatal hypothermia, known as the warm chain (see Box 1.5).

For babies needing **resuscitation** see Chapter 17.

For **examination of the newborn** see Chapter 5.

Breastfeeding. As with labour, it is important for midwives to 'sit on their hands' at this point: try to minimise interruption, giving the mother and baby space to explore each other. Most babies are very alert immediately after a natural birth. They will readily root towards the breast, nuzzle, lick and suckle when they are ready. The first hour after birth is a special time. Some animals are known not to attach to their young unless they are able to lick and smell them immediately after birth (Buckley, 2004b).

Examine the perineum for trauma when the woman is ready. Many will want this to be over as soon as possible so that they can relax and enjoy their baby (see Chapter 4).

Offer analgesia. Multigravid women, in particular, can experience strong afterpains, and all women are vulnerable to perineal and rectal pain, even with an intact perineum. Excessive perineal pain may indicate a haematoma (see Chapter 15).

Records. Carefully record the birth. Computer details are usually also required. This gives the opportunity for a psychological break for the midwife who may have been under intense pressure for some hours. Sensitive midwives will make the mother, not

---

Box 1.5   The warm chain.

```
 (1)  Warm delivery room
 (2)  Immediate drying
 (3)  Skin-to-skin contact
 (4)  Breastfeeding
 (5)  Bathing and weighing postponed
 (6)  Appropriate clothing and bedding
 (7)  Mother and baby together
 (8)  Warm transportation
 (9)  Warm resuscitation
(10)  Training and awareness
```

WHO (1997).

the paperwork or their own tiredness, the priority. Most parents relish being left on their own to explore and enjoy their baby. Others may prefer to have a midwife hovering. Most of the paperwork can be done in the room and so be flexible.

Think about the birth partner. They can feel exhausted, overwhelmed and even traumatised by experiencing birth. Congratulate them on their support; show that you realise their needs are important. Remember they, like their partner, may need time later to recount their story.

Offer food and drink. There is nothing like the smell of tea and toast in the middle of the night to remind you a baby has been born.

Get her settled. The mother should not be hurried to have a bath or move to a fresh bed: some will feel the need to freshen up earlier than others. If the birth is at home, she can have all the time in the world. The 'routine' postbirth bath has become almost a ritual after birth for many midwives: many mothers (and babies) may enjoy the experience but some mothers may be too tired to want to move. It has been suggested that some shivery women may value being warmly wrapped and left for some time (Simkin & Ancheta, 2005): the cooling by evaporation that occurs following a bath may chill them further. Bathing should be optional, not routine practice.

Check that her pulse, temperature, BP and lochia are normal. Record when she has passed urine. On a busy labour ward there is often pressure to transfer the woman quickly to the postnatal area. Sometimes this is just habit, and midwives are pressured to rush even if the labour ward is quiet. Resist this coercion. Sometimes, however, it is necessary for the safety of other mothers who may need a birth room and the midwife's attention imminently. If this is necessary, consider continuing skin-to-skin contact by suggesting that the baby bathes with the mother if she wants a bath, or goes to the father for skin-to-skin contact, and/or tucks inside the mother's or father's clothes for further contact during transfer to the postnatal area. Enthusiastic midwives find innovative solutions.

Summary

Latent phase

- Ideally spent at home
- If PROM:
  - Check for infection: if infection, advises induction of labour with IV antibiotics
  - Wait 24 hours for labour to start: after this time NICE recommend IOL but some women will choose expectant management

Established first stage

- Continuous midwifery support is effective analgesia.
- Make her feel safe: build her a 'nest'.
- Encourage:
  - Mobilisation and position changes
  - Regular bladder emptying, eating and drinking
  - Natural coping methods

- Observe/monitor:
  - Basic vital signs
  - Contractions and her response to them
  - Progress and descent by palpation and VE (if required)
  - FHR intermittently unless concerns
- Avoid:
  - Unnecessary VEs/ARM/other interventions
  - Arbitrary time limits

Second stage

- Observe/monitor:
  - Descent by external signs, palpation and/or VE
  - FHR intermittently unless concerns
- Encourage:
  - Upright posture, non-directed pushing
  - Low lighting and privacy
  - Slow, gentle birth and skin-to-skin contact
- Avoid:
  - Episiotomy
  - Arbitrary time limits if all is well

Third stage

- Physiological management:
  - The woman should have had a normal labour and birth.
  - Leave the cord unclamped if possible (or cut and leave maternal end unclamped).
  - Encourage skin-to-skin contact and breastfeeding.
  - Monitor blood loss: observe for signs of separation. Hands off.
- Active management:
  - Give oxytocic: NICE recommends syntocinon 10 IU IM.
  - NICE recommends immediate cord clamping (but evidence is unclear).
  - Perform controlled cord traction with fundal guarding.

Useful contacts

Association for Improvements in the Maternity Services (AIMS)   Helpline: 0870 765 1433. Website: www.aims.org.uk

Doulas UK   Website: www.doula.org.uk

National Childbirth Trust (NCT)   Enquiry line: 0870 444 8707. Website: www.nct-online.org

Nursing and Midwifery Council (NMC)   Telephone: 020 7637 7181. Website: www.nmc-uk.org

Royal College of Midwives   Website: www.rcm.org.uk

References

Albers, L., Sedler, K., Bedrick, E., Teaf, D. & Peralta, P. (2005) Midwifery care measures in the second stage of labour and reduction of genital tract trauma at birth: a randomised trial. *Journal of Midwifery and Women's Health* **50**, 563–72.

Association of Radical Midwives (ARM) (2000) Association of Radical Midwives Nettalk: checking for cord. *Midwifery Matters* **87**, 28–30.

Baston, H. (2001) Blood pressure measurement: midwifery basics. *The Practising Midwife* **4** (9), 10–14.

Bedwell, C. (2006) Are third degree tears unavoidable? The role of the midwife. *British Journal of Midwifery* **14** (9), 212.

Begley, C. (1990) A comparison of 'active' and 'physiological' management of the third stage of labour. *Midwifery* **63**, 3–17.

Bergstrom, L., Seedily, J., Schulman-Hull, L. *et al.* (1997) 'I gotta push. Please let me push!' Social interactions during the change from first stage to second stage of labour. *Birth* **24** (3), 173–80.

Buckley, S. (2004a) Undisturbed birth – nature's hormonal blueprint for safety, ease and ecstasy. *MIDIRS Midwifery Digest* **14** (2), 203–9.

Buckley, S. (2004b) What disturbs birth? *MIDIRS Midwifery Digest* **14** (3), 353–7.

Burvill, S. (2002) Midwifery diagnosis of labour onset. *British Journal of Midwifery* **10** (10), 600–5.

Caroci, A. & Riesco, M. (2006) A comparison of 'hands off' vs 'hands on' for decreasing perineal lacerations during birth. *Journal of Midwifery Women's Health* **51**, 106–11.

Carroli, G. & Belizan, J. (1999) Episiotomy for vaginal birth. *Cochrane Database of Systematic Reviews*, Issue 3, Art. No. CD000081. DOI: 10.1002/14651858.CD000081.

CEMACH (2007) *Diabetes in Pregnancy: Caring for the Baby After Birth. Findings of a National Enquiry. England, Wales and Northern Ireland.* CEMACH, London. Available at: www.cemach.org.uk (accessed March 2008).

Cheung, Y., Hopkins, I. & Caughey, A. (2004) How long is too long: does a prolonged second stage of labour in nulliparous women affect maternal and neonatal morbidity? *American Journal of Obstetrics and Gynaecology* **191**, 933–8.

Combs, C. & Laros, R., Jr (1991) Prolonged third stage of labor: morbidity and risk factors. *Obstetrics & Gynecology* **77** (6), 863–7.

Crafter, H. (2002) Intrapartum and primary postpartum haemorrhage. In *Emergencies Around Childbirth – A Handbook for Midwives* (Boyle, M., ed.), pp. 113–26. Radcliffe Medical Press, Oxford.

Crowther, C., Enkin, M., Keirse, M., & Brown, I. (2000) Monitoring progress in labor. In *A Guide to Effective Care in Pregnancy and Childbirth*, 3rd edn (Enkin, M., Keirse, M.J.N.C., Neilson, J., Crowther, C., Duley L., Hodnett, E. & Hofmeyr, J., eds), pp. 210–218. Oxford University Press, Oxford.

Davis, E. (1997) *Hearts and Hands: A Midwife's Guide to Pregnancy and Birth*, 3rd edn. Celestial Arts, Berkeley, California.

Department of Health (DoH) (2004) *National Service Framework for Children, Young People and Maternity Services*, pp. 27–9. Department of Health, London.

Downe, S. (ed.) (2004) *Normal Childbirth: Evidence and Debate.* Churchill Livingstone, Oxford.

Dupuis, O., Madelenat, P. & Rudigoz R. (2004) Faecal and urinary incontinence and delivery: risk factors and prevention. *Gynaecology, Obstetrics and Fertility* **32**, 540–48.

Elbourne, D. & Wiseman, R.A. (2004) Types of intra-muscular opioids for maternal pain relief in labour. *Cochrane Database of Systematic Reviews*, Issue 1.

Erlandsson, K., Dsilna, A., Fagerberg, I. & Christensson, K. (2007) Skin-to-skin care with the father after caesarean birth and its effect on newborn crying and prefeeding behaviour. *Birth* **34** (2), 105–13.

Gee, H. & Glynn, M. (1997) The physiology and clinical management of labour. In *Essential Midwifery* (Henderson, C. & Jones, K., eds), pp. 171–202. Mosby, London.

Green, J., Renfrew, M. & Curtis, P. (2000) Continuity of carer: what matters to women? A review of the evidence. *Midwifery* **16** (3), 187–96.

Gupta, J., Hofmeyr, G. & Smyth, R. (2004) Position in the second stage of labour for women without epidural anaesthesia. *The Cochrane database of systematic reviews*, Issue 1.

Hobbs, L. (1998) Assessing cervical dilatation without VEs. *The Practising Midwife* **1** (11), 34–5.

Hodnett, E.D., Gates, S., Hofmeyr, G.J. & Sakala, C. (2004) Continuous support for women during childbirth (Cochrane Review). In *The Cochrane Library*, Issue 3.

Howell, C. (2004) Epidural versus non-epidural analgesia for pain relief in labour (Cochrane Review) In *Cochrane Library*, Issue 1.

Hutton, E.K. & Hassan, E.S. (2007) Late vs early clamping of the umbilical cord in full-term neonates: systematic review and meta-analysis of controlled trials. *JAMA* **297**, 1241–52.

Jackson, K. (2000) The bottom line: care of the perineum must be improved. *British Journal of Midwifery* **8** (10), 609–14.

Jacobsen, B., Nyberg, K., Eklund, G., Bygdeman, M. & Rydberg, U. (1988) Obstetric pain medication and eventual adult amphetamine addiction in offspring. *Acta Obstetrica et Gynecologica* **67**, 677–82.

Jacobsen, B., Nyberg, K., Gronbladh, L., Eklund, G., Bygdeman, M. & Rydberg, U. (1990) Opiate addiction in adult offspring through possible imprinting after obstetric treatment. *BMJ* **301** (6760), 1067–70.

Johnson, C., Keirse, M.J.N.C., Enkin, M. & Chalmers, I. (2000) Hospital practices – nutrition and hydration in labor. In *A Guide to Effective Care in Pregnancy and Childbirth*, 3rd edn (Enkin, M., Keirse, M.J.N.C., Neilson, J., Crowther, C., Duley L., Hodnett, E. & Hofmeyr, J., eds), pp. 255–66. Oxford University Press, Oxford.

Johnston, J. (2004) The nesting instinct. *Birth Matters Journal* **8**, 21–2.

Johnson, M. (1997) TENS in pain management. *British Journal of Midwifery* **5** (7), 400–5.

Kitzinger, C. & Kitzinger, S. (2007) Birth trauma: talking to women and the value of conversation analysis. *British Journal of Midwifery* **15** (5), 256–64.

Kitzinger, J.V. (1992) Counteracting, not re-enacting, the violation of women's bodies: the challenge for perinatal caregivers. *Birth* **19** (4), 219–22.

Lavender, T., Alfirevic, Z. & Walkinshaw, S. (2006) Effect of different partogram action lines on birth outcomes: a randomised controlled trial. *Obstetricas and Gynaecology* **108** (2), 295–302.

Lauzon, L. & Hodnett, E. (2002) Labour assessment programs to delay admission to labour wards (Cochrane Review). In *The Cochrane Library*, Issue 4. Update Software, Oxford.

Leap, N. (2000) Pain in labour. *MIDIRS Midwifery Digest* **10** (1), 49–53.

Leighton, B. & Halpern, S. (2002) The effects of epidural analgesia on labor, maternal and neonatal outcomes: a systematic review. *American Journal of Obstetrics and Gynaecology* **186**, 69–77.

Lemay, G. (2000) Pushing for first time moms. *Midwifery Today* **55**, 9–12.

Levy, V. (1990) The midwife's management of the third stage of labour. In *Intrapartum Care 1–1 A Research Based Approach* (Alexander, J., Levy, V. & Roch, S., eds), pp. 139–43. Macmillan, Basingstoke.

Lieberman, E. & O'Donaghue, C. (2002) Unintended effects of epidural analgesia in labour: a systematic review. *American Journal of Obstetrics and Gynaecology* **186**, 531–68.

Long, L. (2006) Redefining the second stage of labour could help to promote normal birth. *British Journal of Midwifery* **14**, 104–6.

Mainstone, A. (2004) TENS. *British Journal of Midwifery* **12** (9), 578–81.

Mander, R. (2002) The transitional stage – pain and control. *The Practising Midwife* **5** (1), 10–12.

McCandlish, R., Bower, U., van Asten, H., Berridge, G., Winter, C., Sames, L., Garcia, J., Renfrew, M. & Elbourne, D. (1998) A randomised controlled trial of care of the perineum during the second stage of normal labour (HOOP trial). *British Journal of Obstetrics and Gynaecology* **105**, 1262–72.

McNiven, P., Williams, J., Hodnett, E. & Kaufman, H.M. (1998) An early labour assessment program: a randomised controlled trial. *Birth* **25** (1), 5–10.

Mercer, J.C. (2001) Current best evidence: a review of the literature on umbilical cord clamping. *Journal of Midwifery and Women's Health* **46** (6), 402–14.

MIDIRS (2007) *Positions in Labour and Delivery*. Informed Choice Leaflet: Midwives Information and Resource Service, Bristol.

Moore, E., Anderson, G. & Bergman, N. (2003) Early skin-to-skin contact for mothers and their healthy newborn infants. *Cochrane Database of Systematic Reviews*, Issue 2.

National Childbirth Trust (NCT) (2003) *Creating a Better Birth Environment: An Audit Toolkit*. National Childbirth Trust, London.

National Institute for Health and Clinical Excellence (NICE) (2007) *Clinical Guideline 55: Intrapartum Care*. National Institute for Health and Clinical Excellence, London.

NHS Maternity Statistics 2005–2006 (2007) *The Information Centre*. Available at: www.ic.nhs.uk (accessed 3 March 2008).

Nyberg, K., Buka, S. & Lipsitt., L. (2000) Perinatal medication as a potential risk factor for adult drug abuse in a North American cohort. *Epidemiology* **11** (6), 715–16.

Ockenden, J. (2001) The hormonal dance of labour. *The Practising Midwife* **4** (6), 16–17.

Odent, M. (1994) *The Nature of Birthing and Breastfeeding*. Bergin and Garvey, Connecticut.

Odent, M. (1999) *The Scientification of Love*. Free Association Books, London.

Odent, M. (2000) Insights into pushing: the second stage as a disruption of the fetus ejection reflex. *Midwifery Today International Midwife* **55**, 12.

Perez-Botella, M. & Downe, S. (2006) Stories as evidence: the premature urge to push. *British Journal of Midwifery* **14** (11), 636–42.

Prendiville, W. & Elbourne, D. (2000) The third stage of labor. In *A Guide to Effective Care in Pregnancy and Childbirth*, 3rd edn (Enkin, M., Keirse, M.J.N.C., Neilson, J., Crowther, C., Duley L., Hodnett, E. & Hofmeyr, J., eds). Oxford University Press, Oxford.

Prendiville, W.J., Elbourne, D. & McDonald, S. (2004) Active versus expectant management in the third stage of labour. *Cochrane Database of Systematic Reviews*, Issue 1.

Redshaw, M., Rowe, R., Hockley, C. & Brocklehurst, P. (2007) *Recorded Delivery: The Findings from a National Survey of Women's Experience of Maternity Care*. National Perinatal Epidemiology Unit, Oxford. Available at: www.npeu.ox.ac.uk (accessed March 2008).

Roberts, C.L., Torvaldsen, S., Cameron, C.A. & Olive, E. (2004) Delayed versus early pushing in women with epidural analgesia: a systematic review and met-analysis. *British Journal of Obstetrics and Gynaecology* **111** (12), 1333–40.

Robertson, A. (1996) *Empowering Women: Teaching Active Birth in the 90s*. ACE Graphics, Camperdown, NSW, Australia.

Robertson, A. (2006) Nitrous oxide – no laughing matter. *MIDIRS Midwifery Digest* **16** (1), 123–8.

Royal College of Midwives (RCM) (2005) *Campaign for Normal Birth*. Royal College of Midwives, London. Available at: www.rcmnormalbirth.org.uk (accessed November 2007).

Schaffer, J., Bloom, S., Casey, B., McIntire, D., Nihira, M. & Leveno, K. (2005) A randomised trial of the effects of coached vs uncoached pushing during the second stage of labour on postpartum pelvic floor structure and function. *American Journal of Obstetrics and Gynaecology* **192**, 1692–6.

Shorten, A., Donsante, J. & Shorten, B. (2002) Birth position, accoucheur, and perineal outcomes: informing women about choices for vaginal birth. *Birth* **29** (1), 18–27.

Simkin, P. & Ancheta, R. (2005) *The Labor Progress Handbook*. Blackwell Science, Oxford.

Simmons, S.W., Cyna, A.M., Dennis, A.T. & Hughes, D. (2007) Combined spinal-epidural versus epidural analgesia in labour. *The Cochrane Database of Systematic Reviews*, Issue 3.

Simpson, K. & James, D. (2005) Effects of immediate vs delayed pushing during second stage on fetal well-being: a randomised controlled trial. *Nursing Research* **54**,149–57.

Sleep, J., Roberts, J. & Chalmers, I. (2000) The second stage of labor. In *A Guide to Effective Care in Pregnancy and Childbirth*, 3rd edn (Enkin, M., Keirse, M.J.N.C., Neilson, J., Crowther, C., Duley L., Hodnett, E. & Hofmeyr, J., eds), pp. 289–99. Oxford University Press, Oxford.

Smith, C.A., Collins, C.T., Cyna, A.M. & Crowther, C.A. (2006) Complementary and alternative therapies for pain management in labour. *Cochrane Database of Systematic Reviews*, Issue 4, Art. No. CD003521. DOI: 10.1002/14651858.CD003521.pub2.

Soltani, H., Dickinson, F. & Symonds, I. (2005) Placental cord drainage after spontaneous vaginal delivery as part of the management of the third stage of labour. *Cochrane Database of Systematic Reviews*, Issue 4, Art. No. CD004665. DOI: 10.1002/14651858.CD004665.pub2.

Stuart, C. (2000) Invasive actions in labour. Where have all the 'old tricks' gone? *The Practising Midwife* **3** (8), 30–33.

Sullivan, J.R. (1999) Development of father-infant attachment in fathers of preterm infants. *Neonatal Network* **18** (7), 33–9.

Thomson, A. (1995) Maternal behaviour during spontaneous and directed pushing in the second stage of labour. *Journal of Advanced Nursing* **22** (6), 1027–34.

Tiran, D. (2000) *Clinical Aromatherapy for Pregnancy and Childbirth*, 2nd edn. Churchill Livingstone, Edinburgh.

Tiran, D. (2006) Midwives responsibilities when caring for women using complementary therapies during labour. *MIDIRS Midwifery Digest* **16** (1), 77–8.

Torvaldsen, S., Roberts, C.L., Bell, J.C. & Raynes-Greenow, C.H. (2004) Discontinuation of epidural in labour for reducing the adverse delivery outcomes associated with epidural analgesia. *Cochrane Database of Systematic Reviews*, Issue 4, Art. No. CD004457. DOI: 10.1002/14651858.CD004457.pub2.

Walsh, D. (2000a) Evidence-based care. Part 3: assessing women's progress in labour. *British Journal of Midwifery* **8** (7), 449–57.

Walsh, D. (2000b) Evidence-based care. Part 6: limits on pushing and time in the second stage. *British Journal of Midwifery* **8** (10), 604–8.

Wickham, S. (1999) Further thoughts on the third stage. *Practising Midwife* **2** (10), 14–15.

World Health Organization (WHO) (1997) *Safe Motherhood: Thermal Protection of the Newborn: A Practical Guide*. World Health Organization, Geneva.

2 Vaginal examinations and artificial rupture of the membranes

Vicky Chapman

Introduction

Vaginal examinations (VEs) are a common intervention performed during labour with the primary intent of assessing cervical dilatation as well as offering other information. While many clinicians challenge their value, frequency and necessity (Warren, 1999; Crowther *et al.*, 2000; Walsh, 2000a; Royal College of Midwives (RCM), 2005), they do remain a skill that the midwife frequently undertakes.

Incidence and facts

- A study by Lewin *et al.* (2005) of women's experiences of VEs found:
  - Women reported overall an average of three examinations per labour (this is lower than in other studies).
  - 60% of respondents said their permission was sought prior to a VE.
  - 40% felt that they could always refuse a VE; conversely, 42% felt that they could not refuse.
  - 95% felt clearly informed about the subsequent findings.
- Many women find VEs uncomfortable and embarrassing, sometimes traumatic and distressing. They can trigger feelings of sexual intimacy, invasion of privacy and vulnerability and can be especially difficult for women who have been sexually abused (Nolan, 2001).

Accuracy and timing of VEs

'Repeated VEs are an invasive intervention, of, as yet, unproven value. Those who advocate their use thus have the responsibility to test their belief in an appropriately controlled trial' (RCM, 2005 citing Enkin, 1992).

- VEs are relied upon to assess labour progress, and as such they do appear to be a useful guide; however, studies have found that VEs can be an imprecise measure of labour progress particularly when performed by different examiners (Crowther *et al.*, 2000). Where possible, therefore, they should be carried out by the same clinician (RCM, 2005).
- In multiparous women, cervical dilatation does not always correlate to their true labour progress, which is sometimes more accurately reflected in their typical labour behaviour and vocalisation.
- Simkin and Ancheta (2005) describe the importance of additional measures of progress including cervical consistency, thinning and effacement, movement from posterior to anterior and the importance of good cervical application to the presenting part.

VEs are the main focus for assessing progress of labour; Warren (1999) suggests midwives ask themselves, 'What decision has to be made at this time which requires information that can only be obtained from a VE?'

- The timing and accuracy of VEs varies:
  - It is recommended that the timing of VEs in labour should be relevant to each individual woman in order to permit adequate assessment of her progress (and not be performed too frequently or for the sake of 'routine') (Crowther *et al.*, 2000).
  - Conversely, National Institute for Clinical Excellence (NICE) (2007) advocates VEs at routine, fixed 4-hourly time intervals in the first stage of labour.
- Definitions of progress vary (Crowther *et al.*, 2000) but a cervical dilatation of 0.5 cm/hour is advised in the NICE (2007) intrapartum guidelines.
  Labour progress issues are discussed further in Chapter 8.

Information sharing: informed consent or compliance?

A study of women's experiences of VE and information giving in labour found that two thirds of midwives provided good or very good information at this time. The equivalent for doctors was just a third (Lewin *et al.*, 2005).

- Discuss the indication for the examination.
- Check if this is the woman's first VE (often it is).
- Explain what it may feel like and typically how long it may last.
- Offer a chaperone irrespective of the clinician's gender (Royal College of Obstetricians and Gynaecologists (RCOG), 1997).
- In non-English speaking women, ensure an interpreter/advocate is available (RCOG, 1997).

Implied consent (including written consent) may not be sufficient evidence that someone has given *express consent* (GMC, 1998). Many women conform or comply with suggestions for which, when they later reflect, their informed and *express consent* had not actually been sought. Performing a vaginal examination without express consent may constitute assault and has medico-legal implications (RCM, 2005).
  If consent is withheld:

- Remain sensitive, open and accept her decision. (You may have to protect the woman from pressure to comply from particular colleagues.)

- Seek alternative methods of assessing progress in labour as discussed in Chapter 1 under the heading 'Assessing progress in labour'.
- Consider that many women, including survivors of sexual abuse, may not be able to cope with invasive, intimate procedures in labour (see later in this chapter).

Performing a VE

Stewart (2006) found that midwives sanitise their terminology, using abbreviations (a VE) and euphemisms (an 'internal') to distance themselves from intimacy and embarrassment. She comments that some midwives ceremonially prepare a sterile trolley, opening packets and performing a ritualised washing down of the woman's external genitalia as an overt statement of power and an attempt to sanitise the woman's bodily fluids perceived as 'dirty'. Since women are capable of cleaning themselves, this practice, which exposes them to high levels of genital touching and embarrassment, has little basis in necessity. In contrast to this, other midwives use an informal, speedier approach, while maintaining asepsis, by squeezing lubricant inside the opened packet of sterile gloves and donning them discreetly.

Despite VEs being undertaken frequently, the procedure lacks good evidence to guide best practice.

VE procedure

- Ensure the woman's bladder is empty.
- Provide privacy: directly ask any unnecessary people present to leave the room. Never underestimate someone's potential embarrassment or vulnerability even if attending a birth at home. Ensure doors are closed, curtains drawn and in hospital display a 'please knock and wait' sign on the door.
- Cover up the woman's lower half with a sheet/dressing gown.
- Abdominal palpation first! This is a good habit to get into.
- In the absence of useful evidence, it seems prudent if the membranes are not intact, the labour is preterm or prolonged or infection is a possibility, that *sterile* gloves should be worn.
- Evidence suggests a douche or wash down, even using chlorhexidine is of no benefit in reducing ascending infection (Lumbiganon *et al.*, 2004).
- Tell the woman that if she wants you to stop at any point or the VE 'hurts' she can trust that you will respond appropriately.
- Sit next to the woman and encourage her to relax her thighs and bottom before commencing the VE. Use plenty of lubricant and gently advance two fingers inside the vagina.
- Never start a VE during a contraction: it is unnecessary and painful. If the woman has a contraction during the VE (commonly triggered by you touching the cervix), keep fingers still and talk her through or remove them.
- Explain what you are doing, particularly when moving your fingers anteriorly (usually the most uncomfortable and sensitive area) and be aware of the woman's body language; actually ask her if she is okay.
- Be aware of your own body language when performing a VE. Avoid looking disapproving, worried, disappointed or disconnected from what is happening.

For VE findings see Box 2.1 and Fig. 2.1

Following the examination

Always smile and congratulate the woman on how well she coped and discuss the findings. If approached with sensitivity and the findings are good news, this can lift the woman's spirits and reassure her. However, the opposite is also true; if handled insensitively or the news is poor, a VE can be a distressing or negative experience. Try always to find something positive to say, even if there is little change.

- Listen to the fetal heart rate (FHR).
- Offer the woman a sanitary towel and assist her into a comfortable position, ideally upright and off the bed.
- Document your findings.

Box 2.1   Information obtained from a vaginal examination.

Abdominal palpation first

Vulva and vagina
- Healthy or identify potential problems including female genital mutilation/circumcision, genital warts and offensive smelling discharge

Cervix
- Location (posterior, mid, central, anterior or lateral)
- Consistency (soft or firm, thick or thin, rigid or stretchy)
- Application (loosely, moderately or well applied)
- Effacement (uneffaced, partially or fully effaced)
- Dilatation (os closed, 1–9 cm, anterior lip, 10 cm or fully dilated)

Presenting part
- Presentation (cephalic, breech, other)
- Position (see Fig. 2.1, for examples, of various vertex positions)
- Station (ballotable, −3, −2, −1, at spines, +1, +2)
- Caput/moulding (absent or present, approximate amount of caput, degree of overlap of skull bones)

Membranes
- Intact or absent. Artificial rupture of membranes, if performed, give indication
- Liquor absent or present; approximate quantity: +, ++, + + +; colour (if meconium present: light/dark green or black, thick/tenacious or thin, or lumps present)

Documentation
- Findings
- FH

Some common problems

Poor progress

Poor progress can be hard to accept. It can be very demoralising for the woman and creates self-doubt about her ability to labour and birth. It is important to sound optimistic and say something encouraging such as 'the cervix is so much thinner' or 'the baby's in a great position and moving down really well', or similar optimistic news. Chapter 8 considers slow progress in depth.

Anterior lip

This is a small anterior portion of undilated cervix that precedes full dilatation. Multiparous women usually push this away with ease, but in some primigravidae this lip of cervix may take a while to go.

Sometimes when a woman's cervix is fully dilated, the midwife will deliberately suggest it's an 'anterior lip', to allow the woman a longer second stage and therefore increased chance of achieving a normal vaginal birth. This knowledge is something midwives keep among themselves and pass on to their students. Stewart (2007) suggests that because midwives fail to challenge obstetric definitions regarding the 'normal' duration of second stage, these definitions will never stand corrected, and the dominant view remains unchallenged.

Oedematous cervix

This is when the cervix swells anteriorly, feeling tense and enlarged. It is most likely towards the end of the first stage of labour. Some believe that women who push prior to full dilatation have the greatest risk of a swollen cervix. However, Walsh (2000b) suggests that there is no evidence to prove this.

- Walmsley (2000) suggests that a premature urge to push, common in posterior position babies, may be physiologically desirable to rotate the baby into an optimum position prior to full dilatation and descent. In which case midwives may be incorrectly discouraging the woman from pushing.
- If the cervix is oedematous, a common non-evidence-based practice to help a woman resist the powerful pushing urge is to adopt a position which reduces this sensation, such as side lying, all fours or knee-chest positions. Over time the cervix usually dilates or becomes a tight lip which, if not too resistant, some midwives slip over the presenting part during VE.
- If the oedematous cervix will not budge more time and huge support are necessary for the woman to get her to cope with these distressing, expulsive contractions. In some cases an epidural may bring welcome relief.
- Anecdotally, midwives who discover a swollen cervix *midway* through labour suggest it rarely resolves and a caesarean usually becomes necessary (Association of Radical Midwives (ARM), 2000).

A 'shrinking' cervix

This issue has sparked debate among radical midwives to counter the theory that it is always a 'misdiagnosis'. It is possible that the presenting part, or even a bag of membranes, may initially press hard on the cervix, causing it to dilate. If then the bag ruptures, or if the presenting part increases/decreases its degree of flexion during labour, this may alter the pressure on the cervix causing it to appear less dilated at the next VE.

A shrinking cervix has been recognised following delivery of twins sometimes born weeks apart; however, anecdotal evidence suggests that it is more common in occipitoposterior positions and can be a sign of dystocia (ARM, 2000).

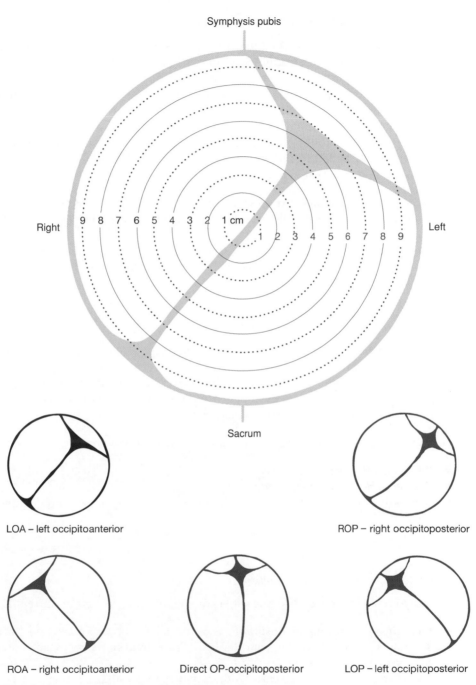

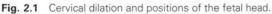

Fig. 2.1   Cervical dilation and positions of the fetal head.

Invasive examinations and sexual abuse

Many women may not disclose if they have been sexually abused as a child or sexually assaulted or raped as an adult. Symptoms associated with sexual abuse survivors are often misinterpreted and women can be labelled as difficult patients. This lack of awareness by health professionals can result in inappropriate treatment, resulting in further damage (Aldcroft, 2001). Women experiencing any intervention have to comply and let someone do something to their body, which may feel invasive, unpleasant and possibly painful. 'Submitting' to the midwife or doctor can be reminiscent of their past abuse. They may be left feeling vulnerable, powerless, violated and dirty (Kitzinger, 1992). Some points to bear in mind include the following:

- Women who have suffered previous sexual abuse are more likely to have a difficult birth experience which results in a higher level of obstetric interventions. (Gutteridge, 2001).
- Sociologists have observed how carers can act in a paternalistic manner, with the woman feeling powerless and childlike, regressed back to her former role as a victim (Kitzinger, 1992).

Phobias and behaviours linked to past abuse

- Fear or obvious dislike of VEs, invasive procedures, needles or going to the dentist.
- History of depression, poor self-esteem and emotional problems (Riley, 1995).
- There is a correlation between women who have been sexually abused as children and psychiatric/emotional dysfunction and postnatal depression (Riley, 1995).
- Disclosure to the midwife of previous abuse.

Behaviour during intimate procedures may include the following:

- 'Shutting off' during the procedure.
- Crying or becoming distressed.
- Regressive or infantile behaviour including talking in a childish voice (Gutteridge, 2001).
- Tensing up or refusing to proceed with the examination.

What can the midwife do to help?

Try not to replicate abuse. Ask yourself, 'Is this VE really necessary?' (Warren, 1999).

- **Give the woman control.** Ensure she is comfortable. Let her know you will stop if she wants you to. Squeezing your free hand as a sign to stop may avoid her having to speak (Aldcroft, 2001).
- **Avoid voyeurism.** The presence of others may replicate abusive situations. So send others out of the room, particularly male midwives/doctors (Kitzinger, 1992).
- **Language.** Avoid patronising or disempowering terms. Even well-intended words can regress women back to their former victim status, with the midwife now as the perpetrator (Mayer, 1995), e.g. 'That's a good girl', 'Open your legs a bit wider', 'Lie still, this won't hurt', 'shhh' (Gutteridge, 2001).

- **Reality check.** Ground the woman in the 'here and now' explaining what is happening as it happens. Keep the situation focused on the cervix, the labour, and the baby, rather than let her return to her former state as a victim (Aldcroft, 2001).

Artificial rupture of the membranes

For the vast majority of women experiencing normal labour, their membranes tend to remain intact throughout the first stage, often rupturing spontaneously around the time of full dilatation, heralding the onset of the second stage. This is physiologically normal and works perfectly well.

The RCM (2005) and NICE (2007) conclude that artificial rupture of the membranes (ARM) is an intervention which should not be considered a routine part of normal labour care. Performing ARM carries risks (see below) including increased FHR abnormalities, increased uterine contractions and is linked to a small increase in caesarean sections. Following ARM, many women feel their contractions worsen and describe feelings of loss of control and self-doubt.

A recent large Cochrane review has found that amniotomy has a smaller effect on labour duration and other outcomes than was previously thought. There was no statistically significant difference between those groups who had an ARM and those who did not. ARM did not appear to affect first stage of labour duration, maternal satisfaction, analgesia use, infection, maternal morbidity or fetal morbidity. It appeared to have little effect on multiparous women, although it resulted in a shorter second stage for some primigravidae. For women with slow progress ARM did not affect further oxytocin use but did seem to have a positive effect on subsequent labour progress and duration (Smyth *et al.*, 2007).

> 'Given the current state of knowledge, it would seem reasonable to reserve ARM for labours which are progressing slowly. Its use then would be as a treatment for dystocia rather than as a prevention' (Rosser & Anderson, 1998).

The RCM (2005) recommends that the decision to ARM should only be taken in direct consultation with the woman, when the evidence is discussed and the intervention justified and not minimised (RCM, 2005). This discussion should not take place just before or during a VE. 'I'm just going to break your waters' is in no way seeking consent.

Benefits of ARM

- If progress is slow ARM appears to improve subsequent labour progress and duration in nulliparous women.
- Allows for visualisation of the colour and quantity of the liquor.

Risks of ARM

- **FHR concerns.** ARM increases the risk of severe, variable FHR decelerations (Goffinet *et al.*, 1997), which may slightly increase the risk of caesarean section (Walsh, 2000a; Smyth *et al.*, 2007). While this has been reported in previous studies, Cochrane found overall this was not statistically significant (Smyth *et al.*, 2007). Some clinicians recommend ARM to observe the liquor if fetal compromise is suspected. However, since ARM may adversely affect the already poor fetal condition, this is a flawed risk assessment.

- **Cord prolapse** is a particular risk only in certain circumstances such as with a high head or malposition. In over 50% of cases of cord prolapse, ARM is a direct cause. Cord prolapse is associated with poor perinatal outcomes (Prabulos & Philipson, 1998).
- **Trauma and pain.** ARM can be an uncomfortable even painful procedure, particularly if the cervix is minimally dilated. It is possible to scratch the mother or baby with the amnistick – the baby is particularly at risk if the midwife makes repeated attempts to rupture membranes which have in fact already ruptured. Following ARM contractions can suddenly increase dramatically, giving the woman no time to 'pace' herself. Many women feel their contractions worsen, and describe feelings of loss of control.

Contraindications to ARM

- Maternal choice.
- A high head, or ballotable presenting part, a second twin, a malposition (e.g. breech) or very preterm infant.
- Placenta praevia.
- ARM is not advisable during the first stage of labour if a baby is particularly susceptible to cord compression or fetal compromise, e.g. preterm, growth-restricted or breech babies (Banks, 1998), a second twin, or if oligohydramnios (Moore, 1996).
- ARM should be avoided in women with a sexually transmitted disease, genital tract infection or in a woman suspected of carrying Group B Streptococcus (or only if the latter is receiving appropriate antibiotic treatment).
- Women who are human immunodeficiency virus (HIV) positive have an increased risk of transmission of HIV to their unborn baby if their membranes rupture, particularly if the rupture exceeds 4 hours (Enkin, 2000). Midwives should bear in mind that not all women know their HIV status, and some will remain undiagnosed.

Summary

- VEs have become routine practice but have not been well researched.
- NICE recommends 4-hourly labour VE; others challenge routine VE.
- Cervical dilatation may not reflect labour progress, especially in multigravidae.
- Remember some women have experienced prior abuse.
- Do
  - Ensure privacy and clear informed consent.
  - Try to ensure an interpreter is present if appropriate.
  - Perform abdominal palpation first.
  - Tell her you will stop if she asks; be aware of your body language.
  - Be gentle.
  - Say something positive and give feedback.
- Don't
  - Start a VE during a contraction.
  - ARM unless there is slow progress and no contraindications: it involves risk.

References

Aldcroft, D. (2001) A guide to providing care for survivors of child sex abuse. *British Journal of Midwifery* **9** (2), 81–5.

Association of Radical Midwives (ARM) (2000) Association of radical midwives nettalk: incredible shrinking cervices. *Midwifery Matters Issue* **87**, 30.

Banks, M. (1998) *Breech Birth Woman Wise*. Birthspirit Books, Hamilton, New Zealand.

Crowther, C., Enkin, M., Keirse, M.J.N.C. & Brown, I. (2000) Monitoring progress in labour. In *A Guide to Effective Care in Pregnancy and Childbirth*, 3rd edn (Enkin, M., Keirse, M.J.N.C. & Neilson, J., eds), pp. 281–8. Oxford University Press, Oxford.

Enkin, M. (2000) Infection in pregnancy. In *Guide to Effective Care in Pregnancy and Childbirth*, 3rd edn (Enkin, M., Keirse, M.J.N.C. & Neilson, J. *et al.*, eds), pp. 154–68. Oxford University Press, Oxford.

GMC (General Medical Council) (1998) *Seeking Patient's Consent: The Ethical Considerations*. Available at: www.gmc-uk.org/guidance/current/library/consent.asp#forms (accessed March 2008).

Goffinet, F., Fraser, W., Marcoux, S., Breart, G., Moutquin, J. M., & Darvis, M. (1997) Early amniotomy increases the frequency of fetal heart rate abnormalities. *British Journal of Obstetrics and Gynaecology* **104**, 548–53.

Gutteridge, K. (2001) Failing women: the impact of sexual abuse on childbirth. *British Journal of Midwifery* **9** (5), 312–15.

Kitzinger, J.V. (1992) Counteracting, not re-enacting, the violation of women's bodies: the challenge for perinatal caregivers. *Birth* **19** (4), 219–22.

Lewin, D., Fearon, B., Hemmings, V. & Johnson, G. (2005) Informing women during VEs. *British Journal of Midwifery* **13** (1), 26–9.

Lumbiganon, P., Thinkhamrop, J., Thinkhamrop, B. & Tolosa, J.E. (2004) Vaginal chlorhexidine during labour for preventing maternal and neonatal infections (excluding Group B Streptococcal and HIV). *Cochrane Database of Systematic Reviews*, Issue 4.

Mayer, L. (1995) The severely abused woman in obstetric and gynaecological care. Guidelines for recognition and management. *Journal of Reproductive Medicine* **40** (1), 13–18.

Moore, T.R. (1996) Oligohydramnios. In *Protocols for High Risk Pregnancies*, 3rd edn (Queenan, J.T. & Hobbins, J.C., eds), pp. 488–95. Blackwell Science, Oxford.

National Institute for Health and Clinical Excellence (NICE) (2007) *Clinical Guideline 55: Intrapartum Care*. National Institute for Health and Clinical Excellence, London.

Nolan, M. (2001) VEs in labour (Expert View). *The Practising Midwife* **4** (6), 22.

Prabulos, A.M. & Philipson, E.H. (1998) Umbilical cord prolapse. Is time from diagnosis to delivery critical? *Journal of Reproductive Medicine* **43** (2), 129–32.

Riley, D. (1995) *Perinatal Mental Health*. Radcliffe Medical Press, Oxford.

Rosser, J. & Anderson, T. (1998) Amniotomy to shorten spontaneous labour: a presentation of the main points from the Cochrane Database review on routine ARM. *MIDIRS Midwifery Digest* **8** (2), 201–202.

Royal College of Midwives (RCM) (2005) *Midwifery Practice Guidelines. Evidence Based Guidelines for Midwifery – Led Care in Labour*. RCM Press. Available at: www.rcm.org.uk (accessed November 2007).

Royal College of Obstetricians and Gynaecologists (RCOG) (1997) *Guidelines on Intimate Examinations*. Available at: www.rcog.uk (accessed March 2008).

Simkin, P. & Ancheta, R. (2005) *The Labor Progress Handbook*. Blackwell Publishing, Oxford.

Smyth, R.M.D., Allderd, S.K. & Markham, C. (2007) Amniotomy for shortening spontaneous labour. *Cochrane Database of Systematic Reviews*, Issue 4. Art. No. CDOO6167.

Stewart, M. (2006) "I'm just going to wash you down" sanitizing the VE. *MIDIRS Midwifery Digest* **16**(1), 30–36.

Stewart, M. (2007) Midwives' and women's discourse about vaginal examination in labour. Unpublished PhD thesis. University of the West of England, Bristol.

Walmsley, K. (2000) Managing the OP labour. *MIDIRS Midwifery Digest* **10** (1), 61–2.

Walsh, D. (2000a) Evidence-based care. Part 3: assessing women's progress in labour. *British Journal of Midwifery* **8** (7), 449–57.

Walsh, D. (2000b) Evidence-based care. Part 6: limits on pushing and time in the second stage. *British Journal of Midwifery* **8** (10), 604–608.

Warren, C. (1999) Why should I do VEs? *The Practising Midwife* **2** (6), 12–13.

3   Fetal heart rate monitoring in labour

Bryony Read

Introduction

Fetal heart monitoring, whether intermittent or continuous, is performed with the intent of assessing the well-being of the fetus and detecting the few who are hypoxic. Continuous electronic fetal monitoring (EFM) became widely popular in the 1970s, often used routinely without evidence of benefit. Iatrogenic intervention frequently resulted. More recently, EFM has been targeted at higher-risk pregnancies, even though its efficacy even in this area remains unproved.

Women may find themselves caught in the centre of this debate, and may be made anxious, often unnecessarily, about the well-being of their unborn baby.

Intermittent auscultation

Intermittent auscultation (IA) is the auscultation of the fetal heart at intermittent intervals, using a pinards stethoscope or a hand-held doppler device. Midwives have traditionally monitored according to the stage of labour and increased the frequency of auscultation when the woman is in established, advanced labour. Unfortunately, there have been no trials to compare the more flexible and individualised time intervals for monitoring the fetal heart rate (FHR), relative to the stage of labour and the degree of risk. In the absence of any randomised controlled trials, National Institute for Health and Clinical Excellence (NICE) (2007) has made recommendations for IA based only on medical expert committee opinion, recommending auscultation after a contraction for 1 minute:

- Every 15 minutes in the first stage of labour
- Every 5 minutes in the second stage of labour

Beech Lawrence (2001) and Spiby (2001) suggest that frequent IA may be as restrictive as continuous EFM.

Using a pinards/hand-held doppler

Effective use of a pinards requires a precise awareness of the baby's position, and indeed it can be used to confirm position. One benefit of the pinards is that it will only pick up the fetal, rather than the maternal heart rate. A pinards can be used throughout labour. Women may find the pressure required for good pinards auscultation uncomfortable. A hand-held doppler device can be placed more lightly on the abdomen and also allows others to hear the fetal heart. A water-resistant device can be used in baths/birthing pools. Some midwives/women may prefer the simplicity of the pinards and are aware that while the use of doppler ultrasound appears to be safe, it has never been proved unequivocally to be so.

To use a pinards, palpate to ascertain the fetal position and place the bell end over the baby's torso. Then press the ear on to the flat end to secure it and let go of the pinards, carefully listen for a muffled thudding, the same sound as putting an ear directly over someone's chest to hear their heart. Midwives can purchase their own wooden pinards from the Association of Radical Midwives (ARM) (listed in the 'Useful contacts' section at the end of this chapter).

If there are any factors of concern regarding the FHR the assessment of variability becomes important. The FHR should vary at least five beats from the baseline rate over a period of 1 minute. However, it is particularly difficult to assess by audibility alone. A hand-held doppler that displays the FHR is useful, as it shows variations of the heart rate.

If there is any deviation from the norm, such as decelerations, bradycardia or tachycardia, then a cardiotocography (CTG) should be commenced, or, if at home, consider transfer to hospital for a CTG. However, FH decelerations often occur in the second stage, and if delivery is imminent a CTG may be impractical and pointless. Hindley *et al.* (2006) explain some midwives find IA difficult to implement because their maternity units promote active management of labour over more conservative approaches to childbirth. Many units still have their own fetal monitoring guidelines (Hindley *et al.*, 2005) which may not always conform to NICE guidelines.

Electronic fetal monitoring

'EFM was introduced with the aim of reducing perinatal mortality and cerebral palsy. This reduction has not been demonstrated in the systematic reviews of randomised controlled trials (RCTs). However an increase in maternal intervention rates has been shown' (NICE, 2007).

Despite the lack of evidence to support EFM, even for women deemed 'high-risk', NICE (2007) continues to recommend its routine use for any woman with a 'risk' factor. For a variety of complex reasons, EFM technology has become part of the hospital-birth culture (Walsh, 2001). As part of this culture, hospital doctors and midwives rely heavily on this form of monitoring as part of their skill base, even if evidence suggests their confidence may be misplaced. It may be difficult for many clinicians to re-skill themselves physically and psychologically and to, therefore, avoid coercing women into accepting EFM. Hindley *et al.* (2006) found that although midwives may state that it is theoretically preferable to use IA, many continue to be reliant on EFM for fear of missing a pathological FH feature. It was also found that EFM continues to be used on busy shifts when one-to-one care is not available.

Units using EFM should have fetal blood sampling (FBS) available before a caesarean section (CS) is performed. This technique allows fetal capillary blood to be tested for its pH values, leading to an indication of action to be taken (for more information see the Appendix and 'Fetal blood tests' in Chapter 23). FBS can, in theory, (a) confirm the need for a CS or (b) reassure and avoid an unnecessary CS which otherwise would have been carried out based on CTG evidence alone. However, Cochrane review found no evidence of higher CS rates when FBS was not available (Alfirevic *et al.*, 2006) and NICE (2007) reports increased instrumental delivery but no difference in outcomes.

NICE (2007) recommends the following:

- The 'admission trace' should be abandoned for low-risk women: they should be offered *intermittent auscultation*.
- EFM should be *offered* to 'high-risk' cases.

Indications for continuous EFM can be seen in the Appendix.

NICE also suggests EFM for:

- Meconium-stained liquor
  - Light staining: *consider* EFM based on assessment of other risks, e.g. stage/progress of labour
  - Significant staining, e.g. thick/tenacious dark green or black staining, or lumps of meconium: advise continuous EFM
- Fresh bleeding in labour
- Oxytocin for augmentation
- Maternal pyrexia: 38°C once or 37.5°C twice 2 hours apart

To perform a CTG:

- Explain to the mother why continuous CTG is being offered. Consent must be obtained.
- Record the indication in the notes and on the CTG.
- Label the CTG with date, the mother's name, hospital number and maternal pulse to differentiate it from the FHR.
- The date and time should be set correctly, and the paper speed should be at 1 cm/min (in the UK).
- Palpate for position and presentation.
- Auscultate using a pinards prior to positioning the FH monitor, as the ultrasound can 'double up' the maternal pulse and show a false FHR.
- Attach the toco (pressure sensitive) contraction monitor around the top of the uterus and the FH monitor over the fetal heart area. Secure with belts.
- Explain simply to the parents the range of the fetal heart and the contraction line. Explain that any 'loss of contact' does not mean that the baby's heartbeat has stopped.
- Undo monitor belts and encourage periodic mobilisation, if possible, to reduce discomfort and complications caused by restricted mobility.
- Consider any external factors that may cause a change in the FHR, e.g. lying flat for an examination, vomiting or pethidine, and note them on the CTG. Usually, a change

of position to left lateral or sitting more upright will resolve any anomalies. Lying flat can cause aortocaval compression, which is the compression of the inferior vena cava and the aorta by the gravid uterus, often producing maternal hypotension and fetal hypoxia.

- Anyone asked to review the trace should note their findings on the trace and in more detail in the maternal notes, along with the date, time and signature.
- Following the birth, the midwife should sign the CTG and write the time and type of birth.
- The CTG should be filed securely in the maternity record. CNST (2006) recommend re-sealable hole-punched envelopes.
- If there is a poor outcome, all CTG traces should be copied as the original is likely to deteriorate in quality and records may need to be examined years after the event.
- Altaf *et al.* (2006) found that a lack of ownership relating to the cleaning and maintenance of CTG machines was a considerable cause of frustration and time wastage for staff.

Fetal scalp electrode

A fetal scalp electrode (FSE) is an accurate but invasive form of monitoring the FHR. Once frequently used, such monitoring is now generally only used where there is significant concern about the FHR with poor contact from the external CTG. It can occasionally cause scarring and/or neonatal infection.

The FSE should not be applied if:

- The woman's consent is not obtained (most women do not like the idea of a clip piercing their baby's skin).
- The baby is <34 weeks gestation or has a bleeding disorder, e.g. haemophilia.
- There is a non-cephalic or non-vertex presentation.
- The woman has an infection, pyrexia, human immunodeficiency virus, hepatitis or any sexually transmitted disease, or the woman is in a high-risk group for these conditions (such as an intravenous drug user).

Classification of fetal heart rate features

The CTG can be classified as normal, suspicious or pathological (see Table 3.1 for a helpful guide).

CTGs can also be documented using the acronym DR C BRAVADO (see Box 3.1).

Box 3.1   DR C BRAVADO CTG documentation.

Determine **R**isk **C**ontractions (frequency and strength) **B**aseline **RA**te **V**ariability **A**ccelerations **D**ecelerations **O**verall assessment

AAFP (2004).

Table 3.1 CTG classification.

	Baseline (bpm)	Variability (bpm)	Decelerations (bpm)	Accelerations (bpm)
Reassuring	110–160	≥5	None	Present
Non-reassuring	100–109 161–180	<5 for 40–90 min	Typical variable decelerations with over 50% contractions for >90 min Single prolonged deceleration up to 3 min	The absence of accelerations with an otherwise normal CTG is of uncertain significance
Abnormal	<100 >180 Sinusoidal pattern ≥10 min	<5 for 90 min	Atypical variable decelerations with over 50% contractions for >90 min, or late decelerations, both for >30 min Single prolonged deceleration >3 min	

CTG classification:

Normal	A FHR trace where *all four* features are classified as reassuring
Suspicious	A FHR trace with *one* feature classified as non-reassuring categories but the remaining features as reassuring
Pathological	A FHR trace with *two or more* features classified as non-reassuring or *one or more* as abnormal.

Reproduced with kind permission from NICE (NICE, 2007).

Positive and negative aspects of EFM

Positive aspects

- The belief underpinning the use of EFM is that it may identify a hypoxic fetus and enable early intervention and delivery.
- In studies reviewed by Grant (2000), parents said that EFM demonstrated that the baby was alive, giving them positive information. Some women and their partners felt reassured by hearing their baby's heartbeat (Sinclair, 2001). This was enhanced if they could see the monitor (Grant, 2000).
- Clinicians often feel reassured that they are doing something physical, measurable and observable when recording a trace of the fetal heart.
- A CTG trace may protect against litigation.
- Although not best practice, there are times on a busy delivery suite where EFM is used to 'keep an eye' on the fetal heart when the midwife is unavailable.

Negative aspects

- NICE (2007) uses the term 'offer' or 'advise' as opposed to 'recommend' when discussing EFM with women. This is presumably because EFM cannot be recommended due to lack of evidence to demonstrate benefit even for 'high-risk' women.
- EFM increases interventions such as FBS, episiotomy, instrumental delivery and CS. While it is associated with a reduction in neonatal seizures, it does not reduce

cerebral palsy, infant mortality or other standard measures of neonatal well-being (Alfirevic *et al.*, 2006; Graham *et al.*, 2006).

- Iatrogenesis is pathology that is caused by medical intervention, which, as Walsh (2001) states, is unacceptable because it is entirely preventable. The iatrogenic risks/complications of EFM are rarely discussed with women. 'Is this because clinicians are unaware of these complications?' questions Wagner (2000), who challenges clinicians by asking 'Is ignorance misconduct?' Many interventions can be unpleasant and stressful, and particularly hard to justify when the delivery is brought forward (e.g. by an episiotomy or an instrumental delivery/CS) and the baby is delivered without evidence of hypoxia. Wagner (2000) poignantly suggests doctors are rarely sued or criticised for unnecessary interventions.

- Beech Lawrence (2001) argues that not all risk is 'high risk' and that some conditions are notoriously misdiagnosed, such as oligohydramnios and growth-restricted babies, and that meconium-stained liquor has degrees of severity from irrelevant to ominous. Preterm infants have different heart from term infants due to the baby's immature autonomic nervous system and evidence that EFM offers any advantage over IA in preterm labours is not forthcoming (Alfrevic *et al.*, 2006).

- Grant (2000) demonstrates women undergoing EFM experience discomfort and restricted movement. NICE (2007) recommends that women are informed that EFM will restrict their mobility. Restricted movement is likely to prolong labour, to increase the need for analgesia and to increase FHR abnormalities (Gupta *et al.*, 2004). Some women feel EFM interferes with their relationship with their partner and caregivers. Women undergoing IA tend to have a more positive labour experience (Grant, 2000).

- The monitor, rather than the mother, can become the focus of attention and interest, and both staff and parents may become overly anxious (Walsh, 2000, 2001).

- The skill of interpreting EFM is of key importance. However, the interpretation of EFM is subject to human error and it is not an exact science. Several studies have highlighted inconsistencies in CTG interpretation both between different practitioners and for the same practitioner on different days (Devane & Lalor, 2005). Altaf *et al.* (2006) report that many midwives feel ambivalent about the use of EFM. Midwives may react to traces, consciously or subconsciously, differently from obstetricians, as identifying a problem may create a shift from midwifery to medical control. Education and training are vital. Midwives and obstetric staff should have regular updates; CNST recommends six monthly updates in CTG analysis (CNST, 2006). Training will help reduce, but not eliminate, differences in interpretation.

Summary

- Most babies go through labour with no problems. FH monitoring aims to detect the few who become hypoxic.
- Some women and their partners find FH monitoring reassuring; however, more report it as an unwelcome distraction and cause of anxiety.
- Express consent must always be obtained for any form of FH monitoring.
- IA is the method of choice for low-risk women in labour.
- There is no evidence to support a 'routine' admission trace.

- Continuous EFM is offered to women who have increased risk factors, although there is no evidence of its efficacy.
  - Units using EFM should have FBS available before a CS is performed.
  - Encourage movement and frequent mobilisation for women having continuous EFM.
  - Always consider the context of a CTG; i.e. what else is happening which might be causing changes to the FHR.
  - CTG traces should be clearly labelled and stored safely.
- Midwives must ensure they can interpret a CTG trace knowledgeably and undertake regular CTG updates.

Useful contact

Association of Radical Midwives (ARM) Suppliers of wooden pinards. Helpline: 01243 671673. Website: www.midwifery.org.uk

References

Alfirevic, Z., Devane, D. & Gyte, G.M.L. (2006) Continuous cardiotocography (CTG) as a form of electronic fetal monitoring (EFM) for fetal assessment in labour. *Cochrane database of Systemic Reviews*, Issue 3, Art. No. CD006066. DOI: 10.1002/14651858.CD006066. Available at: www.thecochranelibrary.com

Altaf, S., Oppenheimer, C., Shaw, R., Waugh, J. & Dixon-Woods, N. (2006) Practices and views on fetal heart monitoring: a structured observation and interview study. *British Journal of Obstetrics and Gynaecology* **113** (4), 409–18.

American Academy of Family Physicians (2004) *Advanced Life Support in Obstetrics (ALSO) Provider Manual*, 4th edn.

Atalla, R., Kean, L. & McParland, P. (2000) Preterm labour and predator rupture of the membranes. In *Best Practice in Labour Ward Management* (Kean, L.H., Baker, P. & Edelstone, D.I., eds), pp. 111–39. WB Saunders, Edinburgh.

Beech Lawrence, B. (2001) Electronic fetal monitoring: do NICE's new guidelines owe too much to the medical model of childbirth? *The Practising Midwife* **4** (7), 31–3.

Clinical Negligence Scheme for Trusts (2006) *Maternity Clinical Risk Management Standards*. NHS Litigation Authority. Available at: www.nhsla.com (accessed March 2008).

Devane, D. & Lalor, J. (2005) Midwives' visual interpretation of intrapartum cardiotocographs: intra- and inter-observer agreement. *Journal of Advanced Nursing* **52** (2), 133–41.

Graham, E.M., Petersen, S.M., Christo, D.K. & Fox, H. (2006) Intrapartum electronic fetal heart rate monitoring and the prevention of perinatal brain injury. *Obstetrics and Gynaecology* **108** (3, part 1), 656–66.

Grant, A. (2000) Care of the fetus during labour. In *A Guide to Effective Care in Pregnancy and Childbirth*, 3rd edn (Enkin, M., Keirse, M.J.N.C., Neilson, J., Crowther, C., Duley, L., Hodnett, E. & Hofmeyr, J., eds), pp. 267–80. Oxford University Press, Oxford.

Gupta, J.K., Hofmeyr, G.J. & Smyth, R. (2004) Position in the second stage of labour for women without epidural anaesthesia. *Cochrane Database of Systematic Reviews*, Issue 1. Art. No. CD002006. DOI: 10.1002/14651858.CD002006.pub2. Available at: www.thecochranelibrary.com

Hindley, C., Wren Hinsliff, S. & Thomson, A.M. (2005) Developing a tool to appraise fetal monitoring guidelines for women at low obstetric risk. *Journal of Advanced Nursing* **52** (3), 307–14.

Hindley, C., Wren Hinsliff, S. & Thomson, A.M. (2006) English midwives' views and experiences of intrapartum fetal heart rate monitoring in women at low obstetric risk: conflicts and compromises. *Journal of Midwifery and Women's Health* **51** (5), 354–60.

National Institute for Health and Clinical Excellence (NICE) (2007) *Clinical Guideline 55: Intrapartum Care.* National Institute for Health and Clinical Excellence, London.

Sinclair, M. (2001) Birth technology. *RCM Midwives Journal* **4** (6), 168.

Spiby, H. (2001) The NICE guidelines on electronic fetal monitoring. *British Journal of Midwifery* **9** (8), 489.

Wagner, M. (2000) Choosing caesarean section. *The Lancet* **356**, 1677–80.

Walsh, D. (2000) Evidence-based care. Part 4: Fetal monitoring should be controlled. *British Journal of Midwifery* **8** (8), 511–16.

Walsh, D. (2001) Midwives and birth technology: a debate that's overdue. *MIDIRS Midwifery Digest* **11** (Suppl. 2), S3–6.

Appendix: Continuous EFM algorithm

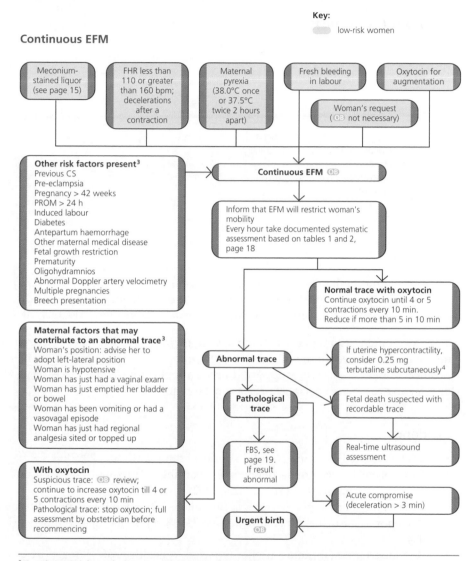

Key:

⬤ low-risk women

Continuous EFM

Meconium-stained liquor (see page 15)

FHR less than 110 or greater than 160 bpm; decelerations after a contraction

Maternal pyrexia (38.0°C once or 37.5°C twice 2 hours apart)

Fresh bleeding in labour

Oxytocin for augmentation

Woman's request (OB not necessary)

Other risk factors present³
Previous CS
Pre-eclampsia
Pregnancy > 42 weeks
PROM > 24 h
Induced labour
Diabetes
Antepartum haemorrhage
Other maternal medical disease
Fetal growth restriction
Prematurity
Oligohydramnios
Abnormal Doppler artery velocimetry
Multiple pregnancies
Breech presentation

Continuous EFM OB

Inform that EFM will restrict woman's mobility
Every hour take documented systematic assessment based on tables 1 and 2, page 18

Normal trace with oxytocin
Continue oxytocin until 4 or 5 contractions every 10 min.
Reduce if more than 5 in 10 min

Maternal factors that may contribute to an abnormal trace³
Woman's position: advise her to adopt left-lateral position
Woman is hypotensive
Woman has just had a vaginal exam
Woman has just emptied her bladder or bowel
Woman has been vomiting or had a vasovagal episode
Woman has just had regional analgesia sited or topped up

Abnormal trace

If uterine hypercontractility, consider 0.25 mg terbutaline subcutaneously⁴

Pathological trace

Fetal death suspected with recordable trace

Real-time ultrasound assessment

FBS, see page 19.
If result abnormal

With oxytocin
Suspicious trace: OB review; continue to increase oxytocin till 4 or 5 contractions every 10 min
Pathological trace: stop oxytocin; full assessment by obstetrician before recommencing

Acute compromise (deceleration > 3 min)

Urgent birth OB

³ These factors (risk factors for women outside the scope of this guideline and maternal factors that may contribute to an abnormal trace) are from 'Electronic fetal monitoring' (NICE inherited guideline C) which this guideline updates and replaces.
⁴ At the time of publication (September 2007), terbutaline did not have UK marketing authorisation for this indication. Informed consent should be obtained and documented.

4 Perineal trauma and suturing

Vicky Chapman

Introduction

'Maternal morbidity caused by perineal trauma can have long term social, psychological and physical health consequences for women. Perineal pain and discomfort may disrupt breastfeeding, family life and sexual relationships' (RCOG, 2004).

Many women sustain perineal trauma when giving birth. Some perineal trauma will heal without intervention, while some will require suturing. The midwife is in a key position to offer advice and support, if necessary performing any necessary suturing or referring to a more specialist professional if required.

Incidence

- 85% UK vaginal deliveries result in perineal trauma (Kettle, 2002).
- Most perineal tears are second degree, varying from small and well aligned to extensive or complicated (Yiannouzis, 2002).
- In the first 3 months postpartum, approximately 23% women report dyspareunia, 19% report some urinary incontinence and 3–10% report faecal incontinence (RCOG, 2004).
- Most long-term symptoms are not reported to health professionals (RCOG, 2004; Bedwell, 2006).
- 0.5–2.5% of women sustain a third- or fourth-degree tear, with a small risk of recurrence in a subsequent vaginal birth of 4.5% (Byrd *et al.*, 2005).

Facts

- Studies on suturing versus non-suturing second-degree tears have found no significant statistical differences between the two groups except on initial healing times (Metcalfe *et al.*, 2006).

- Women report the experience of being sutured as highly unpleasant and those receiving local anaesthetic, as opposed to regional, report high levels of pain throughout the procedure (Saunders *et al.*, 2002).
- The evidence suggests that using the correct repair material and suture technique will significantly reduce postnatal pain (Kettle & Johanson, 2006a, b).
- Performing a rectal inspection and examination *prior* to suturing will improve the detection of third- and fourth-degree tears (Andrews *et al.*, 2005).
- Postpartum faecal and flatus incontinence are commonly (although not exclusively) associated with third- and fourth-degree tears.
- Episiotomy increases the incidence of more serious tearing including third- and fourth-degree tears, faecal incontinence, perineal pain and dyspareunia (Carroli & Belizan, 2004).
- Appropriate training has been linked to increased practitioner confidence, improved evidence-based practice and knowledge of anal sphincter injuries (Andrews *et al.*, 2005) and thus should help reduce morbidity and associated litigation (RCOG, 2004).
- Regular pelvic floor exercises are effective in maintaining or reestablishing urinary continence (Chiarelli & Cockburn, 2002).
- Women appear to prefer their own midwife to conduct the perineal repair (Jackson, 2000).

Reducing perineal trauma

There are few studies on midwifery techniques to protect the perineum during spontaneous delivery (Eason *et al.*, 2000). Factors such as primiparity, episiotomy, instrumental birth (especially forceps) and heavier babies are associated with greater trauma (Dahlen *et al.*, 2006).

There is little practical evidence to inform modern midwifery practice on how to improve perineal outcomes. Evidence suggests that perineal trauma can be reduced by antenatal massage of the perineum in primigravida (Labrecque *et al.*, 1999; Beckmann & Garrett, 2006) and continuous support in labour (Hodnett *et al.*, 2003). There is some evidence of benefit in non-active pushing and a gentle, unhurried birth (Jackson, 2000; Albers *et al.*, 2006), birth at home (Aikins Murphy & Feinland, 1998); also birth position may affect perineal outcome (Shorten *et al.*, 2002) with the lateral birth position having the highest intact perineum rate and upright/squatting postures the lowest (Shorten *et al.*, 2002; Bedwell, 2006). However, upright and hand and knees position (not squatting though) seemed to reduce trauma in one study (Soong & Barnes, 2005). Flexing the head (Bedwell, 2006) and invasive perineal massage in labour does not reduce trauma (Stamp *et al.*, 2001).

(See also Chapter 1, p. 20, for more on prevention of perineal trauma.)

Assessment of perineal trauma

Prior to deciding whether suturing is required (see also Table 4.1), the genitalia should be examined using a good light source. On carefully inspecting the perineum if there is a moderate to large tear, it is thought best practice to perform a *digital* (National Institute

Table 4.1   Classification of perineal trauma.

Anterior perineal trauma
- Injury to the labia varying from painful grazes to deeper – sometimes bilateral – labial lacerations which may require sutures
- Less commonly involves the anterior vagina, urethra or clitoris

Posterior perineal trauma
- **First degree:** Injury to just the skin
- **Second degree:** Injury to the skin, vaginal tissue and perineal muscle. The trauma may be small, medium or large, long and deep; sometimes a branch tear (extending up both sides of the vagina)
- **Third degree:** Injury to skin, perineal muscle and involves the anal sphincter. Sultan (2002) suggests this can be subdivided into:
  - **3a** Partial tear of the anal sphincter
  - **3b** Complete tear of the anal sphincter
  - **3c** Internal sphincter also torn
- **Fourth degree:** Injury to the skin, perineal muscle and extending into the anal sphincter and rectal mucosa

for Health and Clinical Excellence (NICE), 2007) and *visual* inspection of the anus to ascertain any anal involvement.

- Consent must be obtained for this intimate and often uncomfortable examination, and entonox should be offered.
- Be gentle and careful, using wet gauze to part and inspect the labia, then vagina, then perineum, leaving the possible rectal examination until last.
- A third-degree tear may be visualised by parting the perineum where it meets the anus to see if the anal sphincter is intact, nicked or more seriously torn. On rectal examination, gently insert a lubricated, gloved finger into the anus and lift slightly to feel the surface of the rectum and anus, while also checking visually for a tear.

A perineal trauma measuring tool called the Peri-Rule™ has recently been developed. Its inventors suggest that objective assessment of the length and depth of perineal trauma will improve outcomes and reduce litigation (Metcalfe *et al.*, 2006). However, an objective measurement of a tear does not guarantee the quality of the subsequent repair and the Peri-Rule has not been accepted uncritically by midwives.

Labial tears

The labia minora area is very sensitive and vascular: tears tend to heal well without stitches. However, sutures will be required if the tear continues to bleed or the trauma is fairly deep. Bilateral tears or grazes can result in both labia healing together and fusing. Warn the woman about this possibility and, whether or not bilateral trauma is sutured, suggest she gently parts the labia once a day, perhaps in the bath or shower, to minimise the danger of labial fusion.

First- and second-degree tears: to suture or not to suture?

The trend towards not suturing tears has evolved on the strength of limited evidence, and Yiannouzis (2002) suggests several reasons, including increased maternal choice, increased midwifery autonomy and staffing pressures. There have been various small studies involving non-suturing of first- or second-degree tears (Head, 1993; Lundquist *et al.*, 2000; Fleming *et al.*, 2003) and several larger studies (Langley *et al.*, 2006; Metcalfe *et al.*, 2006; Leeman *et al.*, 2007). Midwives and women have strong views on which option they prefer, often resulting in difficulties in recruiting participants and staff compliance. in randomised studies. For example Metcalfe *et al.*'s study noted poor trial compliance: midwives did not suture one third of tears in the group randomised for suturing.

NICE (2007) recommends suturing for the following:

- First-degree tears if the skin is not well opposed.
- All second-degree tears.

However, this advice is based on very limited evidence from one small randomised controlled trial (Fleming *et al.*, 2003). Since then other larger studies have emerged (Langley *et al.*, 2006; Metcalfe *et al.*, 2006; Leeman *et al.*, 2007) and their findings are discussed below.

- All studies found a slower initial healing in the non-sutured groups. This difference was apparent in the immediate short-term period with poorer wound approximation and healing.
- The proportion of women with (subjectively assessed) 'gaping', asymmetrical or open perineal wounds was similar at 6 weeks between the groups in some studies (Langley *et al.*, 2006; Leeman *et al.*, 2007).
- Conversely, Fleming *et al.* (2003) and Metcalfe *et al.* (2006) found poorer wound approximation in some unsutured women at 6 weeks.
- Overall there were few statistical differences in secondary measures of pain, longer-term healing times, pelvic incontinence, infection rates and resumption of sexual intercourse (Langley *et al.*, 2006; Metcalfe *et al.*, 2006; Leeman *et al.*, 2007).

Some clinicians have speculated that leaving the muscle layer unsutured could cause pelvic floor problems later on (McCandlish, 2001). Leeman *et al.*'s study on pelvic floor function found that weak pelvic floor exercise strength was more common with second-degree lacerations compared with an intact perineum, but did not differ between sutured and unsutured groups. Likewise, perineal body or genital hiatus ('gape') measurements did not vary between groups (Leeman *et al.*, 2007).

To date there have been no randomised controlled trials of the quality and size to reach statistical power and draw clear evidence-based conclusions on the non-suturing of second-degree tears. Langley *et al.* (2006) suggest that while the balance of evidence tends towards suturing, it is based on limited and weak trials. So while midwives will no doubt hold a personal preference for a particular choice, it must be the woman who ultimately makes her feelings and preferences known, in light of the limited available evidence.

Non-suturing

- Offers women the opportunity to avoid the pain of being sutured (Lundquist *et al.*, 2000).
- Results in slower initial healing and is more likely to have poor wound alignment.

- Some studies suggest no difference by 6 weeks post-birth; others observe poorer wound approximation in a small minority of non-sutured wounds at 6 weeks (Metcalfe *et al.*, 2006).

Suturing

- Reduces uncertainty as this method is common practice.
- Enables faster initial healing and better wound alignment (Langley *et al.*, 2006; Metcalfe *et al.*, 2006; Leeman *et al.*, 2007).
- Results in no difference in *reported* postnatal pain, but analgesia use is increased (Langley *et al.*, 2006; Leeman *et al.*, 2007).
- Most women find suturing unpleasant, uncomfortable and painful (Saunders *et al.*, 2002). Women may feel they are 'being patched up' but endure it because they believe it to be beneficial (NICE, 2007).

All women should be aware that *suturing remains strongly advisable for* extensive perineal trauma, a large second-degree tear, a third- or fourth-degree tear, if bleeding continues, if the wound is very misaligned/complicated or the result of an unnatural straight-edged cut from an episiotomy. Ultimately, it must remain the woman's choice whether to accept or decline suturing.

Third- and fourth-degree tears

Bedwell (2006) found that a midwife may be stigmatised and overtly or covertly criticised if a third- or fourth-degree tear follows a normal birth. Bedwell's analysis of the evidence found that third-degree tears were not associated with the delivery technique *nor were they preventable* and that although midwives often felt personally responsible, and even guilty, they should be reassured that such tears remain the unavoidable outcome for a tiny percentage of births.

Failure to diagnose third- or fourth-degree tears may be considered substandard care and this contributes to most litigation associated with perineal trauma (RCOG, 2004). Such tears should be properly assessed and sutured by an experienced doctor in theatre, usually under regional anaesthesia. Post-repair care usually involves a catheter, stool softeners and antibiotics (RCOG, 2004).

Due to the impact such trauma can have on a woman's quality of life, the woman should receive clear explanations and obstetric follow-up (Sultan, 2002). The community midwife and general practitioner should also be informed. Webb *et al.* (2007) suggest:

> 'There is no prescribed mode of delivery for any subsequent birth: this will need to be an individualised decision made nearer the time, based on a number of factors including bladder and bowel function and what the woman wishes.'

Providing care for survivors of childhood sexual abuse

Women may not disclose that they have been sexually assaulted as a child or adult. Symptoms exhibited by abuse survivors can be misinterpreted and result in women being labelled as 'difficult patients'. This lack of awareness can result in inappropriate treatment, causing further psychological trauma (Aldcroft, 2001).

For some women the restriction of the lithotomy position makes them feel they are at the mercy of an authoritative figure and are submitting to a painful, invasive and sexually threatening procedure. This can leave them feeling violated and powerless (Kitzinger, 1992) and can have far-reaching psychological consequences. It may affect the relationship with the baby who may inadvertently be blamed for 'putting them through this' (Aldcroft, 2001). (For more information see Chapter 2.)

Suturing procedure

Long-term physical, psychological and social problems may result from incorrect approximation of wounds and unrecognised trauma to the external anal sphincter (RCOG, 2004). The three main factors that influence the outcome of perineal repair are the suturing material, the repair technique and the skill of the operator (RCOG, 2004).

Analgesia

Saunders *et al.* (2002) reported women's experience of pain during perineal suturing: 17% of women reported 'distressing', 'horrible' or 'excruciating' pain. To the reviewers' surprise, women's pain scores did not diminish as the time between suturing and pain reporting increased. In particular, women without regional anaesthetic were found to endure high levels of pain during this procedure. The clinician must be gentle, sensitive and *never* proceed if the woman is inadequately anaesthetised.

- Women may combine entonox and local or regional anaesthetic.
- If the woman has an epidural in situ, the midwife should readily offer a 'top-up' as Saunders *et al.* (2002) found that this offers a superior degree of analgesia compared to local anaesthetic.
- Local anaesthetic takes time to work effectively; the clinician can inject up to 20 ml of 1% Lidocaine/Lignocaine™ (NICE, 2007) and leave it to work prior to preparing equipment for the procedure.
- *Take care to avoid intravascular injection* of Lidocaine/Lignocaine by drawing back on the syringe plunger, to ensure no blood is aspirated which might indicate a vessel has been penetrated. Injection into a blood vessel can cause central nervous system excitatory response leading to confusion, convulsions, respiratory depression, bradycardia and even death (JFC, 2007).

Suturing materials

Current evidence suggests that the suture material of choice for perineal repair is rapid-absorption polyglactin 910 (Vicryl™) and a good second choice is polyglycolic acid as these synthetic sutures are associated with less perineal pain, analgesic use, dehiscence and resuturing, but increased suture removal, when compared with catgut. Catgut suture material has been withdrawn from the UK market since 2002 (RCOG, 2004; Kettle & Johanson, 2006a).

Suturing techniques

Suturing is an aseptic technique. The type of tear may involve different layers (see also Table 4.1) and so will influence the type of suturing technique:

- **Muscle layer.** Current evidence supports using a loose, continuous non-locking technique to suture vaginal tissue and perineal muscle. Subsequent stitch tightness and tension from reactionary oedema are transferred more evenly throughout the whole length of the single knotless suture, which is thought beneficial in reducing short-term pain and subsequent suture removal for tightness and discomfort (Kettle *et al.*, 2002; RCOG, 2004) (See under 'Perineal suturing procedure').
- **Skin layer.** The use of subcuticular continuous suturing is superior to interrupted sutures for the perineal skin (Kettle *et al.*, 2002; Kettle & Johanson, 2006b). All midwives should learn and practice this simple technique as it reduces postnatal pain and constitutes best practice.
- **Skin layer unsutured.** Studies have also evaluated suturing only the vaginal and perineal muscle layers but leaving the skin unsutured. NICE (2007) suggests if the edges are opposed, the perineal skin can remain unsutured. This is also preferable to interrupted sutures to the skin, resulting in a significant reduction in adverse outcomes, but was associated with a slight increase in wound gaping up to 10 days following birth (RCOG, 2004). Petrou *et al.* (2001) suggest leaving the skin unsutured is also cost-effective as it reduces use of healthcare resources.

There has, as yet, been no comparison between subcuticular continuous suturing and leaving the skin unsutured.

Figure 4.1 shows the basic sequence of inserting a stitch and tying a knot.

Suturing at home

Midwives must be resourceful! A good fixed light source is essential. Ensure the woman can lie comfortably with her bottom on the edge of a firm bed with the midwife positioned on the floor or low stool. The woman may find it most comfortable to rest her legs on separate chairs or she can abduct them herself but this is only usually comfortable for a short time. If both the woman and the midwife get on the floor, it is very hard on the midwife's back and visualising/accessing the perineum can be awkward.

Perineal suturing procedure

Following discussion, explanations, reassurance and informed consent, the midwife can prepare everything ready for suturing, including a fixed light source, optional post-suturing analgesia and, in hospital, the call bell within reach (so the woman can summon assistance if required during suturing).

Before starting the repair address the following questions:

- Is the mother as comfortable as possible?
- Does she understand what has to be done and how long it will take?
- Can I see what has to be done?
- Can I do it?

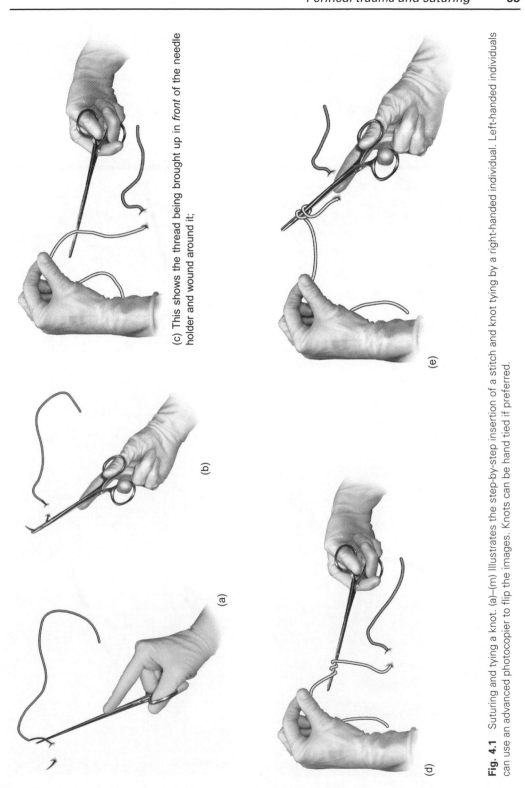

(c) This shows the thread being brought up in *front* of the needle holder and wound around it;

(b)

(a)

(e)

(d)

Fig. 4.1 Suturing and tying a knot. (a)–(m) Illustrates the step-by-step insertion of a stitch and knot tying by a right-handed individual. Left-handed individuals can use an advanced photocopier to flip the images. Knots can be hand tied if preferred.

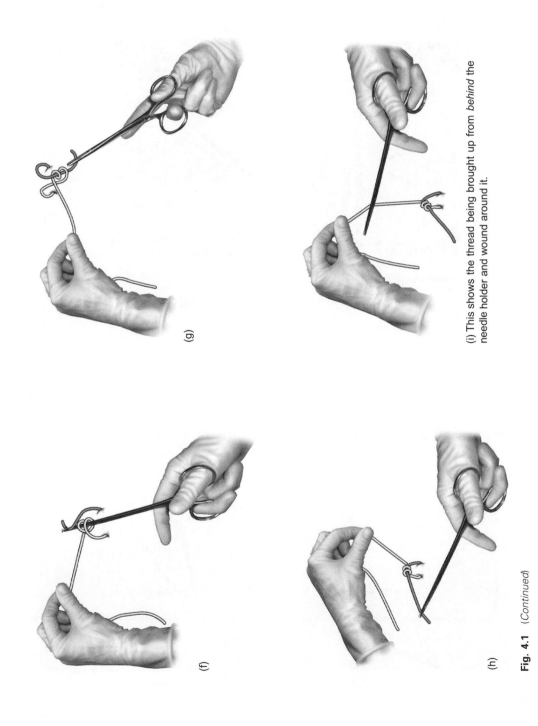

(g)

(f)

(i) This shows the thread being brought up from *behind* the needle holder and wound around it.

(h)

Fig. 4.1 *(Continued)*

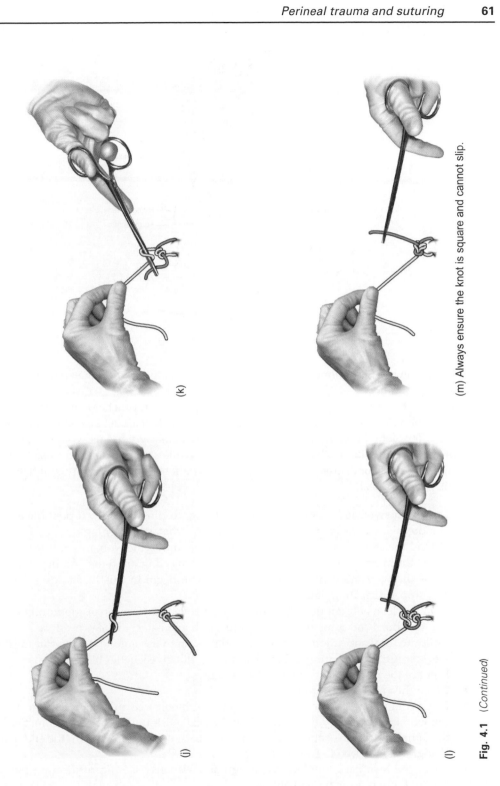

(k)

(j)

(l)

(m) Always ensure the knot is square and cannot slip.

Fig. 4.1 (*Continued*)

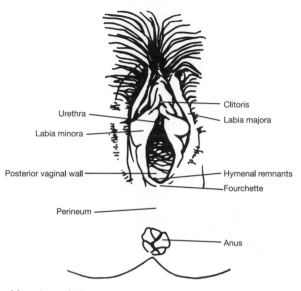

Urethra

Labia minora

Posterior vaginal wall

Perineum

Clitoris

Labia majora

Hymenal remnants

Fourchette

Anus

Fig. 4.2   Anatomy of female genitalia.

An overview of the perineum is shown in Fig. 4.2 to help visualise the anatomy of the female genitalia.

Placing the woman's legs in lithotomy is no longer routine practice in many hospitals. The woman may prefer to just relax her legs apart (Kettle *et al.*, 2002), resting her knees against obsolete lithotomy poles if desired. A particularly nervous woman may feel more in control with her legs resting apart and, while she may need to close them if something hurts or distresses her, the midwife's patience and sensitivity will help her through this ordeal.

- Ensure the woman is comfortable and holding/feeding her baby if possible as she is more likely to relax and pay less attention to what is happening.
- Extend the sterile field by placing a sterile sheet under the woman's buttocks.
- Warn the woman before touching, wiping or injecting anything. As the midwife earns the woman's confidence, the woman will begin to trust her midwife, relax and stop anticipating pain.
- Initially clean only enough of the perineum to inject the local anaesthetic, otherwise this will burn and sting and is, therefore, not a good start to the procedure.
- Infiltrate local anaesthetic (the woman may wish to use entonox) and wait for it to work; infiltration 10 minutes before suturing will give a better block.
- Prepare the instruments and count all swabs.
- Clean the area more thoroughly if required.
- Insert a tampon. This keeps the area below it blood free and visually clear. Warn the woman this is very uncomfortable; she may wish to use entonox again. Secure the tampon string to drapes (if used) or the sheet covering the woman (the end of the string does not need to be sterile).
- Move the tear 'back together' to realign and visualise significant meeting points; ensure there is no anal involvement.

- Locate the apex in the vagina; secure the first stitch just above it.
- Using a continuous suture technique, bring the muscle layers together (see Figs. 4.3a–c).
- If a stitch appears misplaced then unfortunately it will require the needle to be cut free to allow unpicking and then a knot tied. Recommence a new set of continuous stitching from the point left off.
- For the skin: if the edges are opposed after suturing the muscle layer, it can be left unsutured (NICE, 2007). If sutures are required, use a subcuticular continuous suturing technique (Figs. 4.3d–h). Do not insert interrupted stitches.
- Visually inspect the stitches before preparing the woman for the uncomfortable removal of the tampon.
- Inform the woman before checking her rectum. Gently insert a lubricated finger, fleshy side up and slowly withdraw it, checking the anus visually as well as feeling for any stitches that may have gone through, for 'buttonholes' or a tear.
- If the woman wishes (providing there are no contraindications), administer diclofenac 100 mg suppository rectally post-suturing. This reduces additional analgesia use and perineal pain for around 24 hours and even up to 48 hours following administration (Parsons & Crowther, 2007).
- Place a sanitary pad over the perineum and assist the woman back into a comfortable position.
- Count up and account for all needles, swabs and instruments.
- **Document findings** accurately and comprehensively in black ink, including a diagram to illustrate the trauma (RCOG, 2004), the anaesthetic used, suture material and repair technique (e.g. 'continuous, loose non-locking sutures in the vagina and perineal muscle and subcuticular to the skin'). Document anything unusual such as difficulty controlling bleeding, tying off a bleeding vessel (see p. 214), a branch tear, graze, skin flap or awkwardly shaped tear.

Some general information can be shared with the woman during suturing:

- Suggest she tries to pass urine in the bath following suturing, as it is thought to be less painful.
- Discuss sitting, breastfeeding and comfort, pain control (e.g. cool packs) and if sutures become tight or irritating in several days, suggest that, although it may appear daunting, the snipping of the stitch inside the introitus can bring great relief.
- Most women do not have their bowels opened until day 3 postpartum; discuss this topic and explain that she will not 'come undone'. Advise her about hygiene and washing, wiping gently from front to back, supporting the perineum with a pad when having bowels open, etc.
- Around 20% childbearing women suffer from urinary incontinence. Layton (2004) suggests that midwives may not be giving women enough information about this unpleasant and socially embarrassing problem. Suturing can be the perfect time for midwives to communicate to women the importance of regular pelvic floor exercises, explaining that these have been proved to be effective in maintaining continence to a significant degree (Chiarelli & Cockburn, 2002).
- It may be appropriate to discuss the first sexual intercourse after the baby. Suggest the couple both feel relaxed and aroused enough before having full intercourse and consider the use of lubricating jelly.

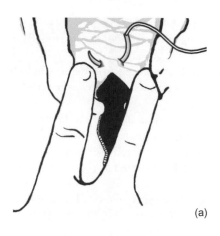
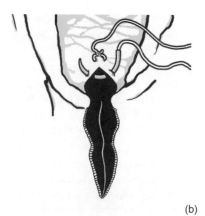

(a)

(b)

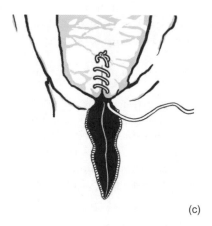
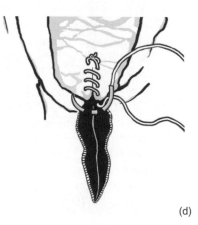

(c)

(d)

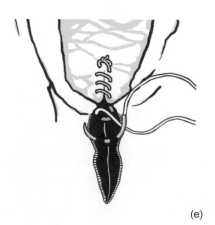
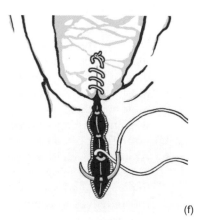

(e)

(f)

Fig. 4.3   Suturing a second-degree tear. Place the first stitch above the apex of the vaginal trauma, in order to secure any deeper bleeding points (a, b). Place the loose, continuous sutures from the apex along the tear. Do not use a locking or blanket stitch, or pull sutures too tight (c). The perineum stitches are placed loosely and deeply in the subcuticular tissue (d–g). Place subcuticular, continuous sutures just under the skin (avoid placing any sutures in the fourchette) (h–k). Finish with the thread in the vagina, where a knot is tied (l).

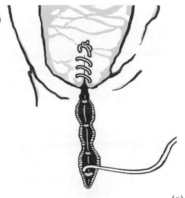

(g)

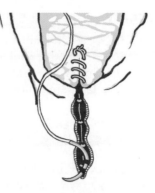

(h)

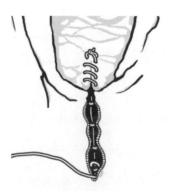

(i)

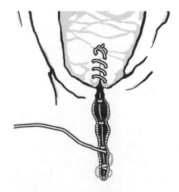

(j)

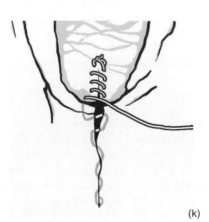

(k)

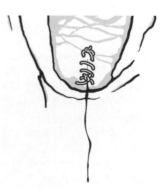

(l)

Fig. 4.3 (*Continued*)

Summary

- There are few studies on midwifery techniques to protect the perineum during birth.
- Suturing is recommended for perineal/labial trauma that is complicated/large/ bleeding/very misaligned/third or fourth degree or from an episiotomy.
- A rectal examination prior to suturing may improve the diagnosis of third/fourth-degree tears, which should be sutured only by an experienced doctor.
- Studies suggest little difference in non-suturing or suturing for second-degree tears; however, these studies are not large enough to reach statistical power.
- It is *the woman's choice* whether to accept or decline suturing.
- Clinicians must be sensitive and responsive to any pain or anxiety expressed.
- Women who have experienced sexual abuse may be especially vulnerable.

Suturing

- Suture using an aseptic technique with effective analgesia
- Rapidly absorbed polyglactin 910 (Vicryl) is the suture material of choice.
- The muscle layer should be sutured with a loose, non-locking, continuous suture.
- The perineal skin can be left unsutured or repaired with continuous (not interrupted) suture technique.

References

Aikins Murphy, P. & Feinland, J.B. (1998) Perineal outcomes in a home birth setting. *Birth* **25** (4), 226–34.

Albers, L.L., Sedler, K.D. & Bedrick, E.J. (2006) Factors related to genital tract trauma normal spontaneous vaginal births. *Birth* **33** (2), 94–100.

Aldcroft, D. (2001) A guide to providing care for survivors of child sex abuse. *British Journal of Midwifery* **9** (2), 81–5.

Andrews, V., Thakar, R., Sultan, A H. & Kettle, K. (2005) Can hands-on perineal repair courses affect clinical practice? *British Journal Midwifery* **13** (9), 562–6.

Beckmann, M.M. & Garrett, A.J. (2006) Antenatal perineal massage for reducing perineal trauma. *Cochrane Database of Systematic Reviews*, Issue 1.

Bedwell, C. (2006) Are third degree tears unavoidable? The role of the midwife. *British Journal of Midwifery* **14** (9), 212.

Byrd, L.M., Hobbiss, J. & Tasker, M. (2005) Is it possible to predict or prevent third degree tears? *Colorectal Disease* **7**, 311–18.

Carroli, G. & Belizan, J. (2007) Episiotomy for vaginal birth. *Cochrane Database of Systematic Reviews*, Issue 1. Update Software, Oxford.

Chiarelli, P. & Cockburn, J. (2002) Promoting urinary continence in women after delivery: a randomised controlled trial. *British Medical Journal* **324** (7348), 1241–4.

Dahlen, H.G., Ryan, M., Homer, C.S. & Cooke, M. (2006) An Australian prospective cohort study of risk factors for severe perineal trauma during childbirth. *Midwifery* **23** (2), 196–203.

Eason, E., Labrecque, M., Wells, G. & Feldman, P. (2000) Preventing perineal trauma during childbirth: a systematic review. *Obstetrics and Gynecology* **95** (3), 464–71.

Fleming, V.E.M., Hagen, S. & Niven, C. (2003) Does perineal suturing make a difference? SUNS trial. *British Journal of Obstetrics and Gynaecology* **110** (7), 684–9.

Head, M. (1993) Dropping stitches. Do unsutured tears to the perineum heal better than sutured ones? *Nursing Times* **89** (33), 64–5.

Hodnett, E.D., Gates, S., Hofmeyr, G.J. & Sakala, C. (2003) Continuous support for women during childbirth (Cochrane Review). In *The Cochrane Library*, Issue 3.

Jackson, K. (2000) The bottom line: care of the perineum must be improved. *British Journal of Midwifery* **8** (10), 609–14.

Joint Formulary Committee (2007) *British National Formulary*, 53rd edn. British Medical Association and Royal Pharmaceutical society of great Britain.

Kettle, C. (2002) Materials and methods for perineal repair. Are you sitting comfortably? Issues around perineal trauma. *RCM Midwives Journal* **5** (9), 298–301.

Kettle, C., Hills, R.K., Jones, P., Darby, L., Gray, R. & Johanson, R. (2002) Continuous versus interrupted perineal repair with standard or rapidly absorbed sutures after spontaneous vaginal birth: a randomised controlled trial. *The Lancet* **359**, 2217–22.

Kettle, C. & Johanson, R. (2006a) Absorbable synthetic versus catgut suture material for perineal repair (Cochrane Review). *The Cochrane Library*, Issue 4. Update Software, Oxford.

Kettle, C. & Johanson, R. (2006b) Continuous versus interrupted sutures for perineal repair (Cochrane Review). *The Cochrane Library*, Issue 4. Update Software, Oxford.

Kitzinger, J.V. (1992) Counteracting, not re-enacting, the violation of women's bodies: the challenge for perinatal caregivers. *Birth* **19** (4), 219–22.

Labrecque, M., Eason, E., Marcoux, S., Lemieux, F., Pinault, J.-J., Feldman, P. & Laperriere L. (1999) Randomised controlled trial of prevention of perineal trauma by massage during pregnancy. *American Journal of Obstetrics and Gynecology* **10** (3), 593–600.

Langley, V., Thoburn, A., Shaw, S. & Barton, A., (2006) Second degree tears: to suture or not? A randomized controlled trial. *British Journal of Midwifery* **14** (9), 550–54.

Layton, S. (2004) The effect of perineal trauma on women's health. *British Journal of Midwifery* **12** (4), 231–6.

Leeman, L.M., Rogers, R.G., Greulich, B. & Albers, L.L. (2007) Do unsutured second-degree perineal lacerations affect postpartum functional outcomes? *Journal of the American Board of Family Medicine* **20** (5), 451–7.

Lundquist, M., Olisson, A., Nissen, E. & Normal, M. (2000) Is it necessary to suture all lacerations after a vaginal delivery? *Birth* **27** (2), 79–85.

McCandlish, R. (2001) Routine perineal suturing: is it time to stop? *MIDIRS Midwifery Digest* **11** (3), 296–300.

Metcalfe, A., Bick, D., Tohill, S., Williams, A. & Haldon, V. (2006) A prospective cohort study of repair and non-repair of second degree perineal trauma: results and issues for future research. *Evidence Based Midwifery* **4** (2), 60–64.

National Institute for Health and Clinical Excellence (NICE) (2007) *Intrapartum Care: Care of Healthy Women and Their Babies During Childbirth. Clinical Guideline 55.* NICE, London.

Parsons, J. & Crowther, C.A. (2007) Rectal analgesia for pain from perineal trauma following childbirth. *The Cochrane Library*, Issue 1. Update Software, Oxford.

Petrou, S., Gordon, B., Mackrodt, C., Fern, E., Ayers, S., Grant, A., Truesdale, A. & McCandlish R. (2001) How cost-effective is it to leave the skin unsutured? *British Journal of Midwifery* **9** (4), 209–14.

Royal College of Obstetricians and Gynaecologists (RCOG) (2004) *Clinical Green Top Guidelines: Methods and Materials Used in Perineal Repair 23.* Available at: http//www.rcog.org.uk/guidelines (accessed October 2007).

Saunders, J., Campbell, R. & Peters, T.J. (2002) Effectiveness of pain relief during suturing. *BJOG: An International Journal of Obstetrics and Gynaecology* **109**, 1066–8.

Shorten, A., Donsante, J. & Shorten, B. (2002) Birth position, accoucheur, and perineal outcomes: informing women about choices for vaginal birth. *Birth* **29** (1), 18–27.

Soong, B. & Barnes, M. (2005) Maternal position at midwife-attended birth and perineal trauma: is there an association? *Birth* **32**, 164–9.

Stamp, G., Kruzins, G. & Crowther, C. (2001) Perineal massage in labour and prevention of perineal trauma: randomised controlled trial. *BMJ* **322**, 1277–80.

Sultan, A. (2002) 'Have I missed a third degree tear?' The identification, treatment and follow-up of women who experience perineal trauma. Are you sitting comfortably? Issues around perineal trauma. *RCM Midwives Journal* **5** (9), 298.

Webb, S., Parsons, M. & Toozs-Hobson, P. (2007) The role of specialised birth plans for women with previous third or fourth degree obstetric anal sphincter injuries (OASIS). *MIDIRS* **17** (3), 353–4.

Yiannouzis, K. (2002) Describing perineal trauma: the development of an assessment tool. Are you sitting comfortably? Issues around perineal trauma. *RCM Midwives Journal* **5** (9), 300–301.

5   Examination of the newborn baby at birth

Caroline Rutter

Introduction

The newborn check, which involves a thorough examination of the baby, is performed in the first few hours after birth and, with experience, is generally quite quick to perform. Once familiar with the appearance of the average newborn, anything unusual is easily noticed. Remember general observation of the baby's condition and behaviour is as important as formal and systematic assessment.

It is important to involve the parents in their baby's check, explaining all actions and reassuring them. If an abnormality is suspected, a clear and simple explanation should be given and a senior paediatrician contacted. Where relevant, transfer to a consultant unit from a midwife-led unit or home may be necessary for paediatric examination and discussion with the parents.

The midwife's assessment of the baby at birth

Most babies are born responding well and these babies should be given straight to their mother for uninterrupted skin-to-skin contact. Occasionally, a baby may be born with an obvious problem requiring a prompt response. The Apgar score is used as one assessment of the baby's condition following birth (Table 5.1). Whilst the Apgar score is well established, it is not uncritically accepted and some have suggested abandoning it. (Patel & Beeby, 2004). The Apgar score may be helpful for deciding if resuscitation is required, but should not be relied on to determine the cause or prognosis of any hypoxic episode. If there are concerns about a baby's condition, then paired (arterial and venous) cord bloods should be analysed which will give a clearer picture of the degree and duration of any labour hypoxia.

Colour

Caucasian babies should appear pink at birth, often with blueish extremities (peripheral cyanosis) for several hours following delivery. Babies with darker skins tend to have a much paler version of their parents' skin tone with lighter extremities.

Possible problems are as follows:

- **Blueness around the mouth and trunk (central cyanosis).** It could indicate a respiratory or cardiac problem. Darker skin babies can look greyish white when cyanosed. If a baby appears cyanosed, oxygen should be administered, respiratory effort and heart rate assessed, and resuscitation should be initiated if required (see Chapter 21). Paediatric support should be requested.
- **Very pale baby.** Cardiac anomalies, anaemia or shock should be considered and resuscitation should be initiated if necessary.
- **Facial congestion.** A petechial rash seen as blue/mauve discolouration of the skin around the baby's face. This can be result from a rapid delivery, cord around the neck or shoulder dystocia. The lips and mucous membranes should be pink. Do not confuse facial congestion with a more generalised rash resulting from thrombocytopenia or congenital infections such as toxoplasmosis, meningitis or herpes (Baston & Durward, 2001).
- **Red baby.** A plethoric appearance may be due to a large transfusion of placental blood, e.g. in twin-to-twin transfusion.
- **Jaundice.** Within 24 hours of birth, jaundice is abnormal and may be due to haemolytic disease/rhesus incompatibility or from a congenital infection, e.g. rubella, toxoplasmosis, herpes, cytomegalovirus or syphilis. Such infections may cause other symptoms including respiratory distress, rash, hypo/hyperthermia, hypoglycaemia and poor feeding (Hull & Johnston, 1999).

Table 5.1 Apgar score.

Score	0	1	2
Colour	Blue or pale	Body pink, limbs blue	Pink
Respiratory effort	Absent	Irregular gasps	Strong cry
Heart rate	Absent	<100 bpm	>100 bpm
Muscle tone	Limp	Some limb flexion	Strong active movements
Reflex irritability	None	Grimace or sneeze	Cry

Apgar score is normally assessed at 1 and 5 min. Some like to record a 10 min score.
The 1 min score is often low: babies often recover quickly and have a good 5 min score.
A poor 5 min score is more indicative of a baby with real problems requiring active resuscitation.
Score at 5 min: 8–10, normal; 5–7, mild asphyxia; ≤4, severe asphyxia.

Respirations and cry

Not all newborns breathe immediately at birth nor do all cry at delivery, particularly if the birthing environment is calm, quiet and relaxed. Indeed anecdotal reports suggest that water birth babies do not always breathe immediately, but if the cord is not clamped and cut and is still pulsating at >100 bpm, the baby is likely to be receiving a good oxygen supply. However, some babies are seemingly inconsolable at birth. Once the baby is in the mother's arms and settled in skin-to-skin, the baby will usually relax and stop crying, often opening its eyes and with patience will eventually root towards the breast.

Possible problems are as follows:

- A baby with persistent tachypnoea (respirations >60/min in a term baby), grunting, nasal flaring or sternal recession is showing signs of respiratory distress. There are many causes including infection, meconium aspiration and cardiac problems. Refer to a paediatrician.
- A very mucusy baby who does not breathe following attempted inflation breaths will require gentle suction. Excessive secretions may be a sign of oesophageal atresia.
- A healthy newborn cry is variable, but a distinctly high pitched or 'irritable' cry could indicate pain or cerebral irritation.

Heart rate

A baby's heart rate can easily be ascertained by placing two fingers on the chest, directly over the heart, or by holding the base of the umbilical stump and counting the pulsating heart rate. Normal heart rate (HR) for a newborn baby should be 110–160 bpm.

Possible problems are as follows:

- *Bradycardia* (HR < 100 bpm) may be due to hypoxia. If other signs are good, the HR can recover quickly. If <60-bpm cardiac massage will be necessary (see Chapter 17).
- *Tachycardia* (HR > 160 bpm) may indicate a healthy response to a hypoxic episode. Again if other signs are good, it can recover quickly. It can however also indicate infection or a respiratory or cardiac problem. Refer for paediatric opinion if it persists.

Muscle tone

The newborn should have good muscle tone as well as normal reflexes and responses, such as opening its eyes and responding to external stimuli and touch. A baby who is floppy with poor muscle tone and little reflex response may have experienced significant hypoxia, or have a congenital abnormality, e.g. Down's syndrome.

Measurements of the newborn

Weight

Following skin-to-skin contact and feeding, the baby should be weighed. The parents may wish to watch and take photographs. Ideally electronic scales are used for greatest accuracy, zeroed after positioning a warm towel. A kg/lb conversion chart is provided in the Appendix.

A baby weighing less than 2.5 kg is usually considered to be of low birth weight; a very low birth weight is below 1.5 kg. Ethnic origin-specific weight charts may be useful in avoiding inappropriately labelling a baby as small for dates (Chung *et al.*, 2003).

A macrosomic or large baby is one with its weight above the 90th centile for its gestational age.

Both small and macrosomic babies are at risk of hypoglycaemia, so this should be noted and blood glucose estimates considered (Newel *et al.*, 1997).

A baby born at <37 weeks is classified as preterm. Some babies may be both preterm and small for dates: these babies are at higher risk of problems, as growth retardation is a sign of placental insufficiency.

Length

Jokinen (2002) suggests, in the light of recommendations from the Joint Working Party on Child Health (Hall & Elliman, 2002), that a baseline length measurement remains important for assessment of a baby's future growth and well-being. Fry (2002) emphasises the possibility of early detection of Turner's syndrome if length measurement at birth is used as a baseline in relation to subsequent growth patterns. Timing of this measurement and equipment used has been under debate. In the first hours after the birth the baby may still be in a fetal position and so this may not be the optimum time to obtain such a measurement. National Institute for Health and Clinical Excellence (NICE) (2007) recommends waiting at least 1 hour after birth. Jokinen (2002) notes that a tape measure has been proved to be unreliable (Wilshin *et al.*, 1999). Various studies have shown that midwives can get improved results if using the more accurate supine length measurement tools, such as a roll-up mat (Jokinen, 2002). The normal range for a term baby is 48–55 cm (Seidel *et al.*, 2006).

Head circumference

The head should be measured around the occipitofrontal circumference. The normal range for a term baby is 32–37 cm (Baston & Durward, 2001). Again there are arguments for delaying this measurement until the head has regained its shape following delivery and for the use of a metric insertion tape specifically designed for this purpose (Fry, 2002).

Vitamin K prophylaxis

Vitamin K is essential for the formation of prothrombin, which enables blood to clot. Haemorrhagic disease of the newborn (HDN) is a rare, potentially fatal, disorder that has been associated with low vitamin K levels. HDN may also be known as vitamin K deficiency bleeding (VKDB) since it can also occur later than the first week of life (Hey, 2003b). HDN/VKDB occurs most commonly in the first week: common bleeding sites are gastrointestinal, cutaneous, nasal and from circumcision (Puckett & Offringa, 2000). Late-onset bleeding occurring after the first week for up to 8 months is often associated with liver disease or malabsorption and is potentially more dangerous (Hey, 2003b).

Incidence and facts

- HDN/VKDB affects:
  1 in 17 000 babies without vitamin K prophylaxis.
  1 in 25 000 to 1 in 70 000 in babies who have had a single oral 1–2 mg dose at birth.
  1 in 400 000 after a single intramuscular (IM) injection at birth (Puckett & Offringa, 2000).

- The incidence of haemorrhagic disease is significantly reduced in those babies receiving vitamin K at birth (Puckett & Offringa, 2000).
- Babies most at risk are those who are premature, unwell or have had traumatic deliveries.
- The Department of Health (DoH) (2005) recommends that all newborn babies are given vitamin K. More than 97% of UK babies currently receive it.
- Golding *et al.* (1992) suggested a tentative link between IM vitamin K and childhood leukaemia. Whilst the uncertainty cannot be completely resolved without a randomised controlled trial (which would be unethical), further studies show no association and it is concluded that Golding *et al.*'s findings were probably coincidental (DoH, 1998; Fear *et al.*, 2003).

Vitamin K controversy

Doubt exists as to the optimal level of vitamin K in the newborn. Wickham (2000) suggests that since most babies have similar levels, this may not be 'low' but physiologically normal and desirable. Wickham proposes that the research suggesting that breast milk was low in vitamin K was carried out when feeds were restricted in length and frequency, resulting in reduced intake of fat-rich colostrum and hindmilk (where fat-soluble vitamin K is mostly found). In the early days and weeks following birth, babies build up a supply of vitamin K from feeding. Vitamin K is added to artificial milk. Totally breastfed babies have been found to be slightly more prone to late-onset haemorrhagic disease. However, it should be noted that in over half of the babies who develop late-onset HDN, there was an underlying cause, such as malabsorption or liver disease, contributing to vitamin K deficiency (Puckett & Offringa, 2000). It is suggested that term breastfed babies are mainly at risk only if early intake is limited or poor (Palmer, 1993; Hey, 2003b).

There is debate over relative benefits of IM or oral administration (Hey, 2003a). Intramuscular administration, although more effective, has the disadvantages of 'trauma' and poor acceptance by parents, as well as potential risks of very high vitamin K levels, whereas the disadvantages of oral preparations include increased cost, reliance on parent compliance and poorer absorption which may also (as the primary concern is HDN babies) affect babies with undiagnosed cholestasis (Sutor *et al.*, 1999).

In conclusion, the RCM (1999) and the DoH (1998) both advocate that newborns should receive supplementary vitamin K but that the choice of administration (oral or IM) and whether to decline it altogether should rest with the parents. NICE (2006) recommends all parents are offered IM vitamin K for their baby and if this is declined should be offered an oral preparation as a 'second-line' option.

Top-to-toe check of the newborn

Each midwife will have a system for checking the newborn baby (top to toe and front to back is one way). Ensure the baby is not exposed naked for too long to avoid getting cold. The check can be performed in the cot or on the bed, wherever the mother is resting, so she can watch.

Head

Newborn babies can have very misshapen heads at birth. Parents should be reassured that the shape does quickly return to normal and that moulding (overriding of the skull bones) and caput succedaneum (oedema of the scalp) are common at birth. A swelling known as a cephalhaematoma (an effusion of blood beneath the periosteum of the cranial bone) is not present at birth but can develop in the hours/days following birth. The parents should be informed that it may take several weeks to resolve and may contribute to jaundice in a few days following birth, but is not usually serious.

Face

The appearance and symmetry of the face can be indicative of various conditions, e.g. Edward's, Down's or Turner's syndromes. Baston & Durward (2001) recommend seeing both parents before commenting on any unusual appearance as the baby may simply have inherited familial traits.

Eyes

The eyes should be clear from discharge or inflammation, which if present within 24 hours of birth should be investigated as it could be a result of a gonococci infection which can lead to blindness. Other infections such as chlamydia and staphylococcal conjunctivitis usually occur a few days after birth. The eyes should be checked for the absence of cataracts (visible as a cloudy cornea), or a translucent iris, which can be a sign of albinism. Subconjunctival haemorrhages (red, crescent-shaped lesions on the conjunctiva) are not uncommon and usually resolve in a matter of weeks.

Ears

As with other areas of the body, the ears may have skin tags. These are usually small and are commonly tied with suture material by a paediatrician, until they drop off. Tags or dimpling are usually of no significance but occasionally indicate renal problems and should be documented and mentioned to a paediatrician. Low set ears can be associated with various disorders such as Patau's/Down's syndrome.

Mouth

Check the mouth for problems such as congenital teeth, which may need removing. A short, square or heart-shaped tongue may indicate tongue tie, i.e. a short tight frenulum. A very small number of babies with tongue tie may need a simple procedure to resolve the problem.

To check for cleft palate, insert a clean finger, fleshy side up and move across the roof of the mouth, and/or inspect with a light which may reveal a sub-mucous cleft, not easily felt (Fig. 5.1). Undetected clefts can cause feeding, and later speech, difficulties. Any baby with milk coming down its nose during a feed when not vomiting may have a cleft palate (Martin & Bannister, 2003).

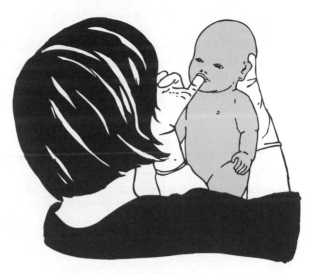

Fig. 5.1 Finger inspection for cleft palate.

A cleft lip can be very distressing for the parents. It may be almost unnoticeable or extensive and may be unilateral or bilateral. Surgery is normally required.

Chest and abdomen

To check for fractures, trace the fingers along the clavicles feeling for irregularities. Breast enlargement is not uncommon in both boys and girls, and the breasts may even secrete a small amount of milk. There should be two nipples.

Check that the umbilical clamp is secure. Protrusions at the base of the umbilicus may indicate exomphalos (herniating bowel). The cord should have one vein and two arteries. The presence of only one artery in the cord can be associated with renal abnormalities.

Sternal recession, particularly with other signs of respiratory distress such as nasal flaring, grunting or tachypnoea, should be reported to a paediatrician.

The abdomen should feel soft. Any hernias should be reported.

Genitalia

The size, normal placement and any skin pigmentation should be noted. Parents who have darker skin may have babies with a darker scrotum or labia. In cases of indeterminate gender avoid guessing the baby's sex, as an incorrect guess can cause subsequent distress. Indeterminate gender is a complex area and very stressful for the parents. Sometimes a paediatrician can clearly determine the gender on close examination by palpating any penile tissue and gonads. More complex cases will involve genetic and endocrine blood tests and possibly scanning for ovaries, usually including specialist referral. This can take some weeks. Blood is often taken for congenital adrenal hyperplasia (CAH) screening, another cause of ambiguous genitalia, and may be repeated several weeks later as initial results are not always conclusive. CAH is a serious condition which can be life-threatening. Treatment is lifelong.

Baby boys

The size of the penis varies greatly. Observing the location of the urethral orifice may reveal hypospadias, where the urethral meatus opens on the undersurface of the penis. This occurs in 8.5 per 10 000 births (Birth Defects Foundation (BDF), 2007). If the baby has a hypospadias, it is important to note the passage of urine, as a dribble instead of a stream could indicate a blockage of the urethra and surgery may be indicated to prevent renal damage. Babies with hypospadias should not be circumcised, as some of the skin may be needed for surgical repair later.

Gently examine the scrotal sack for the presence or absence of testes, which if absent will usually descend by 6 weeks of age. Documentation of their presence is important in case they later move out of the scrotal sac and are then, incorrectly, diagnosed as having not descended.

Some baby boys are born with a large, swollen scrotum, known as a hydrocele. This is fairly common, not serious in the newborn, and resolves spontaneously over the following months.

Baby girls

The labia and clitoris can look large in preterm and small-for-dates newborns. A particularly large labia or clitoris could suggest the baby is of indeterminate sex; testes can sometimes even be felt beneath the 'labia'.

A mucus discharge, which can be blood tinged, may be visible at the vagina and may persist for several days. Parents should be reassured this is normal.

Anus

Check the presence and location of the anus. A misaligned anus can be associated with malformation of the rectum (Baston & Durward, 2001). Note and document any passage of meconium.

Back and spine

Run a finger down the spine to feel for hidden swellings or indentations. Spina bifida can be found anywhere from the neck to the coccyx. Neurological damage (if any) occurs below the level of the lesion:

- Spina bifida occulta: often visible as a dimple. Frequently asymptomatic and of no significance.
- Meningocele: a sac covers the spinal cord. Some degree of disability often results.
- Myelomeningocele: spinal nerves are exposed. This is the most serious form.

Limbs

The limbs should look symmetrical. Fingers and toes may be webbed or overlapping, deformed, fused, missing or extra digits may be present (Fig. 5.2). A single palmer crease may indicate Down's syndrome. These features can be hereditary or features

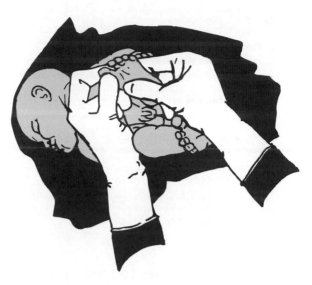

Fig. 5.2 Fingers and toes should be counted and checked for any deformity.

of various syndromes. Fused, malformed or missing digits can also be caused by the formation of amniotic bands in utero.

Talipes presents as the feet being either turned in with the toes pointing down, or out with the heel pointing down. If the foot can be pulled back into position, this is talipes equinovarus or 'positional talipes' and rights itself spontaneously. If the bones within the foot have developed abnormal positions, this 'structural talipes' will need physiotherapy, splinting and occasionally requires surgery. Most babies do very well with treatment and grow up normally, being able to walk, run and play sport (STEPS, 2006).

Skin

Birthmarks may be found; some are more obvious than others. Parents can be naturally quite distressed at large or visible birthmarks, such as those on the baby's face, and will want to know if they are permanent or treatable. Other features such as hyperpigmented macule (formerly known as Mongolian blue spot), rashes, bruising and birth trauma should be discussed and documented. For more information on birthmarks and skin discolouration see Box 5.1.

Box 5.1 Birthmarks and skin discolouration.

Hyperpigmented macule (formerly known as Mongolian blue spot)
- Bluish pigmentation mainly found over the sacrum, but occasionally over the back, shoulders and limbs.
- It is completely benign and tends to fade within a year.
- It is more common in babies with dark skin, but occasionally in pale-skinned babies.
- Documentation is important, as parents have occasionally been accused later of bruising their baby.

Stork marks (naevus simplex)
- Pink/purple pressure marks, usually found on the face and nape of neck.
- One-third of babies have these; they are benign and fade within a year.

Box 5.1 (*Continued*)

Port wine stain/capillary haemangioma
- Deep dense bluish-purple permanent mark present at birth tends to grow with the baby.
- Cosmetic coverage may be sufficient but laser therapy is available.

Pigmented naevus
- Permanent birthmark often extending across a large area: it may have hair growing through it.
- Excision and skin grafting is possible if the area is not too large.

Strawberry naevus
- Pink/purple raised areas of blood-filled capillaries. They are not obvious at birth but develop in the early days of life.
- Most resolve by 8 years of age, so are normally left alone unless very unsightly. Laser treatment or surgery is possible.

Giving upsetting news to parents

Many parents assume that antenatal screening and scans will have picked up any problems with their baby. Therefore, the birth of a baby with an anomaly can come as a profound shock to parents. Grief is commonly felt and many tears may be cried. Feelings are often contradictory: love and protectiveness mixed with revulsion and guilt. Many people ask 'why us?' unable to understand why their baby is physically imperfect when the rest of the world seems full of perfect, healthy children. Parents need to be reassured and told, 'this is not your fault'.

For the midwife who delivers a baby with a problem, it can also be an unexpected shock. The midwife may feel useless and lost for words or ways to make things better. Parents will take their cue from the midwife; if he/she can sound positive without being unrealistic, then they will be less likely to 'reject' their baby. Kelnar & Harvey (1987) suggest talking to both parents together, holding their baby, while the problem is explained simply and clearly. In some situations, the midwife needs to respond immediately to a visible or obvious problem with a baby at birth. In other situations, there will be time to involve the paediatrician, who can check the baby and he or she may be the appropriate person to inform the parents of a problem.

Robb (1999) suggests that there is no perfect way of giving someone upsetting news. However, a few simple guidelines, sensitively followed, can mitigate some of the distress;

- Keep it simple.
- Provide privacy.
- Remember to say something positive about the baby, e.g. 'you have a gorgeous baby...beautiful eyes...he's so strong'.
- Repeat clear and simple explanations as often as necessary.
- Personalise the information to that family and baby. Use the baby's name if he/she has been given one.
- If you do not know the answers to the parents' questions, get a senior paediatrician to come quickly to avoid giving incorrect information.
- Do not forget other colleagues, referrals and early follow-up.

- Written information, support groups and contact numbers are important, but they are no substitute for giving time and explanations.

Robb (1999) recommends that midwives should practise the breaking of bad news amongst colleagues. It is not something that most midwives feel confident doing or do regularly enough to feel that they are proficient at it. Parents are usually shocked and only remember pieces of what they are told. However, they do remember who told them and if it was handled positively or not (Robb, 1999).

Summary

Assess: good colour and tone, responsive to handling, normal respiration and heart rate.

Measure: weight, length and head circumference.

Head and face: observe for symmetry, moulding, caput, haematomas and birth trauma.

Eyes: check for discharge or cloudiness.

Ears: observe for skin tags, shape and position.

Mouth: examine palate and tongue, check for congenital teeth.

Chest: check shape, respiration, nipple location, any fractures.

Abdomen: observe shape, check for herniation. Verify three vessels in the cord, and clamp secure.

Genitalia: examine: in boys check for hypospadias, hydrocele, descended testes. Document if meconium or urine passed.

Back: examine for spina bifida.

Limbs: observe symmetry, count fingers and toes, check palmar creases. Note any webbing, malformation, talipes.

Skin: check for birthmarks, rashes, Mongolian blue spot, bruising and birth trauma.

Refer concerns to a paediatrician.

Document carefully.

Break bad news sensitively.

Useful contacts

Association for Spina Bifida and Hydrocephalus (ASBAH)   Telephone: 01733 555988. Helpline: 08454507755. Website: www.asbah.org

BDF Newlife   The Birth Defects Foundation. Telephone: 01543 468888. Website: www. bdfnewlife.co.uk

Birthmark Support Group   Telephone: 08450454700. Website: www. birthmarksupport-group.org.uk

The Child Bereavement Trust   Telephone: 01494 446648. Website: www. childbereavement. org.uk

Children's Heart Federation   Telephone helpline: 0808 808 5000. Website: www.childrens-heart-fed.org.uk

Cleft Lip and Palate Association (CLAPA)   Telephone: 020 7431 0033. Website: www. clapa.com

Contact a Family.   UK-wide charity providing advice, information and support to the parents of all disabled children. Telephone: 020 7608 8700. Website: www.cafamily.org.uk

Cystic Hygroma and Haemangioma Online Support Group (CHHSG)   Website: www. Cystichygroma.dsl.pipex.com

Department of Health (DoH)   (2005) *The Pregnancy Book*, London: DoH. This has a useful contacts section for many support groups. Website: www.dh.gov.uk

Down's Syndrome Association (DSA)   Telephone helplines: 020 8682 4001/08452300372. Website: www.downs-syndrome.org.uk

Pierre Robin Support Group   Website: www.pierrerobin.org

REACH (The Association for Children with Hand or Arm Deficiency)   Telephone: 0845 1306225. Website: www.reach.org.uk

SCOPE   Advice and support for carers of children with cerebral palsy. Helpline: 0808 800 3333. Website: www.scope.org.uk

SOFT Support Organisation for Patau's Syndrome (Trisomy 13), Edward's Syndrome (Trisomy 18) and Related Disorders   Telephone helpline: 0121 351 3122. Website: www.soft.org.uk

STEPS (National Association for Children with Lower Limb Abnormalities)   Telephone: 0871 717 0044. Website: www.steps-charity.org.uk

References

Baston, H. & Durward, H. (2001) *Examination of the Newborn: A Practical Guide.* Routledge, London.

Birth Defects Foundation (BDF) (2007) BDF Newlife. Available at: www.bdfnewlife.co.uk (accessed August 2007).

Chung, J.H., Boscardin, W.J., & Garite, T.J. (2003) Ethnic differences in birth weight by gestational age: a partial explanation for the Hispanic epidemiologic paradox? *American Journal of Obstetrics and Gynaecology* **189** (4), 1058–62.

Department of Health (DoH) (1998) *Vitamin K for Babies.* PLO/CNO/998/4 Department of Health, London (withdrawn Dec 2003).

Department of Health (DoH) (2005) *The Pregnancy Book.* Department of Health, London.

Fear, N., Roman, E., Ansell, P., Simpson, J., Day, N., & Eden, O. (2003) Vitamin K and childhood cancer: a report from the UK Childhood Cancer Study. *British Journal of Cancer* **8** (7), 1228–31.

Fry, T. (2002) Measuring newborns: yes, size does really matter. *Midwives Journal* **5** (7), 220–21.

Golding, J., Greenwood, R., Birmingham, K. & Mott, M. (1992) Childhood cancer, intramuscular vitamin K and pethidine given in labour. *British Medical Journal* **305**, 341–6.

Hall, D. & Elliman, D. (eds) (2002) *Health for all Children*, 4th edn. Joint Working Party on Child Health Surveillance. Oxford University Press, Oxford.

Hey, E. (2003a) Vitamin K – can we improve on nature? *Midwifery Digest* **13** (1), 7–12.

Hey, E. (2003b) Vitamin K – what, why and when. *Archives of Disease in Childhood Fetal and Neonatal Edition* **88** (2), F80–83.

Hull, D. & Johnston, D. (1999) *Essential Paediatrics*, 4th edn. Churchill Livingstone, Edinburgh.

Jokinen, M. (2002) Measuring newborns: does size really matter? *Midwives Journal* **5** (5), 186–7.

Kelnar, C.J.H. & Harvey, D. (1987) *The Sick Newborn Baby.* Bailliere Tindal, London.

Martin, V. & Bannister, P. (eds) (2003) *Cleft Care – A Practical Guide for Health Professionals on Cleft Lip and/or Palate.* Academic Publishing Services, Salisbury.

National Institute for Health and Clinical Excellence (NICE) (2006) *Routine Postnatal Care of Women and Their Babies*. National Institute for Health and Clinical Excellence, London.

National Institute for Health and Clinical Excellence (NICE) (2007) *Clinical Guideline 55: Intrapartum Care.* National Institute for Clinical Excellence, London.

Newel, S.J., Miller, P., Morgan, I. & Salariya, E. (1997) Management of the newborn baby: midwifery and paediatric perspectives. In *Essential Midwifery* (Henderson, C. & Jones, K., eds), pp. 229–64. Mosby, London.

Palmer, G. (1993) *The Politics of Breastfeeding*. Pandora, London.

Patel, H. & Beeby, P.J. (2004) Resuscitation beyond 10 minutes of term babies born without signs of life. *MIDIRS Midwifery Digest* **14** (3), 391–3.

Puckett, R.M. & Offringa, M. (2000) Vitamin K for preventing haemorrhagic disease (Cochrane Review). *The Cochrane Library*, Issue 4. Update Software, Oxford.

Robb, F. (1999) Congenital malformations: breaking bad news. *British Journal of Midwifery* **7** (1), 26–31.

Royal College of Midwives (RCM) (1999) Position paper 13b: Vitamin K. *RCM Midwives Journal* **2** (8), 252–3.

Seidel, H.M., Rosenstein, B.J., Pathak, A. & McKay, W.H. (eds) (2006) *Primary Care of the Newborn*, 4th ed. Saunders Elsevier, Philadelphia.

STEPS (2006) *National Association for Families of Children with Congenital Abnormalities of the Lower Limbs*. Available at: www.steps-charity.org.uk (accessed March 2008).

Sutor, A.H., von Kries, R., Cornelissen, E.A.M., McNinch, A.W. & Andrew, M. (1999) Vitamin K deficiency bleeding in infancy. *Thrombosis and Haemoststasis* **81**, 456–61.

Wickham, S. (2000) Vitamin K: a flaw in the blueprint. *Midwifery Today* **56**, 39–41.

Wilshin, J., Geary, M., Persaud, M. & Hindmarsh, P. (1999) The reliability of newborn length measurement. *British Journal of Midwifery* **7** (4), 236–9.

Appendix: Weight conversion chart

lb oz	kg	lb oz	kg	lb oz	kg	lb oz	kg
0 1	0.028	3 9	1.616	7 1	3.203	10 9	4.791
0 2	0.057	3 10	1.644	7 2	3.232	10 10	4.819
0 3	0.085	3 11	1.673	7 3	3.260	10 11	4.848
0 4	0.113	3 12	1.701	7 4	3.289	10 12	4.876
0 5	0.142	3 13	1.729	7 5	3.317	10 13	4.904
0 6	0.170	3 14	1.758	7 6	3.345	10 14	4.932
0 7	0.198	3 15	1.786	7 7	3.374	10 15	4.961
0 8	0.227	4 0	1.814	7 8	3.402	11 0	4.990
0 9	0.255	4 1	1.843	7 9	3.430	11 1	5.018
0 10	0.283	4 2	1.871	7 10	3.459	11 2	5.046
0 11	0.312	4 3	1.899	7 11	3.487	11 3	5.075
0 12	0.340	4 4	1.928	7 12	3.515	11 4	5.103
0 13	0.369	4 5	1.956	7 13	3.544	11 5	5.131
0 14	0.397	4 6	1.984	7 14	3.572	11 6	5.160
0 15	0.425	4 7	2.013	7 15	3.600	11 7	5.188
1 0	0.454	4 8	2.041	8 0	3.629	11 8	5.216
1 1	0.482	4 9	2.070	8 1	3.657	11 9	5.245
1 2	0.510	4 10	2.098	8 2	3.685	11 10	5.273
1 3	0.539	4 11	2.126	8 3	3.714	11 11	5.301
1 4	0.567	4 12	2.155	8 4	3.742	11 12	5.330
1 5	0.595	4 13	2.183	8 5	3.770	11 13	5.358
1 6	0.624	4 14	2.211	8 6	3.799	11 14	5.386
1 7	0.652	4 15	2.240	8 7	3.827	11 15	5.415
1 8	0.680	5 0	2.268	8 8	3.856	12 0	5.443
1 9	0.709	5 1	2.296	8 9	3.884	12 1	5.471
1 10	0.737	5 2	2.325	8 10	3.912	12 2	5.500
1 11	0.765	5 3	2.353	8 11	3.941	12 3	5.528
1 12	0.794	5 4	2.381	8 12	3.969	12 4	5.557
1 13	0.822	5 5	2.410	8 13	3.997	12 5	5.585
1 14	0.850	5 6	2.438	8 14	4.026	12 6	5.613
1 15	0.879	5 7	2.466	8 15	4.054	12 7	5.642
2 0	0.907	5 8	2.495	9 0	4.082	12 8	5.670
2 1	0.936	5 9	2.523	9 1	4.111	12 9	5.698
2 2	0.964	5 10	2.551	9 2	4.139	12 10	5.727
2 3	0.992	5 11	2.580	9 3	4.167	12 11	5.755
2 4	1.021	5 12	2.608	9 4	4.196	12 12	5.783
2 5	1.049	5 13	2.637	9 5	4.224	12 13	5.812
2 6	1.077	5 14	2.665	9 6	4.252	12 14	5.840
2 7	1.106	5 15	2.693	9 7	4.281	12 15	5.868
2 8	1.134	6 0	2.722	9 8	4.309	13 0	5.897
2 9	1.162	6 1	2.750	9 9	4.337	13 1	5.925
2 10	1.191	6 2	2.778	9 10	4.366	13 2	5.953
2 11	1.219	6 3	2.807	9 11	4.394	13 3	5.982
2 12	1.247	6 4	2.835	9 12	4.423	13 4	6.010
2 13	1.276	6 5	2.863	9 13	4.451	13 5	6.038
2 14	1.304	6 6	2.892	9 14	4.479	13 6	6.067
2 15	1.332	6 7	2.920	9 15	4.508	13 7	6.095
3 0	1.361	6 8	2.948	10 0	4.536	13 8	6.123
3 1	1.389	6 9	2.977	10 1	4.564	13 9	6.152
3 2	1.417	6 10	3.005	10 2	4.592	13 10	6.180
3 3	1.446	6 11	3.033	10 3	4.621	13 11	6.209
3 4	1.474	6 12	3.062	10 4	4.649	13 12	6.237
3 5	1.503	6 13	3.090	10 5	4.678	13 13	6.265
3 6	1.531	6 14	3.118	10 6	4.706	13 14	6.294
3 7	1.559	6 15	3.147	10 7	4.734	13 15	6.322
3 8	1.588	7 0	3.175	10 8	4.763	14 0	6.350

6 Home birth

Janet Gwillim

Introduction

There is no place like home.

A home birth can be a deeply personal fulfilling experience for the woman, her partner and family.

Until recent years home birth was the natural place of delivery. From the 1940s onwards there has been a trend towards hospital birth without any evidence of its superiority, culminating in the Peel report (Department of Health (DoH), 1970) which stated that the safest place for all women to give birth was in hospital. This biased approach has been vigorously challenged by many, and in the light of positive evidence the Department of Health now recommends that all women are advised that they can choose from an obstetric unit, midwife-led unit or home birth (DoH, 1993, 2004, 2007).

It is the midwife's duty of care to provide support and care for the woman who chooses a home birth, even if the woman's pregnancy is considered outside normal parameters (Nursing and Midwifery Council (NMC), 2004).

Incidence and facts

- Home birth rates vary widely: an average of 2.14% throughout the UK has been recorded, with considerable regional variation (BirthChoice UK, 2006).
- The evidence indicates that the health outcomes of planned home birth for low-risk women are probably as good as, if not better than those for hospital birth, and for many women there are emotional and practical benefits from giving birth at home (Enkin *et al.*, 1995).
- At the antenatal booking all women should be given full information on the options for hospital or home birth (DoH, 1993, 2007), and be aware that they do not have to decide until later in pregnancy and can change their mind if they wish.
- Women with significant health risks may be advised to deliver in an obstetric unit (National Institute for Health and Clinical Excellence (NICE), 2007) but this remains their choice.

- The National Perinatal Epidemiology Unit survey states that 38% of women report being offered home birth compared with 18% 12 years ago (NPEU, 2007).
- Some health trusts are experiencing financial and staffing restraints which have created difficulties offering cover for home births (RCOG & RCM, 2007).

Benefits of home birth

A woman is likely to be more relaxed in her familiar surroundings at home with her partner and perhaps children around her. She is more likely to have an active birth, experiencing less intervention, also to feel more in control. She has more privacy, less risk of infection and more chance of continuity of care from the same midwives (Allen *et al.*, 1997). NICE meta-analysis reports less intervention at home, i.e. less induction of labour, augmentation, epidural, episiotomy and instrumental/caesarean delivery (NICE, 2007). Women are more likely to breastfeed (National Birthday Trust Fund (NBTF), 1997).

Planned home birth neonatal outcomes, including Apgar scores, appear better in some studies (NBTF, 1997) and marginally worse in some low-quality studies (NICE, 2007): they are difficult to measure due to the self-selected population choosing home birth.

The woman is less likely to suffer from postnatal depression (Mind, 1995).

Home birth is not for everyone. Some women and/or partners worry about children or neighbours overhearing the birth, making a mess on beds and carpets and the trauma/perceived danger of any possible transfer to hospital. Those people will be more relaxed in hospital and that is the right decision for them.

Attending home births

Midwives should feel confident when attending home births. Inexperienced midwives may require support from more experienced colleagues. To help gain confidence, midwives should aim to attend regular home birth workshops. Home birth study days are usually inspiring as well as offering the opportunity for knowledge sharing and experience.

All midwives, especially those who practise in the community, need to keep their skills and emergency drills up to date as well as ensuring that they have practised the manoeuvres for breech birth and shoulder dystocia. Midwives must be able to cannulate, resuscitate adults and babies, and should know what to do if a postpartum haemorrhage occurs.

Personal safety checklist

- Know your destination/location and how to access the woman's house/flat.
- If you are attending another midwife's client, and particularly if the woman's home is difficult to find, ensure that you have a map, with adequate landmarks or directions.
- Carry both an Ordnance Survey and an A-Z map of your area. Satellite navigation would be extremely useful.
- Have a system in place for informing your colleagues of your whereabouts both day and night.

- Inform any other relevant people, e.g. labour suite co-ordinator, supervisor of midwives (SOM), general practitioner (GP), should they need or wish to be involved.
- If you feel threatened going somewhere, take a second midwife with you.
- Ensure that mobile telephone battery charged, torch charged and car fuelled.

Supervision issues

Supervision is in place to protect the public by actively promoting a safe standard of midwifery practice. Supervision should be supportive and proactive.

As well as ensuring that the midwife carries out safe practice, the SOM also identifies personal and professional development needs and encourages evidence-based practice (NMC, 2006).

A SOM can be a useful resource for a home birth. SOM support can include attending a home birth with the midwife, especially if the midwife has concerns about a high-risk mother who insists on a home birth. A SOM can also provide a point of contact for the woman who wants a home birth but has been told that she cannot have one.

Build up a good rapport with your SOM, keep them informed of impending births in your area, share and discuss cases.

Midwives working outside the NHS also need supervision and support. These midwives may be working in independent practice, as a midwife teacher or employed by GPs as a midwife. These midwives may or may not have a contract with an NHS trust.

Essential equipment

Preparation by the midwife

For a list of equipment see Boxes 6.1 and 6.2. Always keep equipment stocked, in working order, and make sure drugs and intravenous (IV) fluids are in date. The list appears endless but if equipment is always separated into the appropriate bags and boxes, then colleagues become familiar with them and in an emergency it is much easier to locate the appropriate piece of equipment.

Preparation by the mother

In addition to a midwife's equipment, the woman intending to have a home birth should also make some preparation beforehand.

- **Protective pack.** The woman may want to make a pack to protect her birthing space consisting of a 1 m × 1¼ m sheet of thick polythene, then thick layers of newspapers glued or sticky taped to the polythene, and a top layer of old clean sheeting, glued, sticky taped or sewn. This can be laid on the floor, bed, settee or wherever the woman wishes to give birth and can then be burnt or taken to the hospital incinerator afterwards.
- **Refreshments and home comforts.** Plenty of drinks and snacks for all present at the birth. Pillows, duvet, flannels, bowls, towels for hot and cold compresses. Transcutaneous electrical nerve stimulation (TENS) machine, music, massage oils, beanbag, birth ball and candles. Birthing pool if wanting water for labour and birth.

Box 6.1 Midwifery equipment.

Labour and birth bag	Antenatal/postnatal bag	Emergency bag
Delivery pack (small community pack) – some units combine delivery/suture packs	Thermometer	Intravenous (IV) giving set × 2 (clear fluids and blood)
	Sphygmomanometer	
	Pinards	Grey/large bore cannulae × 4
Suture pack (small suture pack) and suture material	Doppler	
	Urine testing strips	Selection of small cannulae
Tampon	Tape measure	Three-way tap
Urethral catheter	Baby scales	Plaster and IV sterile fixing dressing
Amnihook	Cord clamp remover	
Sterile gloves	Stitch cutters	Sterile gloves
Unsterile gloves	Scissors	Unsterile gloves
Inco pads/sanitary towels	Plastic apron	Label for drug additives
Water based vaginal lubricating jelly	Sterile gloves	Razor
	Unsterile gloves	Pinards
Baby labels (some parents wish to have these)	Glycerine suppositories	Plastic apron
	Speculum	Inco pads/sanitary towels
Syringes and needles	Water-based vaginal lubricating jelly	Blood bottles for haemoglobin, cross-matching and forms
Blood bottles and equipment for Rhesus-negative women		
	Swabs for culture	
Drugs/IV fluids	Torch	IV fluids
Local anaesthetic	Neonatal screening test kits	Normal saline
Syntometrine/syntocinon		Hartmann's solution
Ergometrine	Paperwork for pathology laboratory and notes	Gelofusine/haemaccel
Vitamin K		Essential resuscitation equipment
Plastic aprons	Blood bottles	(see Box 17.2 on p. 240)
Rubbish bag	Sharps container	

- **Warm birthing environment.** Some means of heating may be necessary in the winter to boost the room temperature. Clothes and nappies for the baby. Hot water bottle to warm whatever the woman has chosen to wrap her baby in at birth.
- **Pethidine.** Pethidine is rarely used at a home birth because of its poor pain relieving qualities and unwanted side effects. If the woman wishes to have pethidine 100 mg, she should get it prescribed by her general practitioner and have this dispensed ready for her use. It is the woman's property and the midwife cannot remove it from the house/flat afterwards, but it is advisable to suggest that it is destroyed prior to the midwife's departure.

Box 6.2 Drugs and gases carried by the midwife.

Syntometrine®
Syntocinon® 10 IU & also 40 IU
Ergometrine
Oxytocics (can be kept for about 1 year in high temperatures. Advisable to discard every 6 months (Chua *et al.*, 1993))
Lignocaine 1% 20 ml
Neonatal intramuscular vitamin K (1 mg in 0.1 ml) or neonatal oral equivalent preparation
Naloxone hydrochloride for the baby if using pethidine

Gases
Entonox
Oxygen

Care in labour

The woman and her family are the centre of the care. The care needs to be given *sensitively*. Not all women want to give birth at home and the midwife should support her in her decision and should continue to support her if she changes her mind or the need arises to be admitted to hospital. For the midwife it is an honour to be asked to attend a home birth and it can be a rewarding experience for everyone.

Early labour

- **First call.** When the woman contacts the midwife on call to say she thinks she may be in labour, listen and decide whether to go to her. For independent midwives distance may play its part in the decision about when to attend a woman in labour, as she may not live nearby, and it may be more appropriate to stay once the decision is made to visit. Perform a full check (see Chapter 1). Watch for a while to see how the contractions are progressing before offering a vaginal examination. Think to yourself: 'Is a vaginal examination necessary?' Discuss the woman's plans with her again now that she has started labouring.
- **Advice.** Make sure that the woman and her partner know to call again if she has a spontaneous rupture of membranes or if her membranes are already ruptured and the colour changes, has some heavy bleeding, the contractions become stronger or they are worried. Remember to document everything you have performed and your findings. Arrange a time to go back and review the situation unless she calls you back in the meantime.
- **Return at the time you arranged.** If you are going to be late, make sure you telephone the woman to let her know. You may need to go back two or three times before she needs you to stay. Staying when you are not required does not help a labouring woman and her family.

Labour

- **Staying.** When the time comes for the midwife to stay, make sure you do not dominate the situation. It is the woman's day and *she* is going to birth *her* baby, not the midwife.
- **Equipment.** Try not to have all the equipment in the birthing space but have it handy outside the room ready if you need it. It may be threatening to the woman to see all the 'emergency' equipment ready as if problems are expected. If there is evidence of fetal compromise some midwives do make a discreet newborn resuscitation area in the corner of the room. The mother may then be asked to move towards such an area so that the baby can remain attached to its umbilical cord even if it requires resuscitation.
- **Monitoring the well-being of the woman and baby.** Observations should be performed and documented in the notes. Discuss any deviation from the normal at the time with the woman and her partner, and record this in the notes.
- **Observations performed.** Maternal blood pressure, pulse, temperature, frequent auscultation of the baby's heartbeat. Noting the regularity, strength and length of the contractions and the dilatation of the cervix. Encourage her to drink and empty her bladder frequently. Avoid artificial rupture of the membranes due to the potential

complications that are associated with this intervention although it can be justifiable as a last resort for a slow labour before planning to transfer a woman to a consultant unit (see also Chapters 2 and 8).

- **Blend into the background.** Most women will labour well when they have not had to move elsewhere and are able to remain in their own environment, in a position they wish to be in with their family and friends. Make sure you blend in with the background and enable the woman to labour. This is also recommended by the *National Birthday Trust Report* (Chamberlain *et al.*, 1994).

The birth

- **Second midwife.** Remember to call the back-up midwife before he/she is needed urgently. Independent midwives have challenged the routine of having a second midwife at all home births and only call for back-up if they have a specific concern. Some independent midwives suggest that a second midwife can affect the dynamics of the relationship with the woman. If a second midwife attends, leaving the door on the latch is sensible so that the woman is not disturbed. The second midwife does not have to be present in the room, only somewhere else in the house so as not to intrude.
- **The birth.** Providing the woman feels in control and well supported, a home birth can be a deeply personal experience for her and her partner. Enable the woman to birth her own baby, to make as much noise as she wishes and to lift her baby to her breast and to discover the sex. Give her time to do this; do not overcrowd her but just quietly observe until she is ready to speak.
- **The third stage.** Most babies will naturally search at the breast which encourages the natural release of oxytocin. Allow the woman to expel her placenta when she wishes. If the woman chooses to have a managed third stage of labour then an oxytocic drug should be given intramuscularly and the placenta and membranes delivered by controlled cord traction within a few minutes (see Chapter 1). The placenta is the woman's property and she may want to keep it. If the placenta is to be disposed of by the midwife a placenta bin/bag will be required for transporting it to the hospital incinerator.
- **After the third stage.** The woman may want to celebrate in a variety of ways. She may want to remain very quiet and together with her partner, or she may want to enjoy champagne with her family and friends or share the moment with her other children. She may also be very hungry and want lots of fresh toast and tea. Whatever she chooses, respect her wishes.
- **Prior to leaving the house.** Midwives normally remain in the house after the third stage until the woman and the midwife feel happy that the time has come for the midwife to leave. During this time weighing, measuring and examining the baby can be performed, offering vitamin K, completing the notes and having a cup of tea.
- **On leaving.** Make sure that the woman's uterus is well contracted, her lochia is not excessive and that she has passed urine. The woman and her family need to be given the contact numbers to call a midwife should any problems occur and a time given for the return visit by the midwife. NHS midwives will need to complete hospital paperwork/computer details and all midwives should replenish their equipment. Any colleagues who were informed of the home birth should be informed that the woman and her baby are safely delivered.

Possible transfer to hospital

When things do not go according to plan during labour or after the birth, transfer may be indicated. (See Box 6.3 for a list of possible problems.)

The midwife needs to use his/her judgement. If the woman is very near the onset of the second stage or is in the second stage of labour, especially is if she is not a primigravida, it may not be possible or safe to move to hospital before the birth of the

Box 6.3   Possible problems requiring transfer to hospital.

Pre-labour rupture of the membranes – with no labour after 24 hours (NICE, 2007)

Liquor
- Offensive smell
- Old meconium with associated problems
- Obvious fresh meconium
- Heavily bloodstained

Bleeding
- Bleeding causing concern

Fetal heart rate
- Persistent decelerations with contractions
- Decelerations following contractions
- Persistent bradycardia/persistent tachycardia

Position of baby
- Posterior position with no progress
- Breech position
- Complicated presentation

Maternal observations
- Pyrexia
- Raised blood pressure

Pain
- Women wanting further pain control
- Unusual pain in labour

Choice
- Woman changed her mind

Dilatation
- No progress for a length of time
- Swollen anterior lip of cervix for a long time

Postpartum
- Retained placenta
- Postpartum haemorrhage
- Third-degree tear

Baby
- Any condition causing concern

baby. Think: 'Is an emergency ambulance on the way?' 'Has the hospital delivery suite co-ordinator been informed?'

Emergency transfer to hospital

- **Dial 999.** In an emergency ask the partner to phone the emergency services and ask for a paramedic ambulance. Although the ambulance is alerted immediately and on its way, the control operator will ask other questions.
- **Directions.** Directions given to ambulance control as to how to get to a house/flat can take a long time to explain, especially when it is dark and in rural areas as landmarks do not always show up. The partner can save the midwife's valuable time in making this call so that the midwife is able to be with the woman.
- **Second midwife.** If a second midwife has not already been requested to attend, use a mobile telephone so that the woman is not left unattended. It may not be possible to do this yourself if you are busy sitting cannulas, taking blood, controlling bleeding or resuscitating the baby. Make this the partner's next telephone call.
- **Inform co-ordinator.** The hospital delivery suite needs to be informed; make sure the co-ordinator knows. The co-ordinator is in overall charge of the delivery suite and will assess the situation, get a room prepared and inform the relevant people, for example, consultant obstetrician, registrar, paediatrician, pathology laboratory, theatre, special care baby unit (SCBU) and a supervisor of midwives if necessary to give you support. Working as a team inside and outside the hospital counts. Remember to keep colleagues informed, keep communicating.
- **Record keeping.** Write times down and remember to take the woman's notes to hospital. Take emergency bag, the personal bag and collect together other equipment.
- **Escort the woman.** Go with her in the ambulance, leave the car and get a lift or taxi back to the car later. The hospital will pay the fare.

Non-emergency transfer to hospital

In a non-emergency situation transfer to hospital may be necessary. This may be for a number of reasons. The usual non-urgent reasons are that the woman has changed her mind or that she wishes to have a form of pain relief unavailable to her at home.

Other reasons for transfer are prelabour rupture of the membranes and no labour or slow progress in labour (Davies *et al.*, 1996). Think: 'Is the woman able to travel by car or should she travel by ambulance?' In a non-emergency situation the midwife may be able to travel by car and follow the ambulance to the hospital. With increasing pressure on the ambulance service a non-emergency ambulance may take a long time to arrive, so it may be preferable to travel by car.

The woman and her partner may be extremely upset with the decision to transfer to hospital, even when the decision has been made entirely by themselves. Explain that neither of them have failed; the language used in midwifery about 'failure to progress', 'maternal distress' and the like does not help parents come to terms with their decisions.

They will need to be debriefed very carefully afterwards, with the midwife who cared for them together with the notes.

Remember that the woman does not have to transfer to hospital. If you have a good relationship with her and her partner and they know you would not be suggesting the transfer to them unless you were worried, they are unlikely to refuse. Remember to document everything.

- **Born before arrival (BBA).** Remember in a term pregnancy normally occurs because the woman has a precipitate labour and birth. The midwife will need to use her judgement to decide whether the woman and her baby need to be admitted to hospital for observation. A history of fresh meconium-stained liquor might indicate the need to be admitted. For a preterm birth before 36 weeks, the mother and baby will most likely need to be admitted to hospital. Often these babies are well at birth, but need some extra care when they are a few hours old. Skin-to-skin contact is recommended to keep the baby warm and secure. This is preferable to an incubator should a transfer be indicated (Christensson *et al.*, 1998). New laws on safety and transferring a baby to hospital in a vehicle rests with the driver taking responsibility (DOT, 2006). Local rules may differ.
- **Unplanned home birth.** Unplanned home births also occur because either there is no time to transfer prior to the birth or the mother has changed her mind in labour. These births are, generally, without problems but all relevant people need to be informed.
- **Unplanned breech.** Unplanned, undiagnosed breech birth at home can be a shock if the midwife arrives to find the breech presenting and descending (see Chapter 13). Again all the relevant people need to be informed; the midwife must just get on and deliver the breech. Breech babies are more likely to be temporarily shocked at birth and may need some basic resuscitation.
- **Remember** the same applies to all home births whether planned or unplanned, for NHS midwives: informing the hospital and your colleagues.

Summary

- Know your destination and keep colleagues informed of your whereabouts.
- Always keep equipment stocked, in working order, drugs and IV fluids in date.
- Care as per normal labour (Chapter 1).
- Avoid interventions with potential complications, such as artificial rupture of the membranes.
- Stand back; do not dominate the couple's space. Let the woman labour.
- Discuss and document any need to transfer to hospital fully with the woman and her partner.
- Have a second midwife present for the birth.
- In the event of an emergency call a paramedic ambulance. They can provide prompt, skilled hands for resuscitation and cannulation and can always leave if they are not required. Inform the labour ward coordinator if the woman needs to be admitted to hospital.

Useful contacts

Association for Improvements in Maternity Services (AIMS)   AIMS Helpline: 0870 765 1453. Homebirth Support Co-ordinator 0870 765 1447. Website: www.aims.org.uk
Home birth reference websites   www.homebirth.org.uk and www.birthchoice.com

Independent Midwives Association (IMA)   Telephone: 01483 425833. Website: www.independentmidwives.org.uk

National Childbirth Trust (NCT)   Enquiry line: 0870 444 8707. Website: www.nct.org.uk

Royal College of Midwives (RCM)   Telephone: 0207 3123535. Website: www.rcm.org.uk

References

Allen, I., Bourke, Dowling, S. & Williams, S. (1997) *A Leading Role for Midwives?* Policy Studies Institute, London NW1 3SR.

BirthChoice UK (2006) Home birth rates up, but remain low overall. *Midwives*, May.

Chamberlain, G., Wraight, A. & Crowley, P. (1994) *National Birthday Trust Report – Report of the Confidential Enquiry into Home Births*. Parthenon Publishing Group, London.

Christensson, K., Bhat, G.J., Amadi, B.C., Eriksson, B. & Hojer, B. (1998) A randomized study of skin-to-skin versus incubator care for rewarming low risk hypothermic neonates. *The Lancet* **352**, 1115.

Chua, S., Arulkumaran, S., Adaikan, G. & Ratnam, S. (1993) The effect of oxytocics stored at high temperatures on postpartum uterine activity. *British Journal of Obstetrics and Gynaecology* **100**, 874–5.

Davies, J., Hey, E., Reid, W. & Young, G (1996) Prospective regional study of planned home births. *British Medical Journal* **313**, 1302–306.

Department of Health (DoH) (1970) *Peel Report*. HMSO, London.

Department of Health (DoH) (1993) *Changing Childbirth. Report of the Expert Maternity Group*. Department of Health, HMSO, London.

Department of Health (DoH) (2004) *National Service Framework for Children, Young People and Maternity Services*, pp. 27–9. DoH, London.

Department of Health (DoH) (2007) *Maternity Matters*. Department of Health, London

DOT (2006) *Think Road Safety Leaflet*. Available at: www.thinkroadsafety.gov.uk (accessed March 2008).

Enkin, M., Keirse, J.N.C., Renfrew, M.J. & Neilson, J.P. (1995) *A Guide to Effective Care in Pregnancy and Childbirth*, 2nd edn. Oxford University Press, Oxford.

National Birthday Trust Fund (NBTF) (1997) *Home Births – The Report of the 1994 Confidential Enquiry* (Chamberlain, G., Wraight, A. & Crowley, P., eds). National Birthday Trust Fund. Parthenon Publishing, Lancaster.

National Institute for Health and Clinical Excellence (NICE) (2007) *Clinical Guideline 55: Intrapartum Care*. National Institute for Health and Clinical Excellence, London. Available at: www.nice.org.uk (accessed March 2008).

Nicolson, P. (1995) *Postnatal Depression – Psychology Science and the Transition to Motherhood*. MIND Publications, London.

NPEU (2007) *Recorded Delivery, a Practical Survey of Women's Expectations of Maternity Care 2006*. National Perinatal Epidemiology Unit, Oxford. Available at: npeu.ox.ac.uk (accessed March 2008).

Nursing and Midwifery Council (NMC) (2004) *Code of Professional Standards for Conduct, Performance and Ethics*. Nursing and Midwifery Council, London.

Nursing and Midwifery Council (NMC) (2006) *Standards for the Preparation and Practice of Supervisor of Midwives*. Nursing and Midwifery Council, London. Available at: www.nmc-org.uk (accessed March 2008).

RCOG & Royal College of Midwives (RCM) (2007) *Joint Statement No 2*, April.

7 Water for labour and birth

Vicky Chapman and Cathy Charles

Introduction

Labour and/or birth in water can be a wonderfully relaxing experience for a mother and baby. Deep-water immersion in labour became popular in the 1970s. When women relaxing in water unexpectedly gave birth, it was realised that fears about drowning were unfounded (Odent, 1983), and water birth evolved from there. Research, therefore, has followed, rather than preceded, practice which has drawn some criticism.

Water birth should be regarded as a core midwifery competence, and all midwives should keep informed and observe water births (Royal College of Midwives (RCM), 2000). Some managers and midwives obstruct water birth requests, inventing excuses to deny women use of a pool (Robinson, 2001), and some units have pools sitting virtually unused. It has been suggested that only midwives who are supportive of water birth should be involved in caring for such women because they are less likely to be obstructive and more likely to support the woman. However, potentially a woman may arrive on a delivery suite to be told 'Sorry, there's no one on tonight who can do water births'. Also, midwives who have not learned about water births may be placed in a dangerous position if called upon to assist at a pool birth in the home, birthing centre or large hospital, especially in an emergency. All midwives should be able to assist at a water birth.

Facts

- The actual number of UK water births is unknown as it is poorly recorded: it is certainly many thousands of women. Some birth centres have water birth rates of up to 80% (National Institute for Health and Clinical Excellence (NICE), 2007).

- Women express high levels of satisfaction with use of water immersion in labour (Duffin, 2004), and all women should be offered the opportunity to labour in water (NICE, 2007).
- The National Service Framework requires that 'all staff have up to date skills and knowledge to support women who choose to labour without pharmacological intervention, including the use of birthing pools' and 'wherever possible, allow access to a birthing pool with staff competent in facilitating waterbirths' (Department of Health (DoH), 2004).
- It should be a service requirement to provide continuing professional development for midwives on water births (RCM, 2000).

Benefits of warm water immersion

Research into water immersion/birth is not easy. Often researchers do not clearly distinguish between shallow- or deep-water immersion, and/or confuse *labour* in water with *birth* in water. The much-revered randomised controlled trial is not well suited to this subject (Jowitt, 2001), as women prefer to choose options in labour if and when they are ready for them. Being pressured into or denied water immersion/birth following the opening of a brown envelope (even though a woman may have consented to this in principle) may raise anxiety levels and affect labour progress. Research results should, therefore, be interpreted with caution. NICE (2007), for example, feels that the evidence supports water immersion in labour, but does not prove or disprove the benefits of actual birth in water.

Research/anecdotal accounts tend to suggest that:

- **Beneficial labour hormone levels** in warm water immersion include endorphins and oxytocin, with reduced catecholamine secretion (Odent, 1983; Ockenden, 2001a), which appear to lower pain perception (Ockenden, 2001b).
- **Less analgesia** is needed by women using a pool compared to dry land labour (Garland & Jones, 2000; Otigbach *et al.*, 2000; Burns, 2001; Cluett *et al.*, 2004a). Water in labour appears to be a cost-effective analgesic and is recommended by NICE (2007).
- **Relaxation.** Water offers a peaceful, secure environment, which helps the woman to relax. The woman's buoyancy in the water encourages her to find comfortable positions enabling her to move freely (Ockenden, 2001b).
- **Backache** appears to be eased (Nightingale, 1996).
- **Fewer tears.** Women birthing in water may experience intact perineums or less severe tears compared to similar births on dry land (Garland & Jones, 2000; Burns, 2001; Garland, 2006), but more research is needed (RCM, 2005)
- **Postpartum haemorrhage** rates appear lower in women having water births, although again further research is needed (Garland, 2006). This is interesting because most third stages following water birth tend to be physiological.
- **Slow progress** may be improved by water immersion (Cluett *et al.*, 2004b).
- **No difference in length of labour and 5 min Apgar score** following use of a waterbirth pool (Garland & Jones, 2000; Burns, 2001).
- **No apparent increase in neonatal infection or neonatal intensive care unit admission** (Cluett *et al.*, 2004a) although further research is needed (Royal College of Obstetricians and Gynaecologists (RCOG)/RCM, 2006).

Risks of warm water immersion

- **Premature gasping:** There are anecdotal accounts of babies developing post-birth respiratory distress secondary to water inhalation (Nugyen *et al.*, 2002), but these are not backed up by larger studies. Babies do not appear to gasp or inhale water when born in warm water unless severely hypoxic. Due to fears of premature gasping in cold water, researchers originally suggested that the water should be around body temperature (Johnson, 1996). This has been challenged by Harper (2002) who describes healthy babies born in cold sea as low as 24°C.

- **Hyperthermia.** Fetal temperature is 0.5°C higher than normal (37°C) maternal temperature. If the mother becomes pyrexial, however, there will be a greater relative difference in the mother's and baby's temperatures, i.e. the baby will get considerably hotter and will take longer to cool down (Charles, 1998). If the mother becomes significantly overheated in the pool, the baby can become excessively hot and can become severely asphyxiated (Rosevear *et al.*, 1993).

- **Water embolism.** Early concerns about water embolism are hypothetical: there have been no recorded cases.

- **Infection.** There are theoretical concerns about infection but few recorded cases which could not have been due to chance alone. In 1993 one baby born in a home spa bath died from *Legionella* pneumonia which was isolated from the bath (Nagai *et al.*, 1993). Unlike most birthing pools, spa baths have recesses difficult to access, and it is inadvisable to use these for water births. Confidential Enquiry into Maternal and Child Health (CEMACH) (2004) states that water birth may carry a risk for the mother due to faecal contamination of the perineum and genital tract, but the evidence base is thin.

  Mobile pools normally have a single-use disposable liner. (See later in chapter for pool cleaning recommendations.)

- **Snapped cord.** It has been documented following water birth (Crow & Preston, 2002) and is easily dealt with (see later in chapter).

- **Slow progress.** Women who get in at <5 cm cervical dilation or who stay in >2 hours may find labour slows down (Eriksson *et al.*, 1997; Odent, 1998). This may be due to the absence of the gravity effect, which is known to aid labour progress. The risk may have been overstated since it is easily reversible: i.e. get out of the pool and mobilise. A woman who is very distressed and feeling out of control in early labour may find a period of water immersion an ideal way of relaxing and regaining some control. She also may not want a vaginal examination (VE) prior to entering the pool. Prescriptive restrictions on when a woman should enter the water and how long she should stay in are therefore unhelpful (Garland, 2006). It is just a question of being vigilant to the frequency and strength of contractions, and responding appropriately.

  Interestingly, water immersion may actually help some women with slow progress, possibly due to its relaxing effect, reversing the stress response which inhibits contractions (Cluett *et al.*, 2004b).

- **Midwifery back pain.** This is sometimes an excuse cited by midwives who do not feel comfortable with water birth. In fact, there is rarely any need to lean over the side of the pool, except for fetal heart (FH) auscultation or perhaps briefly to perform a VE. Bend from the hips if you need to lean over. One of the joys of water is that it stops clinicians interfering with the birth process. Like so many labour situations, try to 'sit on your hands' and avoid continually leaning over to peer at the perineum. As discussed later, the birth itself should be 'hands off'. Think about a low stool for sitting alongside the pool.

Criteria for labouring in water

Each unit will have its own criteria for labouring in water but care should be individualised to meet women's requests. Ultimately, the woman makes the decision when she has been presented with all the information.

Criteria include the following:

- Women's informed choice.
- Normal, term pregnancy from 37 weeks (RCM, 2000).
- Singleton, cephalic presentation (RCM, 2000).
- Opioid (e.g. pethidine) given <2 hours ago and the woman is not drowsy (NICE, 2007).
- Spontaneous rupture of the membranes of less than 24 hours (RCM, 2000).
- Arguably, most situations where intermittent monitoring is being performed. If the woman is not having electronic fetal monitoring (EFM), even if clinicians do not agree with her decision, there are few arguments against water immersion in labour.

Relative contraindications

- **Infection.** This is a contentious area, since many trusts may be unhappy to 'permit' water birth for women with infections, e.g. HIV, hepatitis B and group B strep. There is no definitive answer to this, but it should always be remembered that many women have infections we know nothing about, so universal precautions should always be practised. Whilst body fluids obviously cannot be so well contained when birth occurs in water, one might speculate that concentrated blood splash injuries might be fewer, since (a) blood is diluted in large volumes of water; (b) the birth is usually 'hands off': a sudden gush of fluid will be dispersed in the water, rather than splashing the midwife's face; and (c) the baby may be partially cleansed of maternal body fluids as it delivers through the water.
- **Pyrexia.** Any woman with a pyrexia should always be recommended to leave the pool due to risk of infection and fetal hyperthermia (Charles, 1998). She will probably be feeling hot and uncomfortable anyway.
- **Prolonged rupture of membranes.** It risks ascending infection – such women are usually advised not to labour in water. Although since it is safe to have a bath with prolonged rupture of membranes (NICE, 2007) one might question the logic of this.
- **High body mass index.** Larger women may benefit from the buoyancy effects, allowing them to take up otherwise awkward positions, e.g. kneeling, but there is a fear that very large women may be difficult to 'extract' from the pool in an emergency. This is a delicate subject and should be approached sensitively.
- **Need for electronic fetal monitoring.** It is technically possible to monitor continuously during water immersion (Zanetti-Dallenbach *et al.*, 2007) and waterproof cardiotocography (CTG) leads are available (Price, 2001), but many midwives would be horrified at the idea of a water pool being invaded in this way. If a woman has

chosen water birth against advice and EFM would have been recommended, ask her if she would consider as a compromise getting out for an occasional CTG trace. She has every right to refuse.

- **Heavy bleeding/thick meconium liquor.** CTG and closer monitoring would be strongly recommended. Both may result in fetal distress which could cause a baby to gasp prematurely, so water is not advisable. Thin meconium is less of a concern and may not need continuous CTG (NICE, 2007); there is no consensus on this issue.
- **Oxytocin augmentation.** Despite reports of women with an oxytocin infusion labouring successfully in pools (H. Ponette, website; Zanetti-Dallenbach *et al.*, 2007), this is unusual practice in the UK.
- **Previous caesarean section.** If a woman has chosen to have intermittent ausculta-tion for her vaginal birth after caesarean (VBAC) section labour, there is no rea-son to exclude her from water immersion. A number of units now provide water immersion/birth for VBAC women (Garland, 2006). It is possible that since women will not be using epidural anaesthesia in water, they may be more likely to be aware of the pain of uterine dehiscence.
- **Multiple birth/breech.** There are anecdotal accounts of breech and water births. e.g. German midwife Cornelia Enning and Belgian obstetrician Herman Ponette (see Useful contacts); however, such accounts must be read critically. Ponette also protects the perineum, controls the head and even occasionally clamps and cuts the cord underwater (a highly questionable practice).

Preparation

Pools are available in many shapes and sizes, fixed or portable. Fill deeply so the woman's abdomen is covered and she is comfortably buoyant.

Water temperature

There is no clear evidence on optimal pool temperature and local guidelines vary. Burns and Kitzinger (2001) suggest 35–37°C for the first stage and 37°C for the second stage and birth. NICE (2007) recommends ≤37.5°C.

Anderson (2004), however, suggests the mammalian capacity for thermostasis en-sures that women will be uncomfortable if they are too hot or cold and agrees with Harper (2002) who says: 'There is no reason for midwives...to worry over keeping the water at a set temperature other than the mother's physical comfort', but ensure the mother does not become pyrexial (Charles, 1998). The RCOG and RCM support this approach (RCOG/RCM, 2006).

The surface temperature is cooler than deeper down, so stir the water well to mix it before measuring the temperature. Hot water may need to be added regularly.

Cleansing

Local infection control policies should cover waterbirth (RCM, 2000). Following use, the pool should be rinsed of debris and cleaned with a chlorine-releasing agent which is effective against HIV, hepatitis B and hepatitis C (Burns & Kitzinger, 2001). Running hospital pool taps for 5 minutes everyday may minimise infection risk (Woodward

& Kelly, 2004). Consider also running the taps for a while prior to filling the pool, particularly in any setting where the pool is not frequently used.

Equipment

- Thermometer to check water temperature.
- Waterproof fetal heart doppler device.
- Lift or aid to get the woman out of the pool in an emergency (if available).
- Gauntlet gloves and eye protectors (not all midwives use these).
- A small mirror for visualisation of progress during the second stage of labour.
- Low stool or step to help the woman in and out easily. The midwife may sit on this too.
- Plenty of towels, warmed if possible.
- Portable entonox or extended tubing to reach the pool.
- Sieve and bowl to collect any faeces.

Water birth at home

Some NHS trusts rent out pools, and many companies offer pool hire (see end of chapter).

Alternatively a home-made tub can be constructed, including:

- Pool liner (available from water birth companies).
- Submersible pond pump for emptying the pool (available from garden centres). Alternatively jugs or bowls can be used, but these are extremely time-consuming: both staff and birth partners will have better things to do after the birth than spending an hour emptying the tub.
- Plastic sheeting matting (available from garden centres) to cover carpets.

A trial run is advisable. Filling a large pool can take some time and quickly drain a domestic hot water tank. Think about how to maintain a good supply, e.g. ensure when labour starts, the thermostat is set to heat the water at any time of day, and/or consider switching on the immersion heater to the hot water cylinder. Used water should preferably drain down a toilet.

Beware of the danger of water and electricity. Trailing leads and lamps are dangerous. Always have a charged torch to hand.

A structural survey of the floor is rarely indicated, but think about where the pool is to be placed. Be aware that when filled it can weigh up to 850 kg so may be best on the ground floor. Birth pool companies are usually very helpful and have a wealth of experience and literature about home water birth.

Labour care

(See also Chapter 1.)

First stage of labour

- **Check the woman's temperature** hourly (D. Garland, personal communication, 2002).

- **Allow her to drink freely** to avoid dehydration as water immersion has a diuretic effect (Ockenden, 2001b) and the exposed areas of the body will sweat. Encourage birth partners to drink and do the same yourself: humid pool rooms can be enervating for everyone.
- **Measure and record the water temperature.** The frequency may vary with local guidelines, but typically every 30–60 minutes.
- **VEs** are usually performed with relative ease in the pool.

Second stage of labour

- **Keep lights as low as possible** (within the bounds of safety) and **voices quiet.**
- **Monitor maternal and fetal well-being** as per normal labour.
- Think about having a **second midwife** present for the birth (this may be policy in some areas). However, as with all births, try to ensure they do not 'break the spell' and interrupt the birth process. A quiet presence in the background is usually all that is required.
- **Adjust water temperature** to 37°C or a comfortable temperature.
- **Viewing the perineum.** If it is really necessary and the woman does not mind, or wants to see for herself, you can submerge a small, portable mirror to visualise progress (think about infection control – a disposable mirror is probably best). However, do not stand constantly and peer in at the perineum. Think: 'what is being achieved by this?'
- **Have a 'hands off' approach to delivery.** It is thought that touching the fetal head underwater may stimulate the baby to try to breathe, although there is no evidence that this has ever happened. Usually, there is no need for any 'hands on'.
- **Let the head deliver.** The woman will usually tell you (not necessarily in coherent words!) or she may instinctively put her hands down to touch. Sometimes there is a small cloud of blood/liquor as the head pops out. You may be able to see the dark head underwater; if you are really unsure a brief touch will confirm.
- **Do not check for the cord.**
- **Await the next contraction.** The woman will usually then birth the baby. Occasionally a little help may be needed to release the shoulder, but assist only if really necessary. If she wishes, encourage the woman to bring her baby to the surface herself.
- If the woman is on all fours, pass the baby underwater through (not around) her legs and bring it gently up to the surface in front of her (Fig. 7.1).
- **Water babies do not always cry** or breathe instantly (Wickham, 2005). Be calm, and check the baby's colour, and if unsure check the heart rate by placing your fingers on its chest. It may open its eyes, look around and move calmly even though it is not breathing. This can be disconcerting, but is rarely a problem: remember if the cord is pulsating, the baby is getting oxygen. If you are concerned, lift the baby's body briefly into the cool air; this will usually stimulate it to breathe.
- **Ensure the cord is left attached and pulsating.** This can continue for some time. It is sensible to check that the cord is intact, as a snapped cord can be a life-threatening emergency for the baby if unnoticed (Crow & Preston, 2002). (See below under the heading 'Possible problems'.)

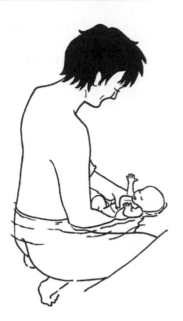

Fig. 7.1 For woman who give birth in the all-fours position, the baby should be passed through the woman's legs so that the woman can receive her baby without the cord becoming caught up or restricted.

Third stage of labour

It is not usually necessary to leave the pool to deliver the placenta unless the woman so wishes. Within a few minutes of birth many women are ready to climb out of the water, which can be by this point a little murky and uninviting.

If the woman chooses to remain in the water, keep the baby warm by submerging the baby's body in the water: only its face needs to emerge.

- **Physiological third stage.** Watch, wait and do nothing (see Chapter 1). Austin *et al.* (1997) cite one isolated case where a baby born in water received a large placental transfusion and developed polycythaemia. Odent (1998) suggests that the cold air would stop the umbilical cord pulsating sooner on dry land (vasoconstriction being caused by exposure to the cold air) and that warm water may delay this from happening. This is a sensible point but others have commented that this is only one case in thousands and anecdotal observation suggests no increased jaundice or polycythaemia. Midwives should be guided by the woman's preference.
- **Active management.** Opinion is divided whether the woman should stay in the pool if she requests active management. If she does, ask her to lift her leg out of the water and cleanse with an alcohol swab prior to giving the oxytocic; *do not give the injection underwater* as this is an infection risk. Some midwives may consider giving an IM injection into the arm, but this may be painful as there is less muscle. Controlled cord traction with fundal guarding is quite possible in birth pools, but ensure that you are happy to do this. If in doubt, suggest the woman leaves the pool.
- **Estimated blood loss.** This is not always easy, although many midwives are adept at assessing the colour of the water: there is usually a moderate visible bleeding as the placenta separates, which tends to sink to the bottom of the tub around the woman. If in doubt, ask her to leave the pool.

Possible problems

In any emergency, home or hospital, call for assistance immediately.

Most common reasons to leave the pool

In a large study by Burns (2001), 47% of primigravidae left the pool at some point in labour, while 53% remained for the birth. Water was consistently rated positively irrespective of whether the woman stayed in the pool for birth or not.

- **Slow progress in the first stage** (see Chapter 8 for suggestions to resolve this).
- **Slow progress during the second stage of labour.** This may often be rectified by the woman leaving the pool or standing up in it, perhaps with one foot up on a stool to widen the outlet. As the baby starts to descend she can get back in the pool for the birth. It may take some time to increase contraction strength. Make sure that the woman does not get cold.
- **Personal choice.** A small minority of women do not enjoy being in the water so do not stay. Others decide to get out just prior to giving birth.
- **Additional analgesia.** While women using the pool are less likely to need additional analgesia (Garland & Jones, 2000; Burns, 2001; Cluett *et al.*, 2004a), some women do request additional pain relief such as pethidine or an epidural and so need to leave the pool.
- **Change in the baby's condition.** Evidence of fetal compromise, such as the fresh passage of meconium or abnormal fetal heart changes.
- **Change in the mother's condition.** Any concern about maternal well-being, e.g. bleeding, pyrexia or hypertension.

Cord entanglement

Most babies with cord entanglement will easily deliver with the cord around the neck or body without the need for any intervention (Association of Radical Midwives (ARM), 2000). You cannot tell if the cord is holding the baby back until the baby fails to deliver. If this happens, confirm the presence of a cord by gentle touch. In the rare eventuality that the cord will not slip over the head, *do not clamp and cut it underwater* but proceed as follows:

- Get the woman out of the water quickly. Standing up may be sufficient, but be ready to catch the baby if necessary.
- Once out of the water apply two clamps to the cord and cut between them; this can be very awkward if the cord is very tight.
- Deliver the baby outside the water.
- Never submerge a baby once it has been born out of the water.

Snapped cord

This rare event is usually uneventful if recognised quickly. However, it is sometimes difficult to visualise a snapped cord due to cloudy water or the position of the baby. Several cases where the problem has gone unnoticed have had serious neonatal consequences (Crow & Preston, 2002).

Always lift the baby carefully into the mother's arms avoiding pulling on a short cord (Garland, 2002).

If the cord snaps, grasp the baby's end of the cord quickly to prevent blood leakage. Apply a clamp securely. Assess the baby and if necessary inform a paediatrician. Post-birth neonatal haemoglobin may be advised.

Shoulder dystocia

If the shoulder is slow to deliver, ask the woman to stand up, perhaps with one foot on a stool to widen the outlet. If this does not help, then the woman must get out of the tub immediately. This in itself often rotates the baby in the pelvis and spontaneous birth then occurs. (See Chapter 16 for further management of shoulder dystocia.)

Postpartum haemorrhage

Some bleeding occurs naturally as the placenta separates. A postpartum haemorrhage is visible as an unnaturally large bright red loss spreading quickly through the water. If you are concerned, ask the woman to leave the pool or pull the plug and drain the pool. The midwife should manage the third stage actively if the woman is haemorrhaging. (See Chapter 15 for more information.)

Loss of consciousness

Very unusually a woman may collapse: usually just a simple faint. It is surprisingly easy to hold a woman who has fainted in the pool, as the water supports her weight and you can hold her head and shoulders comfortably above water. Women tend to recover without any ill effects. However, you may require help, preferably several people, to lift her out. Use a lifting aid or hoist, if available, providing you have time. At a home birth enlist the birth partner to help. Clearly, if the collapse is more serious, further action will be called for once she has left the pool (see Chapter 16).

Practise hypothetical emergency situations with colleagues.

The unresponsive baby

The procedure to follow for an unresponsive baby is to:

- Clamp and cut the cord.
- Transfer the baby in a warm towel to the resuscitaire or prepared resuscitation area if at a home birth.
- Dry the baby vigorously.
- Follow the care for neonatal resuscitation (given in Chapter 17 together with Fig. 17.1 p. 242).

Summary

Maintain a quiet, relaxed atmosphere.
Allow the woman to drink freely.

Keep the water at a comfortable temperature; do not exceed 37.5°C for the second stage.
Monitor maternal temperature hourly and water temperature every 30–60 min.
Suggest she leaves the pool for a while if progress is slow.
Have a hands off birth. Only assist if necessary.
Water babies are often slow to breathe, especially if still attached to a pulsating cord.
Physiological or active management can be conducted in the pool.

Useful contacts

Active Birth Centre Telephone: 020 7281 6760. Website: www.activebirthcentre.com (accessed October 2007).

Association for Improvements in the Maternity Services (AIMS) AIMS Helpline: 0870 765 1433. Website: www.aims.org.uk (accessed October 2007).

Cornelia Enning (a German midwife who has championed water birth) Website: www.hebinfo.de/ (website in German but good pictures).

Dr Herman Ponette (a Belgian obstetrician with a medicalised approach to water birth, but still very interesting) Website: www.helsinki.fi/~lauhakan/whale/waterbaby/p0.html

Splashdown Water Birth Services Ltd Website: www.splashdown.org.uk (accessed October 2007).

Recommended reading

Garland, D. (2002) *Waterbirth: An Attitude to Care*, 2nd edn. Books for Midwives Press, Cheshire.

References

Anderson, T. (2004) Time to throw the waterbirth thermometer away? *MIDIRS Midwifery Digest* **14** (3), 370–74.

Association of Radical Midwives (ARM) (2000) Association of Radical Midwives Netalk: Checking for cord. *Midwifery Matters*, **87**, 28–30.

Austin, T., Bridges, N. & Markiewicz, M. & Abrahamson, E. (1997) Severe polycythaemia after third stage of labour underwater. *The Lancet* **350**, 1445–7.

Burns, E. (2001) Waterbirth. *MIDIRS Midwifery Digest* **11** (3, Suppl. 2), 10–13.

Burns, E. & Kitzinger, S. (2001) *Midwifery Guidelines for Use of Water in Labour.* Oxford Centre for Health Care Research and Development, Oxford Brookes University, Oxford.

Charles, C. (1998) Fetal hyperthermia risk from warm water immersion. *British Journal of Midwifery* **6** (3), 152–6.

Cluett, E., Nikodem, V., McCandlish, R. & Burns, E. (2004a) Immersion in water in pregnancy, labour and birth. *Cochrane Database of Systematic Reviews*, Issue 3.

Cluett, E., Pickering R., Getliffe K. & St George Saunders, N.J. (2004b) Randomised controlled trial of labouring in water compared with standard augmentation for management of dystocia in the first stage of labour. *British Medical Journal* **328** (7), 314–8.

Confidential Enquiry into Maternal and Child Health (CEMACH) (2004) *Why Mothers Die 2000–2002.* The Sixth report of confidential enquiries into maternal deaths in the United Kingdom. CEMACH, London.

Crow, S. & Preston, J. (2002) Cord snapping at a waterbirth delivery. *British Journal of Midwifery* **10** (8), 494–7.

Department of Health (DoH) (2004) *National Service Framework for Children, Young People and Maternity Services*, pp. 27–9. Department of Health, London.

Duffin, C. (2004) Water birth findings reveal high levels of satisfaction. *Nursing Standard* **18** (37), 8.

Eriksson, M., Mattsson, L.A. & Ladfors, L. (1997) Early or late bath during the first stage of labour: a randomized study of 200 women. *Midwifery* **13**, 146–8.

Garland, D. (2002) *Waterbirth: An Attitude to Care*, 2nd edn. Books for Midwives Press, Cheshire.

Garland, D. (2006) 'On the crest of a wave' completion of a collaborative audit. *MIDIRS Midwifery Digest* **16** (1), 81–5.

Garland, D. & Jones, K. (2000) Waterbirth supporting practice through clinical audit. *MIDIRS Midwifery Digest* **10** (3), 333–6.

Harper, B. (2002) Taking the plunge: re-evaluating water temperature guidelines. *MIDIRS Midwifery Digest* **12** (4), 506–8.

Johnson, P. (1996) Birth under water – to breathe or not to breathe. In *Waterbirth Unplugged. Proceedings of the First International Water Brith Conference* (Lawrence Beech, B., ed.), pp. 31–3. Books for Midwives Press, London.

Jowitt, M. (2001) Problems with RCTs and midwifery. *Midwifery Matters* **91**, 9–10.

Nagai, T., Sobajima, H., Iwasa, M., Tsuzuki, T., Kura, F., Amemura, J. & Watanabe, H. (1993) Neonatal sudden death due to *Legionella* pneumonia associate with water birth in a domestic spa bath. *Journal of Clinical Microbiology* **41** (5), 2227–9.

National Institute for Health and Clinical Excellence (NICE) (2007) *Clinical Guideline 55: Intrapartum Care*. National Institute for Health and Clinical Excellence, London.

Nightingale, C. (1996) Water and pain relief – observations of over 570 waterbirths at Hillingdon. In *Waterbirth Unplugged. Proceedings of the First International Water Birth Conference* (Lawrence Beech, B., ed.), pp. 63–9. Books for Midwives Press, London.

Nugyen, S., Kuschel, C., Teele, R. & Spooner, C. (2002) Water birth – a near drowning experience. *Pediatrics* **110**, 411–3.

Ockenden, J. (2001a) The hormonal dance of labour. *The Practising Midwife* **4** (6), 16–17.

Ockenden, J. (2001b) Waterbirth. *The Practising Midwife* **4** (9), 30–2.

Odent, M. (1983) Birth under water. *The Lancet* **2**, 1476–7.

Odent, M. (1998) Use of water during labour – updated recommendations. *MIDIRS Midwifery Digest* **8** (1), 68–9.

Price, S. (2001) Electronic fetal monitoring equipment. *British Journal of Midwifery* **9** (9), 579–82

Robinson, J. (2001) Demand and supply in maternity care. *British Journal of Midwifery* **9** (8), 510.

Rosevear, S., Fox, R., Marlow, N. & Stirrat, G. (1993) Birthing pools and the fetus. *Lancet* **342**, 1048–9.

Royal College of Midwives (RCM) (2000) The use of water in labour and birth. *RCM Midwives Journal* **3** (12), 374–5.

Royal College of Midwives (RCM) (2005) *Evidence Based Guidelines for Midwifery Led Care in Labour: Midwifery Practice Guideline No 1*. Available at: www.rcm.org.uk (accessed March 2008).

Royal College of Obstetricians and Gynaecologists (RCOG)/RCM (2006) *Immersion in Water During Labour and Birth*. Joint statement 1. RCOG, London.

Wickham, S. (2005) Is the Apgar a flexible friend? *Practising Midwife* **8** (7), 35.

Woodward, J. & Kelly, S. (2004) A pilot study for a randomised controlled trial of waterbirth versus land birth. *BJOG: An International Journal of Obstetrics and Gynaecology* **111** (6), 537–45.

Zanetti-Dallenbach, R., Lapaire, O., Maertens, A., Holzgreve, W. & Hosli I. (2007) Water birth: more than a trendy alternative. *Obstetrical and Gynaecological Survey* **62** (4), 222–3.

8 Slow progress and malpresentations/malpositions in labour

Vicky Chapman

Introduction

'Labours wax and wane in intensity and progress: there is no "right length" for a labour. One should be on the lookout for any clinical indications that might suggest fetal distress or other concerns but a longer labour need not, of itself, be seen as a problem' (RCM Campaign for normal birth, 2005).

Labour is a complex process in which psychological and physiological events are intertwined and inseparable. Some women by nature have longer labours than others. Some labours are slowed by a large or awkwardly positioned baby, but still end in a normal birth. Women categorised as having a slow labour should not necessarily require medical intervention. All factors for each individual woman, including her wishes, should be taken into account.

Sometimes slow progress is more serious and indicates a significant problem. Usually with the passing of time, a skilled midwife will identify and refer, those labours truly running into trouble, and avoid unnecessary intervention in labours which are simply progressing slowly but surely.

Current parameters for 'normality' have been defined and imposed on labouring women by obstetricians from a time where practice 'served organisational and management priorities' rather than evidence (Royal College of Midwives (RCM), 2005) and when the views of women were not considered important. Advocates of active management claim shorter labours are better; however, evidence is contradictory and benefits of a slightly shorter labour remain unproved. Diagnosis of slow progress often marks the transfer from 'normality' and 'midwifery care' to one of 'obstetric management' (Cluett *et al.*, 2004). This sometimes highlights cultural friction between two different philosophies of care and illustrates the powerlessness of midwives and childbearing women to challenge obstetric control in 'normal' birth. Debate continues over conservative versus active management in the politics of the medicalisation of birth (Walsh, 2000a; Neilson *et al.*, 2003; Cluett *et al.*, 2004; RCM, 2005; Albers, 2007).

In the quest for preventing long labours, some of the direct iatrogenic effects of the medical model of care – restricted mobility (Gupta *et al.*, 2000), enforced fasting (Johnson *et al.*, 2000), lack of continuity of carer or support in labour (Hodnett *et al.*, 2003) and epidural anaesthesia (Dickersin, 2000) have been overlooked by obstetricians as direct causes of labour dystocia. In ignoring traditional, proven and simple preventative measures, clinicians have instead carried out interventions including routine vaginal examinations, artificial rupture of the membranes (ARM) and oxytocics to 'manage' this fairly common problem with little regard for the woman's individual circumstances or wishes (Albers, 2007).

Incidence

- Slow progress (dystocia) in labour affects mainly primiparas – around 20% (Cluett *et al.*, 2004), however, dystocia is open to interpretation and statistics vary between different practitioners and units (Crowther *et al.*, 2000).
- Outcomes (NHS Maternity statistics, 2007):
  - Two out of three women with a prolonged *first stage* have an emergency caesarean (CS).
  - Two out of three women with a prolonged *second stage* have an instrumental delivery.
- Approximately half of women judged to have a 'slow' labour progress equally well whether or not oxytocic drugs are used (Keirse *et al.*, 2000).

Facts

- Early labour assessment and reassurance by midwives (ideally at home) reduces subsequent interventions, time spent on labour ward, augmentation, analgesia use and epidurals, and women are more likely to report an improved birth experience (McNiven *et al.*, 1998; Walsh, 2000a; Lauzon & Hodnett, 2002).
- During labour women appear to have an altered perception of time and events (RCM, 2005).
- Anxiety and environmental stressors have a negative physiological effect on labour progress.
- Encouraging women to mobilise and remain upright during labour enhances contractions and reduces dystocia.

Prolonged labour

Active management of labour

'Active management of labour has accumulated a number of eminent critics, who assert that the framework for its basic tenets are based on unscientific assumptions' (Regan, 1998).

Active management was claimed to prevent CS in women whose progress was deemed 'slow'. This package of care includes ARM, early recourse to intravenous (IV) oxytocin infusion, continuous CTG, epidural anaesthesia and one-to-one midwifery care.

Neilson *et al.* (2003) state that randomised studies evaluating the efficacy of the whole package of active management are extremely rare. Evidence of any benefit is often contradictory and meta-analysis of the randomised clinical trials on specific components of active management shows that:

- Active management shortens labour by on average 1–2 hours.
- There is no clinical evidence to support any general benefits from a shorter labour (RCM, 2005).
- Claims that active management reduces the instrumental or CS rate are unsubstantiated (Neilson *et al.*, 2003).
- The one consistent reproducible effective component of active management that is often forgotten in debates is the simple, non-invasive effectiveness of continuous one-to-one midwifery support in labour (Thornton & Lilford, 1994). It has been proved to shorten labour, reduce intervention and improve neonatal outcomes and maternal satisfaction (Hodnett *et al.*, 2003; Neilson *et al.*, 2003). This element of active management has consistently been ignored by obstetricians, managers and NHS policy makers.
- Routine ARM has minimal effect length of labour duration, although if used following a diagnosis of slow progress, ARM may improve subsequent labour progress and duration in nulliparous women (Smyth *et al.* 2007).
- Oxytocin augmentation does not improve CS rates, operative vaginal delivery rates or neonatal outcome, and its effect of length of labour remains inconclusive (Thornton & Lilford, 1994; Keirse, 2000).
- Oxytocin increases pain and the risk of hyperstimulation (Keirse, 2000).

Much of the above evidence has been in wide circulation for over 15 years.

Assessing progress in labour and the partogram

The various methods of assessing progress are described in more detail under 'Assessing progress in labour' in Chapter 1.

Midwives use various methods to assess progress including frequency and strength of contractions (Sallam *et al.*, 1999), the woman's response, external signs, abdominal palpation to assess descent of the presenting part (Stuart, 2000) and vaginal examinations (VEs). VEs monitor, amongst other things, cervical dilatation and are the most commonly accepted method for assessing labour progress although they remain unevaluated by research (Crowther *et al.*, 2000). VEs, contraction frequency and abdominal findings can be recorded on a partogram.

The partogram has evolved from Friedman's work in the 1950s on mean time limits for cervical dilatation (Walsh, 2000a). It offers an immediate visual impression of the woman's overall physical condition and has alert and action lines used to record progress. This can be beneficial in hospitals, where midwives may be caring for several women and shifts change regularly. National Institute for Health and Clinical Excellence (NICE) (2007) recommends its use, with a 4-hour action line. However, care may become prescriptive, disregarding the woman's individual circumstances and wishes.

Observational studies (Buchmann, 2000) and a large Southeast Asian trial by the World Health Organization (WHO, 1994) found the partogram helped clinicians recognise, refer and act on prolonged labour. This reduced augmentation, emergency CS and perinatal mortality (Buchmann, 2000). However, some critics cast doubt on the quality of this prospective WHO study (Neilson *et al.*, 2003) as it introduced other variables alongside the partogram (e.g. intensive staff training and a new labour management protocol which included routine ARM in active labour). Neilson *et al.* suggest:

> 'There is only one reliable way of testing whether an intervention improves outcome and that is with a randomized controlled trial. The research method used and additional variables introduced could have been biased and lays the results open to doubt … Even if the results could be relied upon, one could question how applicable they are in other settings in the developed world where women have access to quality care.'

How slow is too slow?

The 'latent' and 'active' phases of labour are artificial constructs defined purely for clinical management purposes (Cluett, 2000); assessing labour onset, defining progress and when to intervene remain subjective and inexact, varying between units, hospitals, regions and countries (Crowther *et al.*, 2000).

- Contractions should become regular and progressively stronger, increasing in frequency and duration.
- Cervical dilatation of 0.5 cm/hour (if there are no other fetal or maternal concerns) may lead to fewer unnecessary labour interventions (Crowther *et al.*, 2000) and has increasingly been adopted in midwifery-led care settings and Wales (All Wales Clinical Pathway, 2004) and forms part of NICE (2007) intrapartum guidelines.
- Simkin and Ancheta (2005) describe the importance of additional measures of progress including cervical consistency, thinning and effacement, movement from posterior to anterior and the importance of good cervical application to the presenting part.

Obstructed labour

Obstruction is the failure of the presenting part to descend in spite of uterine contractions, manifesting itself ultimately as not *slow progress* but *no progress*. Obstruction may be caused by cephalopelvic disproportion (CPD), abnormal lie or presentation, e.g. brow (King *et al.*, 1999). Lack of progress and descent is usually noticeable with the passing of time. What really distinguishes *delay* from *obstruction* is the secondary signs and complications that follow.

Early signs of unresolved obstructed labour:

- Prolonged first and/or second stage
- Severe moulding and caput/high presenting part
- Often fetal heart rate (FHR) abnormalities

Possible late effects (many are usually only seen in developing countries):

- No further descent of the presenting part.
- A rigid retraction band 'Bandl's ring' forms as the lower segment becomes stretched: it can be felt as a transverse ridge across the lower abdomen.
- Bladder damage (often indicated by bloodstained urine).
- Fistulae (usually nulliparous women).
- Ruptured uterus (usually multiparous women).
- Fetal death.
- Maternal shock and sepsis often leading to death. Serious consequences of obstructed labour should never happen where care is adequate (King *et al.*, 1999).

Causes of a prolonged labour

Slow progress can have one or several causes.

Physical causes

- **Fetal presentation/position.** See malpresentations and malpositions in labour later in this chapter.
- **Cephalopelvic disproportion.** CPD is not easily predictable but is usually determined during labour if there is lack of descent of the presenting part (Crowther *et al.*, 2000) with increased caput and moulding (King *et al.*, 1999; Neilson, 2003). Predisposing factors include a small woman with a suspected large baby, maternal diabetes, a macrosomic baby and malposition. Previous uncomplicated delivery of a baby of similar weight is the most reliable predictor of pelvic adequacy (Enkin *et al.*, 2000).
- **Restricted mobility and the semi-recumbent position.** Do midwives cause dystocia? In the UK, three-quarters of women adopt a supine position for labour and birth. This is in part historical and cultural (RCM, 2005) but also due to lack of direction and encouragement from midwives (see also Chapter 1, p. 14).

Upright postures are a simple intervention to ensure adequate uterine contractions preventing dystocia. They open the pelvic outlet by as much as a third (RCM, 2005), reduce the pain felt by women, reduce the duration of second stage (Gupta *et al.*, 2000) the episiotomy rate (Gupta & Hofmeyer, 2004; Nasir *et al.*, 2007) and instrumental deliveries (Roberts *et al.*, 2005; Nasir *et al.*, 2007). Even women with epidural anaesthesia can benefit from adopting non-lying postures (Downe *et al.*, 2004; Roberts *et al.*, 2005).

The RCM (2005) campaign for normal birth acknowledges that *midwives are the key to promoting mobility* throughout labour and that encouraging the use of gravity-enhancing upright postures will help ensure a straightforward birth and may prevent labour dystocia.

Less common physical causes

Usually the following problems will have been identified and discussed prior to labour:

- **Pelvic anomalies**: fractured pelvis, women with significant weight-bearing problems, e.g. from lower limb amputation, spina bifida and spinal injury.
- **Cervical problems** may arise following cervical surgery, e.g. previous cone biopsy. The internal os can feel rough to the touch and the cervix tight and unyielding for a prolonged period (commonly during the latent phase). Simkin and Ancheta (2005) suggest contractions of great intensity may be required to overcome the initial resistance, following which dilatation usually occurs.

Stress response and emotional dystocia

'Dr. Michel Odent advocates "Zee most important thing is do not disturb zee birthing woman." I think we know what he means . . . ' (Lemay, 2000).

- Stress hormones interact with beta-receptors in the uterine muscle to inhibit contractions, slowing labour down (Cluett, 2000). This is most evident in primiparae arriving for the first time on labour ward, where their anxiety response causes their labour to temporarily stop.
- **Psychological stress and anxiety** can be stimulated by many factors. Environmental stress can be caused by arriving on labour ward with its bright lights, unfamiliar noises and lack of quiet privacy, in addition the staff may be busy; a minority even unsupportive or uncaring. (For more information on preparing a good birth environment see Chapter 1.)
- Some women may have personal anxieties such as fear of pain or childbirth and others may have had a previously traumatic delivery or are victims of childhood sexual abuse (Simkin & Ancheta, 2005).

Analgesia

- **Epidural anaesthesia** offers total pain block but can cause reduced mobility, reduced circulating natural oxytocin with poor contractions, malrotation, delay in the first and second stage of labour with associated increased interventions (Dickersin, 2000). Epidural rates vary dramatically between units, suggesting that it is not women who always choose this form of analgesia but those who 'care' for them. If dystocia is to be prevented, alternative methods of pain relief should be explored first and epidural reserved for those women who genuinely request it.
- **Opiates,** e.g. pethidine can make the woman sedated, drowsy and immobile and can indirectly affect progress.
   Conversely, *natural methods of working with pain* (see Chapter 1 for more information) include good one-to-one midwifery support, adopting comfortable positions, soaking in warm water, breathing, relaxation, massage and touch. These not only

encourage pain-relieving endorphin release but are proved effective at facilitating labour progress.

- **Deep warm water immersion** may facilitate the birth process for some women through relaxation and pain-relieving qualities. One small study found that water immersion was as effective a treatment intervention in nulliparas with dystocia as standard augmentation and had fewer associated side effects (Cluett *et al.*, 2004).

Prolonged latent phase

'Some women, having no idea what to expect from early labour, 'over-react', that is they are preoccupied with every contraction and they may rush to use learned coping techniques that are more appropriate for active labour. They often expect to be 5 or 6 cm dilated when they are first checked and are crushed when they are examined and found to be only 1 to 2 cm . . . The caregiver must help to acknowledge the woman's disappointment, giving her some suggestions to reduce the intensity of the contractions and proceed to calm and relax her. She will need help to get her head back to where her cervix is' (Simkin & Ancheta, 2005).

The latent phase of labour sometimes lasts for several days (Burvill, 2002) and does not respond well to interventions such as ARM or oxytocics (Simkin & Ancheta, 2005). In the absence of problems, this stage requires no medical intervention other than effective explanations, reassurance and support. Good support from the midwife and a 'wait and see' course of action will do much to help a woman through a long latent phase.

Midwifery care

A prolonged latent phase can leave the woman exhausted and demoralised as well as doubting her body's ability to continue to labour without problems. One study found that women admitted in the latent phase of labour experienced a need for handing over responsibility for the labour and the well-being of the unborn baby. Reasons identified were the following: longing to complete the pregnancy; having difficulty managing the uncertainty; having difficulty enduring the slow progress; suffering from pain to no avail; and oscillating between powerfulness and powerlessness. The researchers suggest midwives have a vital role in helping women cope by validating their experienced pain and confirming the normality of the slow process, as well as offering information and support (Carisson *et al.*, 2007).

- Women will benefit from their midwife sitting quietly with them through several contractions, chatting, offering empathic acknowledgement of the woman's pain, giving reassurance.
- Discuss practical ideas for coping with contractions such as:
  - Soaking in a warm bath, massage, hot water bottle.
  - Distractions and keeping busy such as going for a walk, cooking, watching a film.
- If it is night time or the woman feels exhausted she should aim to rest and doze for periods (even if she cannot sleep), and keep cosy with a hot water bottle. Suggest side-lying, supported by cushions or a duvet (preferable to lying on her back).

- Before leaving the woman to labour, or discharging her home if in hospital, ensure that she knows how to get in contact with you if she needs to.
- For some women prolonged, persistent pain is hard to bear and a minority request some form of pharmacological analgesia or epidural. Although this has the potential to open the floodgates to medical intervention, it may be the appropriate choice for that woman in her situation. Pethidine may cause contractions to slow down, offering some respite as well as the potential for the woman to doze and relax.
- For more information on the latent phase of labour, see Chapter 1.

Prolonged active first stage

The active phase should see contractions increasing in frequency, strength and pain. It can be useful to ask 'do the woman's contractions seem the same or more frequent, and more painful, than an hour ago?'

It should be standard practice to share the decision-making process with the woman in labour. While some women with slow progress may feel exhausted and demoralised, and welcome assistance, others will be coping well, 'gone into themselves', oblivious to the passing of time.

Midwifery care

Try to identify the cause for slow progress; directly ask the woman if anything is worrying her. Sharing information, explanations and offering possible solutions for specific anxieties can help. Avoid offering 'empty' reassurances, 'don't worry about that, you'll be fine', as this will do little to address her anxieties and even unintentionally suggest that the matter has been discussed and is somehow resolved.

As a midwife you can control the environment: ensure lights dim, doors and curtains drawn, maintain privacy, keep interruptions to a minimum and encourage her partner offer massage, touch and support. It can be useful to also address physical causes: is she hungry or thirsty; when did she last pass urine; have you advised mobilising/upright postures?

In some cases such as a malposition, simple mobilisation and accepting that progress will be slower will help (see 'Malpresentations and malpositions in labour').

(1) It may also be appropriate to try the interventions given in Box 8.1 to increase contractions.
(2) If natural interventions do not help labour progress, then further intervention will be necessary. The next steps are as follows:
   ○ Consider ARM (see Chapter 2)
   ○ VE 2 hours after ARM to check progress (NICE, 2007)
(3) If this does not increase labour NICE (2007) advises:

> 'When delay in the established first stage of labour is confirmed in nulliparous women, advice should be sought from an obstetrician and the use of oxytocin should be considered. The woman should be informed that the use of oxytocin following spontaneous or artificial rupture of the membranes will bring forward her time of birth but will not influence mode of birth or other outcomes.'

Box 8.1   Interventions to improve labour progress.

Support
- Continuous labour support reduces labour duration and interventions (Hodnett *et al.*, 2003).
- 'Lay' attendants are helpful: doulas, female relatives or friends can provide warmth, comfort and care (Simkin & Ancheta, 2005).
- If you are busy, call in additional staff, or suggest getting family/friends to act as additional birth supporters.

Mobilisation and position changes
- Even if the woman is exhausted, upright positions are usually possible and more comfortable than semi-recumbent.
- Gravity-enhancing positions appear to shorten the second stage compared with supine/lithotomy positions which increase fetal heart anomalies, dystocia, epidural use, episiotomy and instrumental delivery (Gupta *et al.*, 2000; RCM, 2005).
- Upright positions appear to help align pelvic bones and the shape/capacity of the pelvis, optimising a 'good fit' between baby and pelvis (Simkin & Ancheta, 2005). Squatting and kneeling significantly widen the pelvic outlet (Borrell & Fenstrom, 1957; Russell, 1982).
- Lying supine may cause the uterus to press on the spine, altering the angle of the uterus, resulting in poor alignment of the baby in the pelvis (Sutton & Scott, 1994).
  (See also p. 14 for evidence of improved clinical outcomes with non-supine positions.)

Comforting touch
- Massage, stroking, hand holding, and close contact in general increases endogenous oxytocin production, thereby stimulating contractions (Simkin & Ancheta, 2005).
- Give partners 'permission' to get in close and hold the woman; encourage attendants to offer comfort and massage and provide privacy for this.
- Touch is very personal; some women do not like it. Use this simple intervention with care.

Acupressure
- Acupressure remains unevaluated, however it is worth considering as it is simple, harm free and may do good. Simkin and Ancheta (2005) describe applying firm pressure for 10–60 seconds over the tibia (4 fingers width up from the inner ankle bone) or to the Ho-ku point of the back of the hand (where the metacarpal bones of the thumb and index finger meet). They suggest this may feel tender but is worth repeating several times if necessary.

Nipple stimulation
- Stimulating the nipples causes natural oxytocin release which enhances contractions (Kavanagh *et al.*, 2005).
- The woman can lightly stroke one or both nipples; most women will naturally require privacy for this.
- Some women may not want to try this intervention which they may find embarrassing, uncomfortable or irritating.

Water/hydrotherapy
- An anxious woman may find a relaxing bath stimulates oxytocin and endorphin release (Ockenden, 2001).
- Water is as effective as standard augmentation in nulliparas with dystocia and reduces epidural use (Cluett *et al.*, 2002).
- Long immersion can sometimes slow labour (Odent, 1998) but this is resolvable by leaving the pool.

Artificial rupture of the membranes (ARM)
Cochrane review found that amniotomy has minimal effect on labour duration and no affect on first stage duration, maternal analgesia use or maternal morbidity or neonatal outcomes (Smyth *et al.*, 2007). (For more information see Chapter 2.)

Box 8.1 *(Continued)*

- For women with slow progress, ARM did not affect further oxytocin use but did seem to have a protective, positive effect on subsequent labour progress and duration (Smyth *et al.*, 2007).
- While multiparous women had no differences overall, nulliparas appeared more sensitive to ARM, and its use appeared to reduce second-stage duration and chances of low Apgar score (7 or less) at 5 min (Smyth *et al.*, 2007).

IV Oxytocin

- Oxytocin is firmly established in labour ward culture as routine practice for managing 'longer than average' labours.
- Evidence of oxytocin effect on length of labour is unclear: many trials suggest it is minimal, and one study showed mobilisation appeared more effective than augmentation (Keirse *et al.*, 2000).
- IV oxytocics may achieve cervical dilatation without improving the outcome (Gee, 2000; NICE, 2007).
- Where there is genuine dystocia, oxytocin will not help. However, Crowther *et al.* (2000) suggest using oxytocics may help avoid a false diagnosis of CPD.
- Women describe oxytocin as 'unpleasant' and more 'painful' and say they would prefer to try without the drug when next giving birth (Keirse *et al.*, 2000).

(See Chapter 18 for more on information on oxytocin administration.)

Following assessment the obstetrician may decide to:

- Wait and see
- Recommend oxytocin infusion (with further VE after 4 hours), possibly with further analgesia (NICE, 2007)
- Offer continuous electronic fetal monitoring (NICE, 2007)
- Proceed to CS if:
  - Oxytocin is contraindicated
  - No further labour progress
  - FHR concerns

Prolonged second stage

Upright maternal birthing position, non-active pushing and avoiding arbitrary second stage time limits are beneficial to improving the spontaneous vaginal birth rate (Walsh, 2000b). There is some evidence that second stage >3 hours increases maternal risk of morbidity (Cheung *et al.*, 2004), and >4 hours increases the risk of more severe perineal trauma, PPH and infection (Myles & Santolaya, 2003). A longer second stage increases the vaginal delivery rate, reduces the CS rate and has no adverse effect on neonatal morbidity, although there is a small increased risk of shoulder dystocia (Myles & Santolaya, 2003).

Terminating a straightforward but slow second stage with an instrumental delivery is a frightening experience for women, it contributes to maternal morbidity and does not benefit infant outcomes (Sleep *et al.*, 2000; Walsh, 2000b).

NICE (2007) diagnoses second stage delay as:

- 2 hours of active second stage for a nulliparous woman: instrumental delivery recommended after 3 hours.

- 1 hour of active second stage for a parous woman: instrumental delivery recommended after 2 hours.
- Women with epidurals are recommended to delay pushing for an hour unless urge present or vertex visible.

Assessing progress

- Increased moulding and caput may feel misleadingly like descent, so always check descent by abdominal palpation (WHO, 2003).
- A total lack of progress in the presence of good contractions indicates more serious problems. Refer to an obstetrician.
- Consider fetal position and station at the onset of the second stage. These factors will help decide the timing of further VE and any obstetric review (NICE, 2007).

Reassess

- NICE (2007) recommend offering a VE after an hour of active second stage, to assess rotation and descent:
  - Refer multigravidae for obstetric opinion if birth not imminent.
  - Offer primigravidae support and encouragement, amniotomy (if membranes intact) and consider further analgesia/anaesthesia. If no birth after another hour (i.e. 2 hours of active second stage) refer to an obstetrician.

Referral

An obstetrician will assess by VE and palpation and may recommend the following:

- 'Wait and see' if birth is approaching
- Consider oxytocin (with CTG)
- Instrumental delivery in the labour room (see Chapter 9) or trial of instrumental delivery in theatre
- CS if no descent at all with pushing

Checklist for slow progress

- Is the cervix fully dilated?
- Is the woman's bladder full?
- Does she have a genuine urge to push? Is she experiencing a latent second phase of labour? If not, pause and await events.
- Is the woman lying down? If so, help her to change her position – upright postures tend to enhance contractions.
- Does she have an epidural (see below)?
- Are contractions adequate? Contractions with a long gap between them will mean that the woman's second stage will be longer and this must be taken into account if augmentation is not being used.
- For inadequate or incoordinate contractions see Box 8.1.

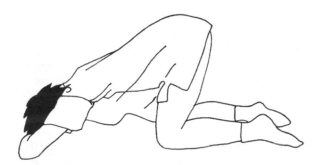

Fig. 8.1   Knee-chest position.

Problem solving

The imminent arrival of the baby may trigger many anxieties in the woman ranging from worries about the baby to a fear of pain and tearing (Simkin & Ancheta, 2005). The midwife may not be able to alleviate the woman's fears, but she should aim to acknowledge them and offer plenty of praise and reassurance, particularly when the woman is pushing (see also Chapter 1 for more on care in the second stage of labour).

Holding back. A woman who is tense and holding back, possibly frightened or inhibited, needs quiet, privacy and a relaxed focus away from her perineum and towards her well-being.

Keep the atmosphere calm, mellow and relaxed. Avoid stimulating the autonomic nervous system with unnecessary noise, lights, distractions, 'white coats' and interruptions. Refrain from shining a spotlight on, or staring at, the woman's perineum with every contraction. If appropriate suggest the woman goes and sits privately on the toilet to push for a while, give her the call bell and be ready close by.

Maternal exhaustion. In contradiction to care for a woman who is inhibited and holding back, a tired, demoralised woman may benefit from stimulation: refreshments (for all), a cool flannel, some music, a position change, a breeze via an open window and for sleepy, tired supporters to rally round, brighten up, wake up and give support.

Reversing the Chi. Lemay (2000) and Parry (2003) describe this: the mother adopts the knee-chest (Fig. 8.1) or side lying (Fig. 8.2) position and tries to literally pull her baby up to her neck for a few pushes.

'This will sound like strange instruction but, if she has learned to trust you, she will give it a whirl. After several contractions in this position with minimal exertion of the mother, the fetal head often appears suddenly at the perineum' (Lemay, 2000).

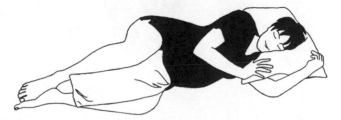

Fig. 8.2   Side lying.

Described by Simkin and Ancheta (2005) as 'abdominal lifting', this intervention possibly lifts and loosens an impacted head. It's worth a go!

Midwife exhaustion. We have all been there after a long night with a primip, exhausted and desperate for our warm bed. A slow second stage can leave tired midwives tempted to call the obstetrician in order to get the baby delivered. Such exhaustion does not always have an easy answer, but asking an energetic trusted colleague to assist you or relieve you to get something to eat and sit down for 10 minutes will help refresh your batteries and is preferable to making poor clinical decisions.

Survivors of childhood sexual abuse. It may help to focus the women in the present, offering gentle reassurance that what they can feel is their baby soon to be born. Chapter 2 provides information on counteracting, and not re-enacting, abuse.

Effective positions for a slow second stage

General mobilisation or upright and frequent position changes should help poor contractions and aid fetal descent.

- **Frequent change of position** is a simple intervention and yet can be the solution to delay in the second stage.
- **A supported squat or asymmetrical postures** can prove beneficial in malpositions/asynclitism (see Figs. 8.3–8.7). Radiological evidence illustrates that the pelvis moves and widens during birth and that the outlet diameters can increase by nearly a third in the squatting or kneeling positions (Borrell & Fenstrom, 1957; Russell, 1982).

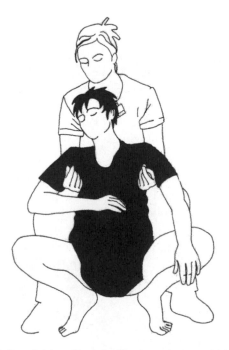

Fig. 8.3   Supported squat. Beneficial positions for the second stage of labour (see also Figs 8.7 and 8.8).

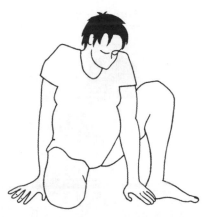

Fig. 8.4 Asymmetrical posture. Postures like this can be useful for poorly positioned babies, e.g. OP or asynclitism. Give the woman plenty of reassurance and encourage her to try different positions to see which she finds most effective.

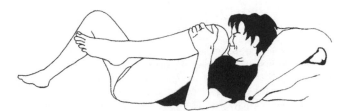

Fig. 8.5 On back with one leg raised. Also an asymmetrical posture (see Fig. 8.4).

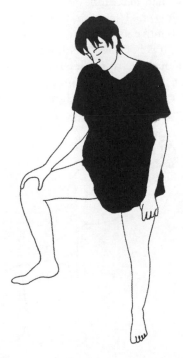

Fig. 8.6 Asymmetrical posture.

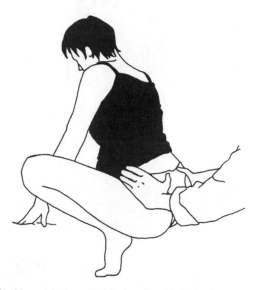

Fig. 8.7   Pelvic press. Simkin and Archeta (2005) describe this in the following way: the woman squats with her birth partner kneeling behind her. The partner places the flats of their hands over the woman's iliac crests and presses them very firmly towards each other during a contraction. Within three to four contractions there should be some evidence of rotation or descent. Do no try this if the woman has an epidural or if this causes any joint pain. Many women with backache find the pelvic press eases their back pain.

- **Encouraging the woman to 'climb'** on, over and off the bed a couple of times, or step on and off up a low stool (try stairs at home – an old midwifery trick). This may cause a stuck baby to move its position and free the lumbar spine.
- **Lithotomy position.** It is not uncommon for women prepared for an instrumental delivery to spontaneously deliver when their legs are abducted and placed in lithotomy as per Fig. 8.9. This position should be used sensitively and with caution as it has potential risks to the mother (including risk of DVT and perineal trauma). It

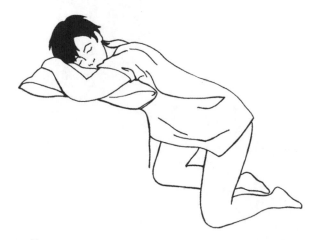

Fig. 8.8   Kneeling position.

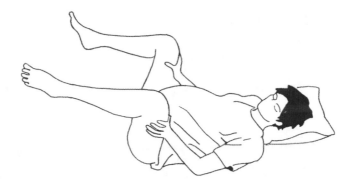

Fig. 8.9 Lithotomy style. Lithotomy style, or lying back, with legs up on to lithotomy poles can be useful to move a stuck baby. This position can be uncomfortable for some women and disempowering if not used sensitively and appropriately.

is dangerous for midwives' backs to support woman's legs on their hips and it can put stress on the woman's pelvis.

Epidural anaesthesia is associated with an increase in instrumental deliveries; however, spontaneous vaginal births with epidurals have been attributed to:

- **Delayed pushing** for around 1 (NICE, 2007) or 2 hours, or until the head is visible at the introitus (Fraser *et al.*, 2000; Roberts *et al.*, 2004)
- **Maternal position.** Second-stage duration is shorter, and instrumental delivery is less likely if the woman in the second stage adopts an upright, all fours or side lying position compared to a semi-recumbent position (Downe *et al.*, 2004; Roberts *et al.*, 2005).
- **Urinary retention** can result from an epidural, and a full bladder can impede progress; consider a catheter.
- **Direction.** Women who have a dense block may need direction and encouragement as to when and how to push.
- **Do not let the epidural wear off** as it does not improve the rate of spontaneous birth and is distressing for the woman. (NICE, 2007.)
- **Reassess.** If there is slow progress after an hour or two of pushing:
  - ○ Consider a VE and abdominal palpation for re-assessment of descent/progress.
  - ○ Refer to an obstetrician for review if necessary.

Malpresentations and malpositions in labour

A *malposition* is the vertex in an abnormal position. The diameter of the skull (see Fig. 8.10) in relation to the pelvic opening is greater than normal (Chadwick, 2002), e.g. the occipitoposterior (OP) position, or asynclitism, where the fetal head is tilted laterally so that the parietal bone presents first (see Fig. 8.11).

Malpresentations are non-vertex presentations, e.g. breech (see Chapter 13), face or brow presentation and transverse lie/shoulder presentation (see Figs. 8.12–8.16).

Malpositions and malpresentations commonly cause progress to be slower than usual but sometimes other complications can arise including deep transverse arrest, operative delivery and increased maternal and neonatal morbidity (Chadwick, 2002; Coates,

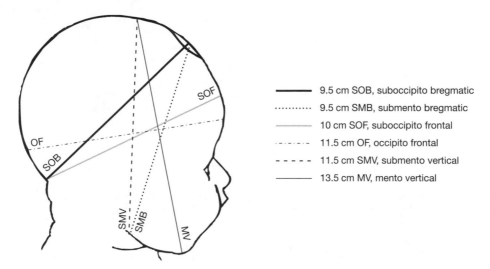

Fig. 8.10   Diameters of the fetal skull.

2002). There is the potential for the woman to be exhausted and the uterus less able to contract efficiently following birth, increasing the potential for postpartum haemorrhage. Women need a great deal of positive encouragement and support to help them through a potentially prolonged and difficult labour (Chadwick, 2002).

Home birth/birthing centre

With malpositions labour can be slower and birth have a variety of outcomes, any of which may necessitate transfer to a consultant unit. Some malpresentations, such as

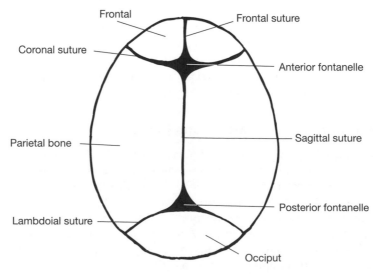

Fig. 8.11   The vault of the fetal skull.

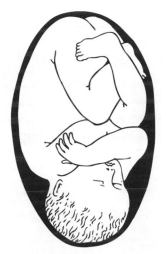

Fig. 8.12 Occipitoposterior position.

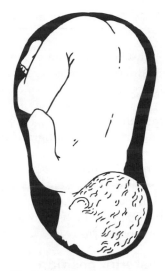

Fig. 8.13 Face presentation.

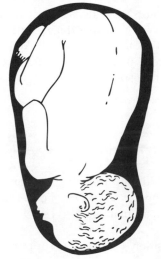

Fig. 8.14 Brow presentation.

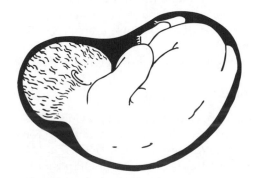
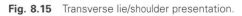

Fig. 8.15 Transverse lie/shoulder presentation.

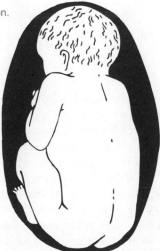

Fig. 8.16 Breech presentation (see Chapter 13 for more information).

a brow presentation, occur or are usually diagnosed during the second stage, and are associated with a high caesarean rate.

Midwives need to be vigilant for presentations or complications, which may necessitate transfer to a consultant unit.

Malposition can result in a longer labour and more difficult birth, although some women (particularly multigrividae) may not need to transfer. Discretely prepare an area for neonatal resuscitation or postpartum haemorrhage as a precaution.

Malpresentation can be serious and risky at home and transfer is usually advisable. However some malpresentations may occur (e.g. brow), or are diagnosed, only during the end of the second stage making transfer less feasible or safe. Shoulder presentation is the most serious: this is an obstetric emergency requiring urgent midwifery response and immediate transfer (see later in the chapter).

Occipitoposterior position

The most common malposition is the OP position. The fetus lies with its back against the mother's, the occiput in the posterior part of the pelvis and the head is deflexed (Coates, 1999). Gardberg and Tuppurainen (1994b) found that the OP position was linked to an increase in maternal morbidity and a higher prevalence of abnormal heart rate patterns in labour, but with no difference in Apgar scores or birth asphyxia.

Incidence and facts

- More common in primigravidae.
- 15% prevalence in labour but most rotate with only 5% persistent OP at birth (Gardberg & Tuppurainen, 1994b).
- Two-thirds of persistent OP positions are said to develop from malrotation from occiptoanterior (OA) to OP during labour (Gardberg *et al.*, 1998). Coates (2002) suggests that current thinking does not reflect this, as many midwives believe OP positions establish during pregnancy.
- An anterior placenta is more common with OP position (Gardberg & Tuppurainen, 1994a).
- Fraser *et al.* (2002) found increased risk of difficult delivery in women with epidurals who started second stage with a high head/OP.

Midwifery diagnosis

OP is usually evident from the classic signs (described below) including 'splitting backache' and contractions pattern.

Abdominal palpation. The fetal back is against the maternal spine, creating a dip around the woman's umbilicus which marks the space between the baby's arms and legs. The FHR is clearest far over to the side of the woman's uterus (Sutton, 2000). The woman may find abdominal palpation deeply uncomfortable as she has to lie back and such a posture usually causes intense back pain/discomfort.

Vaginal examination may confirm the anterior fontanelle in the anterior of the vagina if the head is deflexed (which it often is) but can also detect the posterior fontanelle posteriorly if there is reasonable flexion. Caput and moulding may also be present and make the diagnosis of landmarks on the fetal skull difficult (Chadwick, 2002).

Characteristics of OP labour and birth

- **Spontaneous rupture of the membranes** is common before the onset of labour due to the ill-fitting presenting part (Gardberg & Tuppurainen, 1994b; Sutton, 2000).
- **Deep back pain** during labour with intense back pain during contractions (Sutton, 2000; Coates, 2002).
- **Contractions can be irregular**, often coupling with a lengthy gap before the next (Sutton, 2000; Simkin & Ancheta, 2005), and labour is long and protracted (Sutton, 2000; Coates, 2002).
- **Involuntary pushing is more common** before the cervix is fully dilated (Walmsley, 2000) and can be very distressing for a woman, particularly if her carers are discouraging her from bearing down (Bergstrom *et al.*, 1997). Walmsley (2000) suggests that a premature urge to push, common in OP babies, may be physiologically desirable because it forces the presenting part to flex, then rotate, optimising its position, prior to full dilatation.
- **Second stage labour progress can be slow** due to the wide diameter of the presenting part, which also causes gaping of the vagina before the vertex is visible.
- A **'shrinking' cervix**, or an **oedematous cervix**, can be associated with the deflexed head of the OP baby (Association of Radical Midwives (ARM), 2000).

Midwifery care

Despite practice recommendations to improve or correct fetal misalignment by rotating the fetal head to OA (Sutton, 2000), some authors stress that there is not always a 'quick fix' solution for the baby presenting in the OP position (Walmsley, 2000; Coates, 2002). Walmsley (2000) suggests that preparing the woman for a labour of indeterminate length and providing good midwifery support, may be the most effective midwifery intervention.

External version/internal rotation to OA is described by some authors (Davis, 1997; Coates, 2002). Coates suggests this practice could carry risks, and Gardberg and Tuppurainen (1994b) found that 87% rotate naturally to OA for birth. However, it takes time for a baby to rotate from OP to OA, labour is usually longer and progress can be slow. Medical augmentation is not necessarily indicated. The woman's general condition, her ability to cope and her wishes are all important factors here. Huge support, praise and words of encouragement are necessary to help the woman cope and keep a positive frame of mind.

- **Eat and drink** as desired to avoid dehydration, ketoacidosis and subsequent slow progress (Johnson *et al.*, 2000).
- **Keep the bladder empty** and ensure regular trips to the toilet.
- **Avoid ARM.** Some authors suggest that, if labour is slow, rupturing the membranes can be detrimental as it encourages sudden descent, which may possibly preclude the baby from rotating into a more favourable position and predispose the baby to a deep transverse arrest (Chadwick, 2002 citing El Hata, 1996).

Back pain/painful contractions

- **Heat** can be applied locally to the woman's lower back by the use of a hot water bottle or a microwavable heat pack (Simkin & Ancheta, 2005).

- **Firm, lower-back massage** or direct pressure centrally over the sacrum as directed by the woman can help ease discomfort.
- **Pelvic press** can bring relief as it alters the shape of the pelvis and may help the baby to shift its head and descend (see Fig. 8.7) (Simkin & Ancheta, 2005).
- **Abdominal lifting** may improve fetal alignment and relieve backache. The woman places her hands under her abdomen and lifts it up during a contraction while keeping her knees slightly bent and her pelvis tilted forward (Simkin & Ancheta, 2005).
- **An epidural** may bring welcome relief and help the woman continue with a difficult labour. It may however prolong OP labour and increase the risk of a difficult delivery (Fraser *et al.*, 2002).

Mobilisation and upright postures

Sutton (2000) suggests 'as a rule of thumb; when a woman's knees are lower than her hips she is allowed ample room in her pelvis for the baby to enter'. Women should draw benefits from adopting positions of comfort, being assisted to following their own instincts, inclinations and personal comfort.

- **Mobilising** encourages greater contractions, prevents dystocia and increases spontaneous births (Gupta *et al.*, 2000).
- **Swaying the hips** from side to side, stepping on and off a small stool or marching on the spot are advocated by some.
- **All fours/kneeling/forward leaning postures** usually bring the greatest relief from back pain and are commonly promoted by midwives. All fours reduces pain, improves women's feelings of control and comfort, and if tried specifically in OP labour improves rotation to OA and reduces instrumental delivery rate (Stremler *et al.*, 2005).
- **Lying on alternate sides** is useful for tired women or those with an epidural. Sutton (2000) recommends that if the baby is left occipitoposterior (LOP), the woman lies on her left side, and if the baby is right occipitoposterior, she lies on her right side. This, she suggests, facilitates rotation of the fetal trunk and occiput with the aid of gravity to pull into the correct position (see also Fig. 8.2). One Chinese study confirmed Sutton's side lying approach as statistically significant at converting more OP to OA, with improved birth outcomes (Wu *et al.*, 2001).
- **Avoid semi-recumbent or sitting back postures.** Conversely, some women adopt a 'flat on the back' legs abducted position. Providing the fetal heart is satisfactory, and this is what the woman wants to do, then this may well be the ideal position for the woman.

Face presentation

When the face presents the head is hyperflexed so the occiput is in contact with the fetal back and the mentum (chin) is the denominator. A face presentation can develop from an OP position during the second stage of labour (Chadwick, 2002). The majority of face presentations are in the mentoanterior and are usually unproblematic. Mentoposterior is uncommon and is rarely deliverable vaginally (Gaskin, 1990; American Academy of

Family Physicians (AAFP), 2004) because the fetal neck is shorter than the maternal sacrum, and therefore cannot stretch to the hollow of the sacrum (Chadwick, 2002).

Incidence and facts

- 0.1–0.2% of vaginal births (AAFP, 2004).
- >50% are diagnosed during the second stage of labour (Bhal *et al.*, 1998).
- Two-thirds of face presentations are in multiparous women (Bhal *et al.*, 1998) and are more prevalent in women of black ethnicity possibly due to pelvic shape (Shaffer *et al.*, 2006).
- Associated factors include prematurity (Shaffer *et al.*, 2006), short cord (Gaskin, 1990) and rarely cranial vault abnormalities such as anencephaly (Bhal *et al.*, 1998).
- Shaffer *et al.* (2006) found CS was less common in mentoanterior (only 14% CS rate) than mentoposterior presentation (85% CS rate). However, most authors suggest that mortality and morbidity are not increased in face presentation.

Characteristics of a face presentation

- The presenting part is usually high (Gaskin, 1990).
- Facial features can be felt. The mouth and two mallar prominences can be felt as a triangle. Care must be taken not to damage the baby's eyes on VE (Chadwick, 2002).
- First-stage cervical dilatation may be slower in a face presentation but second-stage progress is usually good (Gaskin, 1990).

Midwifery care

Spontaneous vaginal delivery usually occurs with relative ease (AAFP, 2004). Such births are uncommon and may attract an audience; it is the midwife's duty of care to protect the woman's privacy and to stop uninvited people from coming into the room. The parents should be prepared and reassured that their baby will have a bruised and swollen face at birth and that this will improve significantly in the hours and days following birth.

- Manipulation to convert the presentation to OA or the use of a fetal scalp electrode or vacuum (ventouse) extraction is contraindicated in face presentation (AAFP, 2004).
- IV oxytocin is usually avoided (AAFP, 2004).
- At birth be prepared: there could be a tight, entangled or short umbilical cord and although unlikely anencephaly is a possibility.

Brow presentation

The baby presenting by the brow has its head partially extended, with the widest diameter presenting in the mentovertical (see Fig. 8.10). A brow presentation is an *unstable presentation* and will usually convert to a face or vertex presentation prior to birth (AAFP, 2004). The wide diameter of a persistent brow can prove very difficult to birth but vaginal delivery is possible (Gaskin, 1990). AAFP (2004) suggests more guardedly that a brow is undeliverable under 'normal conditions' and requires a small baby or a roomy pelvis. If the head does not convert to a vertex presentation and becomes obstructed, a CS is required (AAFP, 2004).

Gaskin (1990) suggests that this position can be associated with the cord wrapped around the baby's neck several times. Other authors confirm this, e.g. Bhal *et al.* (1998) who also noted higher incidence of FHR abnormalities, meconium-stained liquor and lower Apgar scores in brow and face presentations.

Incidence

- 0.2% of vaginal births (AAFP, 2004).
- >50% are diagnosed or occur during the second stage (Bhal *et al.*, 1998).
- More common in primigravida.

Characteristics of a brow presentation

- Labour may be slower, more difficult and felt by the woman as a 'back pain' labour (Gaskin, 1990).
- The VE can be difficult to interpret due to oedema and the unfamiliarity of the presenting features (AAFP, 2004).
- Anterior fontanelle and frontal sutures can be felt on one side of the pelvis, orbital ridges on another; the eyes and root of the nose may also be felt (Chadwick, 2002).
- The presenting part is usually very high and the presenting diameter feels unusually large (Gaskin, 1990).

Midwifery care

Gaskin (1990) suggests that the pelvic press (see Fig. 8.7) during the second stage of labour, as well as adopting an upright or squatting posture, will improve the chances of a spontaneous birth.

A CS may become necessary if progress is poor in the second stage.

Transverse lie (shoulder presentation)

Shoulder presentation is undeliverable vaginally and occurs when the baby lies transverse with the shoulder as the denominator (acromion process or dorsum).

External cephalic version (ECV) may be successful. Some doctors then attempt a controlled ARM. However, this is in itself is risky, particularly in early labour, as this risks cord prolapse if the woman is lying flat with an unengaged presenting part.

Incidence and facts

- 0.3% deliveries (AAFP, 2004).
- Of those babies presenting as transverse near term, only 17% will remain in a transverse lie at the onset of labour (Gimovsky & Hennigan, 1995).
- Most shoulder presentations occur in multiparous women (Gimovsky & Hennigan, 1995).

- Predisposing factors include multiple pregnancy, polyhydramnios, placenta praevia, macerated fetus, weak abdominal muscles and uterine abnormality (Coates, 1999).

Characteristics of a transverse lie/shoulder presentation

- The uterine shape appears wide, fundal height is lower than would be expected and the head is palpable on the one side – buttocks on the other and usually nothing in the pelvis (AAFP, 2004). The lie is occasionally oblique but it usually becomes transverse during labour (Coates, 1999).
- VE will firstly detect a high presenting part, and sometimes the distinctive pattern of the ribs may be felt or the shoulder, arm or hand.

Midwifery care

The midwife who detects a shoulder presentation during labour should summon help. If at home, or birthing centre, immediate transfer to hospital is indicated. In an emergency it may be necessary for the midwife to attempt external and, if necessary, internal cephalic version (AAFP, 2004). A VE should only be performed if placenta praevia has been excluded (Coates, 1999).

External cephalic version. Attempting to turn the baby externally by ECV, even if labour has started, can often be successful. AAFP (2004) notes that a second twin who presents as transverse at full dilatation can be turned easily, as the uterus is initially relaxed and accommodating following delivery of the first twin.

Internal cephalic version is often considered hazardous for the baby, and CS is often the preferred option. However, in an emergency (such as a second twin presenting transverse and the cervix fully dilated) internal version may be undertaken (AAFP, 2004). This requires the clinician to perform a VE, grasp the baby's feet and pull the baby into a breech position.

Indications for immediate CS:

- Cord prolapse
- Rupture of membranes
- Unsuccessful ECV
- Long labour (uterine rupture is a serious complication)

Summary

Slow progress in labour

- Preoccupation with strict time definitions in labour are not evidence based
- There is no clinical evidence to support any general benefits from a shorter labour
- Prevention of dystocia is better than cure

Interventions that increase uterine contractibility

- Continuous presence and support from the midwife
- Mobilisation/position changes

- Comforting touch
- Nipple stimulation
- Hydrotherapy/warm bath/water tub
- ARM
- Oxytocin

Malpositions and malpresentations

- **Malpositions** e.g. OP tend to result in longer labours, backache and increased intervention.
- There is often no quick fix for a malposition but upright postures, positive reassurance and huge support will often get a woman through a difficult labour
- **Malpresentations** are non-vertex presentations sometimes associated with prematurity, short/entangled cord or fetal malformations.
- Labour can be slow, often with back pain and a higher prevalence of fetal distress.
- Certain malpresentations e.g. brow or mentoposterior face may not be deliverable vaginally.
- A shoulder presentation constitutes an emergency situation.

Recommended reading

Lemay, G. (2000) Pushing for first time Moms. *Midwifery Today* **55**. Available at: http://www. midwiferytoday.com/articles/pushing.asp (accessed March 2008).

Royal College of Midwives (RCM) (2005) *Campaign for Normal Birth*. Royal College of Midwives. Available at: http://www.rcmnormalbirth.org.uk (accessed March 2008).

Simkin, P. & Ancheta, R. (2005) *The Labor Progress Handbook*. Blackwell Publishing, Oxford.

Walsh, D. (2000) Evidence-based care. Part 3: assessing women's progress in labour. *British Journal of Midwifery* **8** (7), 449–57.

References

Albers, L. (2007) The evidence for physiologic management of the active phase of the first stage of labor. *Journal of Midwifery & Women's Health* **52** (3), 207–15 .

All Wales Clinical Pathway for Normal Labour (2004) Available at: http://www.wales. nhs.uk/sites3/home.cfm?orgid=327 (accessed November 2007).

American Academy of Family Physicians (AAFP) (2004) *Advanced Life Support in Obstetrics*, 5th edn. Course Syllabus Manual. American Academy of Family Physicians, Leawood, Kansas.

Association of Radical Midwives (ARM) (2000) Nettalk: incredible shrinking cervices. *Midwifery Matters* **87**, 28–30.

Bergstrom, L., Seedily, J. & Schulman-Hull, L. (1997) 'I gotta push. Please let me push!' Social interactions during the change from first stage to second stage of labour. *Birth* **24** (3), 173–80.

Bhal, P.S., Davies, N.J. & Chung, T. (1998) A population study of face and brow presentation. *Journal of Obstetrics and Gynaecology* **18** (3), 231–5.

Borrell, U. & Fenstrom, I. (1957) The movements of the sacroiliac joints and their importance to changes in the pelvic dimensions during parturition. *Acta Obstetrica et Gynaecologica Scandinavica* **36**, 42–57.

Buchmann, E.J. (2000) Monitoring progress in labor. In *A Guide to Effective Care in Pregnancy and Childbirth*, 3rd edn (Enkin, M., Keirse, M.J.N.C., Neilson, J., *et al.*, eds), pp. 281–8. Oxford University Press, Oxford.

Burvill, S. (2002) Midwifery diagnosis of labour onset. *British Journal of Midwifery* **10** (10), 600–605.

Carisson, I.M., Hallberg, L.R. & Odberg Petterson, K. (2007) Swedish women' experiences of seeking care and being admitted during the latent phase of labour: a grounded theory study. *Midwifery* (online 27 June 2007).

Chadwick, J. (2002) Malpositions and presentations. In *Emergencies Around Childbirth* (Boyle, M., ed.), pp. 76–9. Radcliffe Medical Press, Abingdon.

Cheung, Y., Hopkins, I. & Caughey, A. (2004) How long is too long: does a prolonged second stage of labour in nulliparous women affect maternal and neonatal morbidity? *American Journal of Obstetrics and Gynaecology* **191**, 933–8.

Cluett, E. (2000) The onset of labour. 2: implications for practice. *The Practising Midwife* **3** (7), 16–19.

Cluett, E.R., Nikodem, V.C., McCandlish, R.E. & Burns, E.E. (2002) Immersion in water in pregnancy, labour and birth. *The Cochrane Database of Systematic Reviews*.

Cluett, E.R., Pickering, R.M. & Getliffe, K. (2004) Randomised controlled trial of labouring in water compared with standard of augmentation for management of dystocia in first stage of labour. *BMJ* **328** (7435), 314. Available at: http://www.bmj.com (accessed November 2007).

Coates, T. (1999) Malpositions of the occiput and malpresentations. In *Myles Textbook for Midwives*, 13th edn (Bennett, R. & Brown, L.K., eds), pp. 507–37. Churchill Livingstone, Edinburgh.

Coates, T. (2002) Malpositions and malpresentations of the occiput: current research and practice tips. *MIDIRS Midwifery Digest* **12** (2), 152–4.

Crowther, C., Enkin, M., Keirse, M.J.N.C. & Brown, I. (2000) Monitoring progress in labor. In *A Guide to Effective Care in Pregnancy and Childbirth*, 3rd edn (Enkin, M., Keirse, M.J.N.C., Neilson, J., *et al.*, eds), pp. 281–8. Oxford University Press, Oxford.

Davis, E. (1997) *Hearts and Hands: A Midwife's Guide to Pregnancy and Birth*, 3rd edn. Celestial Arts, Berkeley, California.

Dickersin, K. (2000) Control of pain in labor. In *A Guide to Effective Care in Pregnancy and Childbirth*, 3rd edn (Enkin, M., Keirse, M.J.N.C., Neilson, J., *et al.*, eds), pp. 313–31. Oxford University Press, Oxford.

Downe, S., Gerrett, D. & Renfrew, M.J. (2004) A prospective randomised trial on the effect of position in the passive second stage of labour on birth outcome in nulliparous women using epidural analgesia. *Midwifery* **20** (2), 157–68.

Enkin, M., Keirse, M.J.N.C., Crowther, C., Duley, L., Hodnett, E. & Hofmeyr, J. (2000) *A Guide to Effective Care in Pregnancy and Childbirth*, 3rd edn. Oxford University Press, Oxford.

Fraser, W.D., Cayer, M., Soeder, B.M., Turcot, L. & Marcoux, S. (2002) Risk factors for difficult delivery in nulliparas with epidural analgesia in second stage of labor. *American Journal of Obstetrics and Gynecology* **99** (3), 409–18.

Fraser, W.D., Marcoux, S., Klauss, I., Douglas, J., Goulet, C. & Boulvain, M. (2000) Multicenter, randomized, controlled trial of delayed pushing for nulliparous women in the second stage of labor with continuous epidural analgesia. The PEOPLE (Pushing Early or Pushing Late with Epidural) Study Group. *American Journal of Obstetrics and Gynecology* **182** (5), 1165–72.

Gardberg, M. & Tuppurainen, M. (1994a) Anterior placental location predisposes for occiput posterior presentation near term. *Acta Obstetrica et Gynaecologica Scandinavica* **73**, 151–2.

Gardberg, M., Laakkonen, E. & Salevaara, M. (1998) Intrapartum sonography and persistent occiput posterior presentation: a study of 408 deliveries. *Obstetrics and Gynecology* **91**, 746–9.

Gardberg, M. & Tuppurainen, M. (1994b) Persistent occiput posterior presentation – a clinical problem. *Acta Obstetrica et Gynaecologica Scandinavica* **73**, 45–7.

Gaskin, I.M. (1990) *Spiritual Midwifery*. The Book Publishing Co., Summertown, Tennessee.

Gee, H. (2000) Abnormal patterns of labour and prolonged labour. In *Best Practice in Labor Ward Management* (Kean, L.H., Baker, P.H. & Edelstone, D.I., eds), pp. 65–79. WB Saunders, Edinburgh.

Gimovsky, M. & Hennigan, C. (1995) Abnormal fetal presentations. *Current Thinking in Obstetrics and Gynaecology* **7** (6), 482–5.

Gupta, J.K. & Hofmeyer, G.J. (2004) Positions for women during the second stage of Labour. *The Cochrane Database of Systems Review*, Issue 1.

Gupta, J.K., Hofmeyr, G.J. & Smyth, R. (2000) Position in the second stage of labour for women without epidural anaesthesia. *Cochrane Database of Systematic Reviews*, Issue 1, Art. No. CD002006.

Hodnett, E.D., Gates, S., Hofmeyr, G.J. & Sakala, C. (2003) Continuous support for women during childbirth. *The Cochrane Database of Systems Review*, Issue 3.

Johnson, C., Keirse, M.J.N.C., Enkin, M. & Chalmers, I. (2000) Hospital practices – nutrition and hydration in labor. In *A Guide to Effective Care in Pregnancy and Childbirth*, 3rd edn (Enkin, M., Keirse, M.J.N.C., Neilson, J., Crowther, C., Duley L., Hodnett, E. & Hofmeyr, J., eds), pp. 255–66. Oxford University Press, Oxford.

Kavanagh, J., Kelly, A. & Thomas, J. (2005) Breast stimulation for cervical ripening and induction of labour. *Cochrane Database of Systematic Reviews*, Issue 3.

Keirse, M.J.N.C. (2000) Prolonged labour. In *A Guide to Effective Care in Pregnancy and Childbirth*, 3rd edn (Enkin, M., Keirse, M.J.N.C., Neilson, J., Crowther, C., Duley L., Hodnett, E. & Hofmeyr, J., eds), pp. 332–40. Oxford University Press, Oxford.

Keirse, M.J.N.C., Enkin, M.W. & Lumley, J. (2000) Social and professional support in childbirth. In *A Guide to Effective Care in Pregnancy and Childbirth*, 3rd edn (Enkin, M., Keirse, M.J.N.C., Neilson, J., Crowther, C., Duley L., Hodnett, E. & Hofmeyr, J., eds), pp. 247–54. Oxford University Press, Oxford.

King, M., Bewes, P.C., Carns, J. & Thornton, J. (1999) Online edition. *Primary Surgery: Non-Trauma*, Vol. 1. Oxford Medical Publications. Available at: www.meb.uni-bonn.de/dtc/primsurg (accessed March 2008).

Lauzon, L. & Hodnett, E. (2002) Labour assessment programs to delay admission to labour wards. *The Cochrane Database of Systems Reviews*, Issue 4.

Lemay, G. (2000) Pushing for first time Moms. *Midwifery Today* **55**. Available at: http://www.midwiferytoday.com/articles/pushing.asp (accessed November 2007).

McNiven, P., Williams, J., Hodnett, E., Kaufman, K. & Hannah, M. (1998) An early labor assessment program: a randomised controlled trial. *Birth* **25**, 5–10.

Myles, T.D. & Santolaya, J. (2003) Maternal and neonatal outcomes in patients with a prolonged second stage of Labor. *Obstetrics & Gynecology* **102**, 52–8. Available free from www.greenjournal.org/cgi/content/full/102/1/52

Nasir, A., Korejo, R. & Noorani, K.J. (2007) Childbirth in the squatting position. *Journal of the Pakistan Medical Association* **57** (1), 19–22.

National Institute for Health and Clinical Excellence (NICE) (2007) *Clinical Guideline 55: Intrapartum Care.* National Institute for Health and Clinical Excellence, London.

Neilson, J.P., Lavender, T., Quenby, S. & Wray, S. (2003) Obstructed labour: reducing maternal death and disability during pregnancy. Oxford University Press. *British Medical Bulletin* **67**, 191–204. Available at: http://bmb.oxfordjournals.org/cgi/content/abstract/67/1/191 (accessed March 2008).

NHS Maternity Statistics England 2005/6 (2007) Information Center for Health and Social Care. Available at: www.ic.nhs.uk/webfiles/publications/maternity0506/ NHSMaternityStats England200506.pdf (accessed March 2008).

Ockenden, J. (2001) The hormonal dance of labour. *The Practising Midwife* **4** (6), 16–17.

Odent, M. (1998) Use of water during labour – updated recommendations. *MIDIRS Midwifery Digest* **8** (1), 68–9.

Parry, D. (2003) Reversing the Chi. *Midwifery Matters.* Issue 98, Autumn. Available at: www.radmid.demon.co.uk/Chi.htm (accessed November 2007).

Regan, M. (1998) Active management of labour: the Irish way of birth. *AIMS Journal* **10**, 2.

Roberts, C.L., Algert, C.S., Cameron, C.A. & Tovaldsen, S. (2005) A meta-analysis of upright positions in the second stage to reduce instrumental deliveries in women with epidural analgesia. *Acta Obstetricia et Gynecologica Scandinavica* **84** (8), 794–8.

Roberts, C.L., Torvaldsen, S., Cameron, C.A. & Olive, E. (2004) Delayed versus early pushing in women with epidural analgesia: a systematic review and met-analysis. *British Journal of Obstetrics and Gynaecology* **111** (12), 1333–40.

Royal College of Midwives (RCM) (2005) Campaign for normal birth. Royal College of Midwives. Available at: http://www.rcmnormalbirth.org.uk (accessed November 2007).

Russell, J.G.B. (1982) The rationale of primitive delivery positions. *British Journal of Obstetrics and Gynaecology* **89**, 712–5.

Sallam, H.N., Abdel-Dayem, A., Sakr, R.A., Sallam, A. & Loutfy, I. (1999) Mathematical relationships between uterine contractions, cervical dilatation, descent and rotation in spontaneous vertex deliveries. *International Journal of Gynaecology and Obstetrics* **64**, 135–9.

Shaffer, B.L., Cheng, Y.W., Vargas, J.E., Laros, R.K., Jr, & Caughey, AB. (2006) Face presentation: predictors and delivery route. *American Journal of Obstetrics and Gynecology* **194** (5), e10–12.

Simkin, P. & Ancheta, R. (2005) *The Labor Progress Handbook*, p. 91. Blackwell Publishing, Oxford.

Sleep, J., Roberts, J. & Chalmers, I. (2000) The second stage of labor. In *A Guide to Effective Care in Pregnancy and Childbirth* (Enkin, M., Keirse, M.J.N.C., Neilson, J., Crowther, C., Duley L., Hodnett, E. & Hofmeyr, J., eds), pp. 289–99. Oxford University Press, Oxford.

Smyth, R.M.D., Allderd, S.K. & Markham, C., (2007) Amniotomy for shortening spontaneous labour. *Cochrane Database of Systematic Reviews*, Issue 4, Art No. CDO06167. DOI: 10.1002/14651858.CD006167.pub2.

Stremler, R., Hodnett, E., Petryshen, P., Stevens, B., Weston, J. & Willan A (2005) Randomised controlled trial of hands knees positioning for occipitoposterior position in labour. *Birth* **32** (4), 243–51.

Stuart, C. (2000) Invasive actions in labour. Where have all the 'old tricks' gone? *The Practising Midwife* **3** (8), 30–33.

Sutton, J. (2000) Occipito posterior positioning and some ideas about how to change it. *The Practising Midwife* **3** (6), 20–22.

Thornton, J.G. & Lilford, R.J. (1994) Active management of labour: current knowledge and research issues. *BMJ* **309**, 366–9.

Walmsley, K. (2000) Managing the OP labour. *MIDIRS Midwifery Digest* **10** (1), 61–2.

Walsh, D. (2000a) Evidence-based care. Part 3: assessing women's progress in labour. *British Journal of Midwifery* **8** (7), 449–57.

Walsh, D. (2000b) Evidence-based care. Part 6: limits on pushing and time in the second stage. *British Journal of Midwifery* **8** (10), 604–608.

WHO (2003) *Managing Complications in Pregnancy and Childbirth: A Guide for Midwives and Doctors*, pp. 61–2. Publication Dept of Reproductive Health & Research. World Health Organisation, Geneva.

Wu, X., Fan, L. & Wang, Q. (2001) Correction of occipito-posterior by maternal postures during the process of labor. Article in Chinese: Zhonghua Fu Chan Ke Za Zhi **36** (8), 468–9. Abstract available in English: www.ncbi.nlm.nih.gov/sites/entrez (accessed November 2007).

9 Assisted birth: ventouse and forceps

Cathy Charles

Introduction

With good labour support, most women will experience a spontaneous vaginal delivery. Some women, however, for a variety of reasons, will not. For those women the options are either an instrumental delivery or a caesarean section (CS). An instrumental delivery carried out competently, in a supportive atmosphere, can still be a triumph for a woman, and a source of celebration. However, there is an increased risk of morbidity and reduced maternal satisfaction with assisted delivery, particularly with a forceps delivery. Clinical competence is of course vital, but emotional support through assisted delivery is equally important.

Incidence and facts

- 11% of births in England were instrumental deliveries in 2005–2006 (National Health NHS, 2007).
- Ventouse is much preferred to forceps: it was used for only 17% of instrumental deliveries in 1989 but has risen in popularity to 63% in 2002–2003 (NHS, 2007).
- There are significant morbidity risks following instrumental delivery, but CS in second stage also carries high morbidity risk and has implications for subsequent births (Royal College of Obstetricians and Gynaecologists (RCOG), 2005).

Avoiding an instrumental delivery

The incidence of a forceps or ventouse delivery varies widely in different settings. Good labour practice is likely to reduce the incidence of instrumental delivery and will include the following:

- Continuous support in labour especially by a non-staff carer (Hodnett *et al.*, 2004).
- Appropriate food and drink in labour (Johnson *et al.*, 2000).
- Encouraging mobilisation/upright position (Gupta *et al.*, 2004).
- Avoidance of epidural (Hodnett *et al.*, 2004), although if instrumental delivery is performed, this is the most effective analgesia.
- Avoidance of continuous cardiotocograph (CTG) monitoring for low-risk women (National Institute for Health and Clinical Excellence (NICE), 2007).
- Avoidance of arbitrary second-stage time limits if progress is being made (Sleep *et al.*, 2000). There is some evidence that maternal morbidity increases after 3 hours in the second stage (Cheung *et al.*, 2004), but there is known maternal morbidity with instrumental delivery (Sleep *et al.*, 2000; Dupuis *et al.*, 2004).
- Use of intravenous (IV) oxytocin in a slow second stage, particularly for primigravidae with poor contractions (NICE, 2007).
- Delaying pushing for women with epidurals for 1–2 hours reduces mid-cavity or rotational deliveries (Roberts *et al.*, 2004), and allowing up to 4 hours for second stage (NICE, 2007) and non-supine position increases the spontaneous delivery rate (Downe *et al.*, 2004). There is no evidence that discontinuing an epidural for the pushing stage speeds delivery and it increases pain (Torvaldsen *et al.*, 2004).

Indications for an instrumental delivery

- Failure to progress/maternal exhaustion in second stage. NICE (2007) guidance suggests that primigravida should be delivered within 3 hours of start of active phase, and a parous woman within 2 hours.
- Fetal distress (non-reassuring CTG, possibly in conjunction with fetal blood sample pH <7.20).
- Elective shortening of the second stage for fetal or maternal benefit (there are few absolute indications as obstetricians differ in their views on this subject).

Choice of instrument

Johanson and Menon (2002a) conclude that ventouse is the method of choice for assisted delivery because:

- A ventouse delivery is less likely to end in a CS, possibly due to the higher effectiveness of ventouse in, for example, the deflexed occipitoposterior position. However, some attempted ventouse deliveries will end in a forceps delivery.
- Forceps are more likely to succeed than ventouse, mainly because it is possible to pull harder.
- A ventouse birth causes fewer serious maternal injuries and fewer neonatal facial and cranial injuries. There are more reports of cephalhaematoma and retinal haemorrhage in ventouse births, but these do not appear to have long-term complications.

- No difference in 1-min Apgar score with a trend towards a lower 5-min Apgar score in ventouse births.
- A ventouse delivery may be difficult if there is marked caput, as suction may be hard to maintain. Following repeated fetal blood sampling attempts, ventouse may be inadvisable due to the risk of scalp trauma.
- Ventouse requires maternal effort. Some clinicians prefer forceps, or resort to them when ventouse fails.

NICE (2007) concludes that the decision should be made according to the clinical situation and the experience of the practitioner.

Care of a woman undergoing instrumental delivery

A calm and sensitive manner towards a woman undergoing instrumental delivery is crucial. Explanations need to be clear and informative, with plenty of support given to the woman and her birth partner(s), for whom such an experience may be a frightening ordeal.

Communication

Debating options at this stage of labour is not always easy. Some women may be feeling very much in control. Others may be exhausted, in extreme pain, and not receptive to discussion. If there are concerns about the condition of the baby, staff may feel under pressure to press on with an assisted delivery and limit debate. It is easy to talk glibly of 'informed choice'; many distressed women in labour will consent to almost anything that offers them a way out.

Birth partners can feel extremely stressed and tired; they may display anger or aggression, as they try to cope with their own and the woman's distress. It may be the partner, rather than the woman, who asks questions at this point. Conversely they may block discussion, saying 'Just get on with it, she's been through enough'.

Ensure that a woman is prepared for the possibility of CS, should the instrumental attempt fail.

Reducing fear

'As fluorescent lights go on, the room fills with people, she hears the metallic clang of lithotomy poles, the sound of tearing paper as instrument packs are opened, the loud voices of people issuing instructions. She may feel disorientated, as the bed is pumped higher, she is tilted back, moved down the bed, legs uncomfortably suspended. As well as these sounds and sensations, she senses the anxiety levels of her attendants (there is something very dramatic about to happen here, so no matter how much pain I'm in now, it is about to get a whole lot worse)' (Charles, 2002).

One obvious fact about instrumental deliveries is that they are frightening for women. Preferably one staff member should focus solely on the emotional needs of the woman and her birth partner(s). If another midwife is not available, this might be a maternity auxiliary/health care assistant.

Resist the urge to put all the lights on: a sudden flood of fluorescent light is frightening, increases the atmosphere of drama and may make a woman feel naked and vulnerable. Perineal illumination and 'spot' areas of lighting, where necessary, are quite sufficient.

The two most painful moments for the mother, apart from the birth itself, are the forceps blades/ventouse cup insertion and subsequent checking of the instrument's position. Ensure that someone is there to prepare and support her through these painful procedures.

Analgesia

NICE (2007) recommends that instrumental birth should have tested effective analgesia. This is the woman's decision, guided by professional advice. Some women would rather get the birth over with quickly, rather than wait for further analgesia. Theoretically, ventouse delivery pain is not significantly greater than from spontaneous birth, since the cup, unlike forceps, takes up no space alongside the head. Pain mainly results from initial cup insertion, followed by the usual delivery sensations. However, fear may increase pain perception.

- Epidural analgesia may be advisable for a forceps delivery. Ensure that it is adequately 'topped up' prior to delivery. Some doctors may instead administer a pudendal block.
- Some women may prefer to use entonox instead of, or in addition to, other methods of analgesia. Ensure that sufficient entonox has been inhaled prior to starting the procedure.
- Perineal lignocaine infiltration prior to ventouse cup insertion may help; there may also be a placebo effect from having given 'something' prior to the procedure.
- It is helpful to explain to a woman undergoing ventouse delivery that her urge to push is important, as this birth will be a collaboration.

Use of IV oxytocin

If the contractions are weak, then oxytocin augmentation may considered. NICE (2007) cautions against oxytocin for the second stage, but does not give any rationale for this. It will be an individual clinical decision and local guidelines may apply. Oxytocin for other stages of labour is normally started low and increased gradually; but if used for instrumental delivery a fairly high dose of oxytocin is usually started immediately. This prevents time being wasted in gradually increasing the dose, and since the delivery is now imminent, any fetal effects are likely to be transitory.

Positioning

- Following explanations and consent, the woman's legs should be gently and symmetrically lifted and supported in an adducted hip position. Lithotomy is not essential although some women may be comfortable in this position, particularly if staff experiment with pole height and adjust the position of the woman's buttocks relative to the poles.
- It is quite possible to carry out an instrumental delivery with two helpers supporting the heels (Charles, 2002).

- For ventouse, other positions such as left lateral or squatting have been suggested (Johanson, 2001). Most professionals will prefer to apply the cup with the woman in a semi-recumbent position. Once applied, there is no reason why a woman should not take up a lateral or squatting position. Squatting is known to increase the pelvic outlet diameter. Having said this, many professionals are more comfortable working with the method they are accustomed to and may resist alternative suggestions.
- Think aortocaval occlusion. Often this is forgotten during instrumental delivery. Create a small lateral tilt from a wedge or pillow.

Bladder care

Most women produce little urine in the second stage and/or have difficulty micturating. Catheterisation was once routine prior to instrumental delivery. Vacca (1997) however states: 'A catheter need only be passed if the woman is unable to void or if the bladder is visibly or palpably distended'. In the absence of substantial research, professionals should use clinical judgement or adhere to local protocol. An indwelling catheter should be removed or the balloon deflated before delivery (RCOG, 2005).

Episiotomy

This should not be a routine intervention performed with every instrumental delivery (Vacca, 1997; American Academy of Family Physicians (AAFP), 2004) or done simply to prevent a tear. An episiotomy is usually only indicated for severe fetal distress (Sleep *et al.*, 2000; Hartmann *et al.*, 2005), although as forceps take up space alongside the head, there may be an increased indication during a forceps delivery for access to apply forceps. A mediolateral rather than midline episiotomy appears to reduce third- and fourth-degree tears following forceps deliveries (Riskin-Mashiah *et al.*, 2002; Viswanathan *et al.*, 2005).

If indicated it should only be performed when the perineum has been stretched thin by the descending head. Clinical judgement should be exercised, taking into account the flexibility of the perineum. Early episiotomy increases maternal morbidity, blood loss and haematoma formation, extension to the anal sphincter or rectum, and postpartum pain (Sleep *et al.*, 2000).

Consent for instrumental delivery should not imply that consent is given for episiotomy without further discussion.

Assisting at an instrumental delivery

Mutual staff support

Instrumental deliveries are stressful for everyone. Staff are often intimidated by the 'medicalised' atmosphere, but should try to avoid appearing rushed. Usually there is reasonable time to prepare. Even if the intervention is for fetal distress, remember that if this were a CS the time from problem diagnosis to delivery would be longer.

The doctor or midwife delivering the baby may appear calm but will be under pressure. Rudeness and roughness towards the woman, however, should not be tolerated. Positive attitudes and efficiency in opening packs, preparing equipment and communicating information will help ensure a safe birth and give the mother confidence in her helpers.

Interestingly, when asked who delivered their baby, 11% of women delivered by forceps and 40% by ventouse reported that both the doctor and the midwife delivered the baby: surely an example of teamwork (Redshaw *et al.*, 2007).

Equipment preparation

To an extent, this will depend on local practice:

- The vulva is cleansed and, usually, draped.
- Relevant sterile instrument packs are opened, and the delivering professional assisted, as requested.
- Incidence of shoulder dystocia and postpartum haemorrhage increases with instrumental delivery. Anticipate this and be prepared.
- For a ventouse birth, an assistant may need to attach the suction tubing to the machine and control the pressure. Leaks are usually due to poor tubing attachment or the release pedal having been left depressed following a previous delivery. Soft cups are more likely to fail than metal cups but are less likely to cause scalp injury (Johanson & Menon, 2002b).
- There are single-use complete hand-held 'Kiwi' ventouse systems available which do not require a separate vacuum machine and can be operated by one person. Their size may make them appear less intimidating to the woman; however, there appears to be a higher failure rate compared to silastic and metal cups (Attilakos *et al.*, 2005).

Instrumental procedure

Once packs are opened, the clinician normally performs a forceps delivery without further direct help.

For a ventouse delivery using a suction machine, the delivering professional gives instructions. Normally pressure starts at 0.2 kg/cm^2 and then increases to 0.8 kg/cm^2 in one step. There is no evidence that slowly increased pressure is of any benefit (Vacca, 1997).

The head should descend with each pull. The procedure should be abandoned if there is no evidence of progressive descent with each pull or if delivery is not imminent after three pulls by an experienced clinician (RCOG, 2005). AAFP (2004) suggests the procedure should be abandoned following three ventouse cup detachments or if there is no progress for three consecutive pulls. Experienced midwives and doctors often recognise when a head will not deliver after just one pull, and will abandon the attempt immediately. CS is then normally indicated.

Advocacy/accountability

Whilst the delivering professional is responsible for their own practice, midwives continue to have a duty of care towards their client and are still accountable for their practice. If a midwife feels that further analgesia is required, or that the delivering professional is having difficulties, they must speak out, acting as an advocate for the client. This is not an easy position to be in.

Post-procedure care

- A midwife should record any aspects of the birth, for example, start of procedure and fetal heart auscultation to ensure an optimal written record of events.
- Once the baby is born, if all is well, events should follow just as if the woman had delivered unaided; skin-to-skin contact and early breastfeeding should be encouraged in the normal way. Parents should be aware that the baby's head may appear marked or moulded, but that this should disappear within hours.
- Diclofenac 100 mg given rectally (PR) following delivery/suturing is the drug of choice (Dodd *et al.*, 2004). There is no evidence that prophylactic antibiotics reduce post-instrumental delivery infections (Liabsuetrakul *et al.*, 2004).

Midwife instrumental delivery

Some midwives now carry out instrumental deliveries, following formal training and assessment, under specified criteria. Many midwives may be uncomfortable with the idea of midwife ventouse/forceps practitioners, feeling that it is a way of saving money and may erode the concept of a midwife's involvement in normal birth (Davies & Iredale, 2006). Others suggest that a woman may get better care from a midwife (Charles, 1999; Alexander *et al.*, 2002). Midwife ventouse practitioners have been successfully practising low-risk ventouse deliveries for over 10 years in the UK with good maternal and neonatal outcomes (Awala *et al.*, 2006).

Do midwife practitioners bring anything special to instrumental birth?

Here are some speculations on how a midwife instrumental practitioner may improve a woman's experience:

- Midwives have a philosophy of promoting normal birth, which means practitioners may not always rush to perform instrumental birth when asked, but make other practical, tested suggestions to facilitate a spontaneous birth.
- Midwives may be more aware of the importance of a relaxed birth environment, e.g. calm atmosphere, low lighting and minimal noise.
- They may use their awareness of a woman's fear and loss of control to make the experience less stressful.
- They may be more likely to consider slow delivery of the head and selective (rather than routine) episiotomy, thus reducing perineal trauma.
- They may be more receptive than other clinicians to ideas such as ventouse in lateral or squatting positions.

Of course, none of the above will be true if the wrong kind of midwives become instrumental practitioners. Midwives are not mini-obstetricians. They should be recruited for training by midwives and selected for attitude as much as clinical skills. We do not need midwives who are by their nature interventionist or 'drama queens (or kings)'.

Criteria for a midwife instrumental delivery

The criteria may vary according to local protocol.

- Fully dilated cervix.
- Occipitoanterior (OA) position (but not necessarily direct OA), well flexed.
- No asynclitism.
- Head no longer palpable (i.e. fully engaged) abdominally.
- Head below the level of the ischial spines.
- No/minimal caput or moulding.
- Good contractions.
- Verbal maternal consent obtained.
- If fetal distress occurs in a stand-alone midwife-only unit and a ventouse/forceps midwife is called in, it is sensible to call an ambulance as well. If the circumstances are inappropriate for instrumental delivery, or the attempt fails immediate transfer is necessary.

Preparation

History

Review the antenatal and labour history, note parity; length of labour and fetal position during labour. Always beware of a slow 7–10 cm cervical dilatation interval. Slow second-stage progress, particularly in multigravidae, may indicate disproportion or malpresentation.

Assessment

An instrumental delivery should not be attempted unless the criteria given above are met. It is important to remain focused and analytical throughout, and not be swayed by the enthusiasm of other staff, or parents, to achieve delivery. It is particularly hard in stand-alone midwife-only units to decline an instrumental delivery because this means transfer to another unit. However, transfer following failed instrumental delivery, with the fetal compromise that may result, is worse.

An abdominal and a vaginal examination should be performed, with consent. Do not rely on the opinion of others, even if several staff reassure you that 'It's definitely OA ...'. Check for yourself.

Monitor the contractions; if poor strength and/or frequency, then IV oxytocin may be advisable.

Communication

Prior to physical examination, the midwife should introduce him/herself to the woman and partner. Attitude at this time is extremely important, and gaining a woman's confidence is crucial. In cases of presumed fetal distress, this discussion may have to be brief, but most people understand and under such circumstances will want actions rather than words.

It is important to acknowledge the woman's hard work so far. Explain the situation and confirm the woman's (and her partner's) understanding. Try to present options; for example, 'If I confirm that the baby is in the right position for ventouse delivery, then we can either do it now, or see how your pushing goes over the next 15 minutes ... ', giving the woman the choice. Some women, however, may be too distressed to make such choices, or may perceive this as indecision. Midwifery judgement should be used, as with all women in labour, to decide the level of information given.

Remember that most post-birth emotional trauma appears to be associated with poor information giving and perceived loss of control (Green, 1990). Never underestimate a woman's capacity to make choices, however distraught she may appear.

Please read the preceding section entitled 'Care of a woman undergoing instrumental delivery' for general comments on instrumental delivery, including *analgesia*, *positioning* and *bladder care*. The following section describes aspects specific to midwife ventouse or forceps delivery.

Midwifery ventouse delivery

Midwife ventouse deliveries are normally performed using silc, or hand-held plastic, cups. Check the suction by applying the cup to your hand. (See also the section entitled 'Assisting at an instrumental delivery' above.)

- Cup insertion is often painful, but with increasing experience, it can be performed smoothly and gently. Entonox may help.
- Immediately following a contraction (warn the woman what is about to happen), insert the squeezed, externally lubricated cup by gently slipping two fingers of the other hand into the introitus, retracting the perineum and sliding the cup into the space created.
- The cup is manoeuvred into the optimal position. Vacca (1997) describes the flexion point which, in a well-flexed OA position, is typically around 3 cm from the posterior fontanelle. This is the point of the vertex where the cup should be applied (see Fig. 9.1).
- If the cup is correctly applied so that it lies over the flexion point, with the sagittal suture running centrally down, then traction will result in the smallest diameter of the fetal head (the suboccipitobregmatic and biparietal) being drawn through the birth canal (see also p. 122, Chapter 8, for diameters of the fetal skull). This minimises traction, thus increasing the likelihood of a successful birth and reducing trauma to mother and baby. In practice maternal tissue often inhibits cup positioning, so then the cup is simply placed as near as possible to the posterior fontanelle.

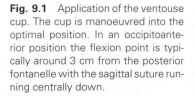 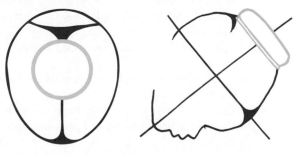

Fig. 9.1 Application of the ventouse cup. The cup is manoeuvred into the optimal position. In an occipitoanterior position the flexion point is typically around 3 cm from the posterior fontanelle with the sagittal suture running centrally down.

- The woman is often distressed following cup application, so reassure and congratulate her that the cup is now in place, and she has got through an unpleasant moment.
- Apply 0.2 kg/cm^2 pressure, and then check the position and ensure that no maternal tissue is trapped in the cup. The process of feeling round the cup is another painful moment, especially anteriorly where space is tight, so warn the woman and proceed gently. If satisfactory, increase to 0.8 kg/cm^2 in one step.
- Await the next contraction. Encourage the woman to get her breath back and focus on the coming need to push. Sometimes it helps to smile, get eye contact, and encourage an atmosphere of controlled excitement, 'It really won't be long now . . . '. This may recharge the atmosphere, giving the woman more energy. Beware though: a 'high adrenaline' environment may scare some women.
- With the contraction, encourage the woman to push and apply steady traction perpendicular to the cup. As the head comes under the symphysis and extends, the cup will rise from horizontal to almost vertical.
- As already discussed, it is not essential to perform an episiotomy for a ventouse delivery (Vacca, 1997; AAFP, 2004); clinical judgement should be exercised and consent obtained, as with any birth.
- Overexcited staff may be tempted to deliver the head quickly. Unless there is good reason to hurry, resist this urge. Remember how slowly a primigravid woman normally delivers; fast perineal stretching will cause increased pain and tissue trauma. Once the head is guided to the perineum, the woman's expulsive urge may do most of the rest of the work. Some midwives will hardly pull at all, as the perineum slowly distends. Such births can be true collaborations between midwife and mother. There are reports of women who believe they had only minimal help (Charles, 1999) and deny they have truly had an instrumental delivery.

Midwife forceps delivery

- Ensure that the woman has adequate analgesia: forceps are usually more painful than ventouse.
- Check the blades lock before using them (they may not be a matching pair).
- Lubricate the blades well.
- Immediately after a contraction (warn the woman what you are about to do) insert the left blade with the shank initially vertical, protecting the left vaginal wall with two fingers of the right hand.
- The blade should slide fairly easily in to lie parallel to the fetal head axis. If not, abandon the procedure.
- The second blade should be similarly inserted, and the blades locked. Depressing the handles slightly can help lock the blades.
- Check for correct application (see Fig. 9.2):
  ○ The posterior fontanelle should be midway between the shanks and 1 cm above them.
  ○ The sagittal suture should be in the midline (try to palpate the lambdoidal sutures to confirm this).
- With a contraction encourage the woman to push: perform traction by pulling on the blades with one hand and pressing down on the shanks.

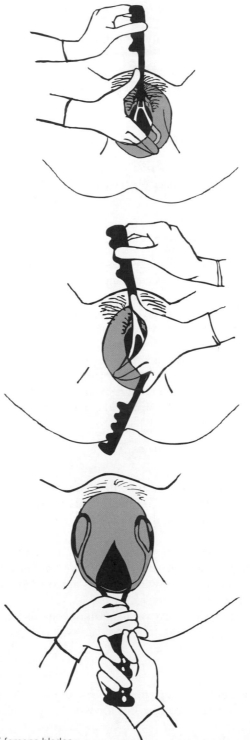

Fig. 9.2 Application of forceps blades.

- The traction axis will change as the head descends along the J-shape of the birth canal.
- Consider episiotomy, especially for primigravidae, as forceps take up space alongside the head.
- As the head crowns traction becomes vertical. Remove the blades before the head is completely out to decrease perineal tension. Think about slow delivery of the head (see ventouse delivery above).

Advocacy/accountability

See also the earlier section 'Care of a woman undergoing instrumental delivery'. Remember: you are a midwife, not an obstetrician. Do not be drawn into making decisions outside your remit.

Post-birth discussion and care

Most ventouse/forceps midwives discuss the birth with the parents afterwards, congratulating the mother on her courage and endurance, and giving an opportunity for questions and explanations. Sometimes this is practicable only immediately following the birth. It is helpful to inform a woman that any subsequent birth is unlikely to require another assisted delivery. Some women and partners may find discussion supportive and reassuring. Others may be too shocked by events to be ready to 'revisit' them or too preoccupied by their new baby to care. Sensitivity should be shown in this, as in all, birth matters.

Postnatal exercises have been shown to improve urinary continence at 3 months postpartum in women who had instrumental deliveries and/or babies >4000 g (Ciarelli & Cockburn, 2002).

Records

Indications and assessment for instrumental delivery, details of procedure and outcome should be recorded. Instrumental midwives may wish to keep a logbook of deliveries (see the Appendix 1) and periodically review their practice, e.g. numbers of failed deliveries.

It is helpful to log any instrumental deliveries that, after assessment, the midwife decides not to perform, and the subsequent outcome. These 'declined deliveries' may indicate a ventouse/forceps midwife's skill as much as the successful births achieved (see the Appendix 2).

Logbooks may form part of an overall audit of ventouse/forceps midwife deliveries in some locations.

Summary

- Ventouse is the mode of choice for most instrumental deliveries.
- Instrumental deliveries are stressful for women, partners and staff. Sensitivity is vital.
- Consent should always be sought before any intervention.

- Warn a woman of the possibility of CS if instrumental delivery fails.
- Midwives are accountable for their own practice, even when another professional has taken over the delivery. Although difficult, voice any concerns about suboptimal care.
- Midwife ventouse/forceps deliveries may be carried out under specified criteria.
  - The midwife should ensure adequate analgesia.
  - Avoid aortocaval occlusion.
  - Routine catheterisation/episiotomy is unsupported by evidence.
  - Prepare a woman for the pain of ventouse cup/forceps insertion.
  - Encourage slow head delivery to minimise perineal trauma.
  - Anticipate shoulder dystocia and postpartum haemorrhage.
  - Midwife ventouse/forceps practitioners are not obstetricians: refer abnormalities.
    Give post-delivery analgesia (e.g. diclofenac 100 mg PR).
    A post-birth discussion may be helpful for a woman and her partner.
    Encourage postnatal exercises.

References

Alexander, J., Anderson, T. & Cunningham, S. (2002) An evaluation by focus group and survey of a course for midwifery ventouse practitioners. *Midwifery* **18**, 165–72.

American Academy of Family Physicians (AAFP) (2004) *Advanced Life Support in Obstetrics (ALSO). Course Syllabus Manual*, 4th edn. American Academy of Family Physicians, Leawood, Kansas.

Attilakos, G., Sibanda, T., Winter, C., Johnson, N. & Draycott, T. (2005) A randomised controlled trial of a new handheld vacuum extraction device. *International Journal of Obstetrics and Gynecology* **112** (11), 1510–15.

Awala, A., Nethra, S., Walker, D. & Charles, C. (2006) The midwife ventouse: a safe practice. *MIDIRS* **16** (2), 181–3.

Charles, C. (1999) How it feels to be a midwife ventouse practitioner. *British Journal of Midwifery* **7** (6), 380–82.

Charles, C. (2002) Practising as a midwife ventouse practitioner in an isolated midwife-led unit setting. *MIDIRS Midwifery Digest* **12** (1), 75–7.

Cheung, Y., Hopkins, I. & Caughey, A. (2004) How long is too long: does a prolonged second stage of labour in nulliparous women affect maternal and neonatal morbidity? *American Journal of Obstetrics and Gynaecology* **191**, 933–8.

Ciarelli, P. & Cockburn, J. (2002) Promoting urinary continence in women after delivery: randomised controlled trial. *British Medical Journal* **324** (378), 1241–7.

Davies, J. & Iredale, R. (2006) An exploration of midwives' perceptions about their role. *MIDIRS Midwifery Digest* **16** (4), 455–60.

Dupuis, O., Madelenat, P. & Rudigoz, R. (2004) Faecal and urinary incontinence and delivery: risk factors and prevention. *Gynaecology, Obstetrics and Fertility* **32**, 540–48.

Dodd, J., Hedayati, H., Pearce, E., Hotham, N. & Crowther, C.A. (2004) Rectal analgesia for the relief of perineal pain after childbirth: a randomised controlled trial of diclofenac suppositories. *An International Journal of Obstetrics and Gynaecology* **111** (10), 1059–64.

Green, J.M. (1990) Expectations, experiences and psychological outcomes of childbirth: a prospective study of 825 women. *Birth* **17** (1), 15–23.

Gupta, J., Hofmeyr, G. & Smyth R. (2004) Position in the second stage of labour for women without epidural anaesthesia. *The Cochrane Database of Systematic Reviews*, Issue 1.

Hartmann, K., Viswanathan, M., Palmieri, R., Gartlehner, G., Thorp, J. & Lohr, K. (2005) Outcomes of routine episiotomy: a systematic review. *JAMA* **293**, 2141–8.

Hodnett, E., Gates, S., Hofmeyr, G.J. & Sakala, C. (2004) Continuous support for women during childbirth. *The Cochrane Database of Systematic Reviews*, Issue 3.

Johanson, R. (2001) The baby lifeline B.I.R.T.H. series. Interactive educational video series. Baby Lifeline Trading, Coventry. Reviewed by V. Tinsley. *MIDIRS* **11** (2), 284–5.

Johanson, R.B. & Menon, V.J. (2002a) Vacuum extraction vs forceps for assisted vaginal delivery (Cochrane Review). *The Cochrane Library*, Issue 4. Update Software, Oxford.

Johanson, R.B. & Menon, V. (2002b) Soft versus rigid vacuum extractor cups for assisted vaginal delivery. *Cochrane Database of Systematic Reviews*, Issue 2, Art. No. CD000446. DOI: 10.1002/14651858.CD000446.

Johnson, C., Keirse, M.J.N.C., Enkin, M. & Chalmers, I. (2000) Hospital practices – nutrition and hydration in labor. In *A Guide to Effective Care in Pregnancy and Childbirth*, 3rd edn (Enkin, M., Keirse, M.J.N.C. & Neilson, J., eds), pp. 255–66. Oxford University Press, Oxford.

Liabsuetrakul, T., Choobun, T., Peeyananjarassri, K. & Islam, M. (2004) Antibiotic prophylaxis for operative vaginal delivery. *Cochrane Database of Systematic Reviews*, Issue 3, Art. No. CD004455. DOI: 10.1002/14651858.CD004455.pub2.

National Health Service (NHS) (2007) *Maternity Statistics 2005–6. The Information Centre.* Available at: www.ic.nhs.uk (accessed March 2008).

National Institute for Health and Clinical Excellence (NICE) (2007) *Clinical Guideline 55: Intrapartum Care.* National Institute for Health and Clinical Excellence, London.

Redshaw, M., Rowe, R., Hockley, C. & Brocklehurst, P. (2007) *Recorded Delivery: The Findings from a National Survey of Women's Experience of Maternity Care.* NPEU. Available at: www.npeu.org.uk (accessed March 2008).

Riskin-Mashiah, S., O'Brien Smith, E. & Wilkins, I. (2002) Risk factors for perineal tear: can we do better? *American Journal of Perinatology* **19**, 225–34; reprinted in September 2007 *MIDIRS* **384**.

Roberts, C.L., Torvaldsen, S., Cameron, C.A. & Olive, E. (2004) Delayed versus early pushing in women with epidural analgesia: a systematic review and met-analysis. *British Journal of Obstetrics and Gynaecology* **111** (12), 1333–40.

Royal College of Obstetricians and Gynaecologists (RCOG) (2005) *Operative Vaginal Delivery: Clinical Guideline 26.* Available at: www.rcog.org.uk (accessed October 2007).

Sleep, J., Roberts, J. & Chalmers, I. (2000) The second stage of labor. In *A Guide to Effective Care in Pregnancy and Childbirth*, 3rd edn (Enkin, M., Keirse, M.J.N.C., Neilson, J., *et al.*, eds), pp. 289–99. Oxford University Press, Oxford.

Torvaldsen, S., Roberts, C.L., Bell, J.C. & Raynes-Greenow, C.H. (2004) Discontinuation of epidural in labour for reducing the adverse delivery outcomes associated with epidural analgesia. *Cochrane Database of Systematic Reviews*, Issue 4, Art. No. CD004457. DOI: 10.1002/14651858.CD004457.pub2.

Vacca, A. (1997) *Handbook of Vacuum Extraction in Obstetric Practice.* Vacca Research, Albion, Queensland, Australia.

Viswanathan, M., Hartmann, K., Palmieri, R., Lux, L., Swinson, T., Lohr, K., Gartlehner, G. & Thorp, J. (2005) The use of episiotomy in obstetrical care: a systematic review. *Evidence Report/Technology Assessment* **112**, 1–8.

Appendix 1: Midwife ventouse practitioner log book record

Midwife ventouse practitioner log book record

Ventouse Practitioner name .... Unit ....
Case no .... Date................ Time of delivery ....
Client name.................................. Reg no .... Age.............
Address ....
Gestation .... Gravida/Para ....
Induction: Yes/No   Method...............
Augmentation: 1st stage .... 2nd stage ....
INDICATION FOR VENTOUSE ....
Abdo palpation .... Fifths palpable per abdo ....
Contractions ....
Vaginal examination: Dilatation.......... Station .... Caput .... Moulding ....

A

R ( ) L

P

Analgesia .... Catheterised pre-procedure: Yes/No
Type of ventouse (e.g. silc/Kiwi)..................... Number of pulls ....
Traction required: Easy/ Moderate/ Strong
Perineum: Intact/ 1st / 2nd / 3rd / 4th degree tear / episiotomy
COMMENTS ON DELIVERY:

EBL................   Baby: Male/female   Birth weight.............
Length of labour: 1st stage...............   Meconium at delivery? Yes/No
                     2nd stage   APGARS..........................
                     3rd stage   General condition of baby....................

Appendix 2: Decision to decline midwife ventouse delivery

It is recognised that midwife ventouse practitioner (MVP) skill may be determined not just by successful ventouse deliveries achieved, but also by declining to attempt ventouse extraction on unsuitable cases. MVPs should complete this form whenever asked to do a delivery which, following assessment, they decide not to perform.

An MVP may decide against a ventouse delivery for any reason. It is understood that decision making, particularly in an isolated community unit, is not always easy.

This form merely aims to monitor MVP decision making. It should in no way inhibit midwives from calling in an MVP for an opinion.

Please note: if an MVP *actually starts* a ventouse delivery, which is then abandoned, s/he should not complete this form, but fill in the existing MVP log book form, and complete a risk-management form, in the usual way.

Do not file this form in client's maternity notes. Please retain a copy for your ventouse practitioner log book.

MVP name:................................. **Maternity Unit:** ....
Date:................................
Client name: .... **Hospital no:** .... **Age:** ....
Address: .... **Gravida/Para:** .... **Gestation:** ....

History/reason for ventouse request:..

Abdo palpation:................................. **Contractions:**.................................
Cervical dilatation:................. **Station:**................. **Moulding:**............. **Caput:**.............
Position:..

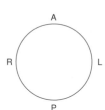

Reason for declining ventouse and action taken:

Outcome:

10 Caesarean section

Cathy Charles

Introduction

Some women readily choose caesarean section (CS); some are reluctantly persuaded to undergo CS, and some have CS thrust suddenly upon them with, realistically, little chance to make any informed choice.

CS can save the life of a mother and/or baby. The problem is that it is often performed unnecessarily. This largely lies in the domain of obstetric decision making, outside the power of the midwife. However, the midwife still has some degree of influence, in supporting a woman's right to choose, and on occasions in challenging the rationale behind the decision.

Incidence and facts

- The CS rate has risen from 9% in 1980 to 24% in England for 2005–2006 (National Institute for Health and Clinical Excellence (NICE), 2004; NHS, 2007) and is expected to continue rising.
- Stated reasons for CS are 22% fetal distress, 20% failure to progress, 11% breech. Over 50% are emergency CS (Thomas & Paranjothy, 2001).
- This rising CS rate has not improved neonatal outcomes and increases maternal morbidity and mortality risk (National Collaborating Centre for Women's and Children's Health (NCCWCH), 2004).
- Whilst there is no accepted optimal CS rate in the UK, the WHO (1985) has stated that a rate <10–15% confers no additional health benefits.
- A safe decision-to-decision interval for emergency CS for presumed fetal distress is not known; NICE (2004) recommend 30 min.

- Regional anaesthesia is recommended for CS. All recent UK maternal anaesthetic deaths have been under general anaesthetic (GA) (Confidential Enquiry into Maternal and Child Health (CEMACH), 2004).

Risks and benefits of CS

Benefits

The overwhelming reason for CS is obviously to prevent mortality and morbidity in mothers and babies. The WHO (1985) believes that a CS rate of around 10–15% reflects appropriate intervention.

- CS may be the only means of delivering a baby in truly obstructed labour. The alternative is fetal, and ultimately maternal, death.
- There may be a reduction in cerebral palsy. However, only around 10% cerebral palsy appears to be birth related, and CS appears to make no difference (NICE, 2004).
- CS may reduce some (but not all) urinary incontinence and uterovaginal prolapse. It makes no difference to faecal incontinence (NICE, 2004).
- Prevention of perineal pain (NICE, 2004) unless the woman has a CS following failed instrumental birth. Abdominal scar pain is of course unavoidable.
- Some women have a morbid fear of childbirth, which counselling may not dispel. CS may give them a sense of control and reduce fears.
- Some may perceive that elective CS offers them a sanitised birth experience: witness the 'celebrity cult' of elective CS. These women are labelled in the popular press as the 'too posh to push' brigade.
- A small number of women with pelvic problems, e.g. congenital hip dislocation, may benefit from CS, but most can be helped to have a normal birth.
- Convenience (if elective CS): the parents know the date of their baby's birth. This may be relevant for parents who wish to avoid a baby being born on a dead sibling's birthday.
- CS can assist in the resuscitation of a mother who has experienced cardiac arrest (see Chapter 17).
- Perceived protection of clinicians from litigation: believing they will be judged to have done their best if a CS is performed, even if the outcome is no better, or even worse (see Chapter 22).

Risks

CS carries risks to mothers and babies particularly in the second stage of labour (see the Appendix for NICE CS algorithm). CS is more likely than vaginal birth to result in (NICE, 2004):

- Abdominal pain. Some unlucky women who have a failed instrumental delivery may also have perineal trauma to cope with.
- Bladder and ureter injury, hysterectomy, but no difference in genital tract injury.
- Increased length of hospital stay, readmission and return to theatre.
- Implications for further pregnancies are placenta praevia uterine rupture and antepartum stillbirth. Women are less likely to have more children following CS than after vaginal birth.

- Thromboembolic disease, intensive therapy unit admission.
- Maternal death. CEMACH (2004) states: 'Further research is needed to estimate more robustly what, if any, is the increased risk of maternal deaths associated with CS, particularly those undertaken without a clinical indication.'
- Neonatal morbidity: babies may have adverse respiratory outcomes particularly after elective CS, and low blood sugar and poor temperature regulation (NICE, 2004; Kolas *et al.*, 2006). Babies of mothers undergoing elective CS are twice as likely to be admitted to neonatal intensive care unit than following vaginal delivery (Kolas *et al.*, 2006).
- It has been speculated that elective CS in particular results in lower maternal hormone levels (oxytocin, endorphins, catecholamines and prolactin) which can affect postnatal mood, self-esteem and breastfeeding (Buckley, 2005).
- Post-traumatic stress disorder can result from any birth (Kitzinger & Kitzinger, 2007), but there are many accounts of post-traumatic stress disorder following emergency CS (BTA website). This 'anecdotal' evidence may be dismissed by some clinicians. It may not be so much the CS itself, but the sense of loss of control and poor support that causes psychological trauma.
- CS (including postnatal stay) costs double that of instrumental delivery and 2–3 times more than spontaneous vaginal birth (Henderson *et al.*, 2001). For every 800 births conducted as CS instead of normal birth without complications, the NHS spends an extra £1 million, costing the NHS £2 billion a year.

Stemming the flow

There is a wide-ranging debate about the reasons for the current steep rise in the CS rate (Odent, 2004; NHS Institute, 2007). Numerous birth initiatives aim to stem this epidemic including the RCM campaign for normal birth (Royal College of Midwives (RCM), 2007) and the National Service Framework (DoH, 2004). The NHS Institute has published *Pathways to success – a self-improvement toolkit* (NHS Institute for Innovation and Improvement, 2007) aimed at enabling trusts to assess their performance and make practice changes to reduce CS rates and offer better care to those women who have CS.

CS may be reduced by the following:

- Home birth (NICE, 2004).
- Supporting women who choose vaginal birth after caesarean section (VBAC) (NICE, 2004): giving women who have had previous CS unbiased, factual information improves uptake of vaginal birth (see Chapter 11).
- Offering continuous support in labour (Hodnett *et al.*, 2004).
- Offering induction of labour after 41 weeks gestation (NICE, 2001) (see Chapter 18).
- Use of a partogram with a 4-hour action line (NICE, 2004) but this is controversial (for more information on partograms, see Chapter 8, p. 109). Inappropriately early diagnosis of 'slow progress' may lead to intervention, which may in fact increase CS.
- Avoidance of continuous cardiotocograph (CTG) monitoring for low-risk women (NICE, 2007). Some would even question its value in high-risk women, since Cochrane review can find no evidence that it improves outcomes (Alfirevic *et al.*, 2006).

- Performing fetal blood sampling (FBS) prior to CS for abnormal CTG (NICE, 2004). However, Cochrane review found no evidence of higher CS rates when FBS was not available (Alfirevic *et al.*, 2006).
- Involving consultants in the decision regarding CS (NICE, 2004).
- Performing high quality instrumental deliveries by experienced clinicians.
- Addressing doctors' lack of awareness of their influence on women's decision making. Studies show the obstetrician's experience, gender, workplace practices and whether working privately or NHS affects decision making regarding mode of delivery (Thomas & Paranjothy, 2001).

This chapter does not aim to address the debate about the appropriateness of CS in detail; hopefully much of the rest of this book, in promoting good midwifery care, will do this. Instead, this chapter aims to help the midwife assist a woman who is, for whatever reason, undergoing CS.

Indications for elective CS

NICE (2004) lists the following:

- **A term singleton breech (if external cephalic version is contraindicated or has failed)** – however see Chapter 13 for further discussion.
- **A twin pregnancy with first twin breech** although NICE can offer no research to support this, but instead say it is 'common practice' (see Chapter 14 for further discussion).
- **HIV** as it reduces the risk of mother–baby transmission.
- **Primary genital herpes in third trimester** as this decreases neonatal infection.
- **Grades 3 and 4 placenta praevia.**

NICE (2004) states that CS should not be routinely offered to women with the following:

- **Twin pregnancy when the first twin is cephalic at term.**
- **Preterm birth.** There is no evidence that CS improves the already high morbidity for this group.
- **Small for gestational age babies** for the above reason.
- **Hepatitis B or hepatitis C.**
- **A recurrence of genital herpes.** As long as this is not a primary outbreak, there is no evidence of high risk of transmission.
- **Maternal request.** Further discussion recommended; offer counselling if fear of childbirth is identified.

Maternal request

The issue of elective CS for maternal request creates hot debate, with one lobby stating that a woman has the right to choose the birth of her choice while others feel that no one should have the right to choose unnecessary major abdominal surgery which absorbs scarce resources (Dimond, 1999; Dodwell, 2002).

NICE (2004) states that maternal request alone is not an indication for CS and that further clarification should be sought and counselling offered.

The experience of CS

CS may come as a blessed relief to a woman after an arduous pregnancy and/or labour. Conversely, she may feel deeply disappointed that she has been unable to give birth naturally. If the CS is an emergency she may be frightened and apprehensive as her birth plans fall apart and events move out of her control. Choice can disappear as the quiet birthing room is invaded suddenly by noise, light and unknown people. She and her partner may even believe that she or their baby might die. Good care and support are critical in helping the woman achieve a positive experience whatever the circumstances and greet her baby with joy.

The principles of care are broadly the same whether a woman is undergoing elective or emergency CS, although the urgency of emergency CS will increase stress levels for everyone. Even if an elective CS, the woman's decision may not have been easy, and she is likely to have the same fears as anyone else undergoing CS.

Elective CS birth plan

It is interesting to speculate why so few women undergoing elective CS write a birth plan. Perhaps they do not feel they have any control over this highly medicalised procedure. Although it is not common practice, it is perfectly possible for a woman to write down her preferences (Lowdon & Chippington Derrick, 2007). The process of enquiring/imagining what may happen may help her and her partner prepare for the event. A written birth plan may also be harder for staff to disregard. Responding to individual preferences may take some staff out of their comfort zone and remind them that there is a person at the centre of the proceedings, not a series of formulaic actions to be performed.

'Women's preferences for the birth, such as music playing in theatre, lowering the screen to see the baby born, or silence so that the mother's voice is the first the baby hears, should be accommodated where possible' (NICE, 2004).

Midwifery care for CS

Consent. Whilst some would question the quality and objectivity of information given to many women considering CS, consent for elective CS is comparatively straightforward. An emergency situation however may be quite different. A competent woman has the right to refuse CS even if she or her baby's health would clearly benefit (DoH, 2001). The midwife may have to support a woman's right to refuse in the face of strong opposition, occasionally even that of her partner.

Written consent is advisable, but in an emergency not essential, as long as the mother has verbally consented (or is not well enough to consent). Informed consent is *not* achieved when a distressed, frightened woman is forced to sign a piece of paper she can barely focus on, while a junior SHO gabbles out the risks of a CS which the woman may believe is now essential to save her baby's life. Such 'consent' will have little validity in a court of law under questioning by any competent lawyer.

Question the obstetrician politely and calmly if you feel there is not a good indication for CS. If there is an abnormal fetal heart rate pattern in the first stage, FBS should be offered first, if technically possible and not contraindicated (NICE, 2004), although disappointingly FBS does not appear to affect CS rates (Alfirevic *et al.*, 2006) or neonatal outcomes (NICE, 2007). Junior/middle grade doctors should not be making the final decision. A consultant obstetrician should be involved in any decision to offer a CS which will depend on evidence of clinical benefit to mother and baby (DoH, 2004). (In practice this 'consultation' can consist of a quick phone call to a consultant saying 'I'm doing a CS, Are you happy?') Be sensitive to the difficult position the obstetrician may be in: pressure from parents (and sometimes midwives!) to perform a CS, along with fears of an adverse outcome, criticism and litigation, can make their job very hard.

Give emotional support. If CS is elective, or occurs for slow labour progress, women usually have time to prepare emotionally. The woman may feel relieved that things are finally drawing to an end and/or distressed that she has been unable to have a vaginal birth. All women need support, but an emergency CS for 'fetal compromise' can be particularly frightening. Hold the woman's hand, give her eye contact and show her warmth: let her know that her baby will be here soon, that she is doing her very best in difficult circumstances, and that the birth will be a triumph no matter what. Birth partners can be tired and emotional too – don't forget to support them. Partners may appear angry. Sometimes they say 'I knew this was going to happen'; following vaginal birth they may forget these transient negative thoughts, but when emergency CS occurs, they feel the bad experience was almost foreseeable.

Accept your own feelings. Midwives may feel disappointment in realising their care has not been enough to achieve a vaginal birth. You are no longer the lead caregiver and may feel disempowered and frustrated, perhaps especially so if you do not agree with the decision for CS. Do not let this affect your behaviour towards the woman: it is not her fault, and she needs your support more than ever.

Physical preparation

- **Full blood count result.** It is sensible to have this prior to any birth, but particularly CS, as 4–8% women lose >1000 ml at CS (NICE, 2004).
- **Site intravenous cannula.** A preload of crystalloid/colloid is recommended if CS under regional anaesthesia (NICE, 2004).
- **Give antacids** or similar drugs pre-CS to reduce gastric volume and acidity (NICE, 2004).
- A **catheter** is normally sited for a regional block due to potential bladder dysfunction (NICE, 2004), and possibly to ensure a full bladder does not obstruct surgery/risk bladder damage, although the routine use of catheters for CS has been questioned (Ghoreishi, 2003). 4% women develop a urinary tract infection following CS with an indwelling Foley catheter despite antibiotic prophylaxis (Horowitz *et al.*, 2004). If there is time, ask the woman if she would prefer to have the catheter sited in theatre or in her room first.
- **Shave.** A lower segment CS will often be at or below the pubic hair line, so a shave is normally performed. Again this can be done in theatre or the woman's room. An electric shaver with disposable head is probably the most comfortable option. Disposable single-use razors are uncomfortable if used dry; soap and water or shaving foam is considerate.

In theatre

Anaesthesia: The Royal College of Anaesthetists recommends that CS should usually be performed under regional anaesthesia (e.g. spinal/epidural). Thomas and Paranjothy (2001) found 77% emergency CS and 91% elective CS are performed under regional anaesthesia in the UK. If the mother is having a GA, her birth partner may not be allowed in the theatre. It is not clear why this is often the case, and this archaic practice is being challenged in more progressive hospitals where staff recognise that it should be up to the couple to decide what is best for them and their baby. Whether the partner is present or absent for the birth, he may wish to cuddle the baby at the earliest opportunity and perhaps offer skin-to-skin contact (SSC) until the mother is awake.

Environment. Do not be intimidated by the number of other staff in theatre and avoid picking up on anyone else's negativity. Sometimes when the team is stressed, individuals may appear irritable, withdrawn or cold. Do not let this become infectious. Keep a relaxed and warm manner towards the woman, even if yours is the only smiling face in the room. She may like to have music playing, a running commentary, or silence so her voice is the first her baby hears. She may want the lights dimmed briefly for the moment of birth and/or photographs taken. These things are easier to plan and implement for an elective CS, but even in an emergency many choices can still be fulfilled. Blithely ignore any staff who cast their eyes to heaven at your strange requests: the mother is the centre of events and the staff are there for her, not the other way around.

Temperature. Make sure the theatre is warm. CS babies are more prone to hypothermia (NICE, 2004). Theatres are large rooms with a constant airflow and staff often notice that they are cold (Ellis, 2005). Put on the resuscitaire as soon as possible (its heater will also help warm the room), although hopefully it will not be needed, as SSC is advised, and a well baby will not need to be separated from its parents.

A screen may protect the mother and partner from seeing too much, but some parents wish to watch their baby being born. Always ask: never assume.

Scrubbing to assist. Some hospitals require midwives to scrub to assist the obstetrician, but others have theatre staff to do this. Midwives may have views on this, feeling they are there to be 'with women', not 'with obstetrician'; if scrubbing is necessary, try to ensure that there is someone free to be with the woman. Anaesthetists are, however, usually very good at connecting with woman and their partners. It is not so much the *quantity* of staff, but the *quality* of care that is important.

Prophylactic antibiotics are recommended after CS (NICE, 2004).

Cord blood analysis. Paired venous and arterial samples will be required following emergency CS (see Chapter 23).

Resuscitation. If fetal compromise is suspected, or following general anaesthesia, a practitioner trained in advanced newborn resuscitation should be present (NICE, 2004) (see Chapter 17).

Skin-to-skin contact. SSC can be achieved with the baby delivered immediately onto the mother's chest (see Chapter 1 for benefits). If the mother is feeling unwell or does not want this, partners may wish to offer initial SSC; babies given SSC with their fathers following CS cry less and appear calmer (Erlandsson *et al.*, 2007). There should be no rush to weigh and measure the baby – this special time is important. Erlandsson concludes:

'The father can facilitate the development of the infant's prefeeding behaviour in this important period of the newborn infant's life and should be regarded as the primary caregiver . . . during the separation of mother and baby.'

Postnatal care

Recovery room. Women should be observed on a one-to-one basis until they are stable, have regained airway control and can communicate (NICE, 2004). This should be done by trained theatre staff.

Breastfeeding can be started in the recovery room. CS mothers are less likely to start breastfeeding in early hours after birth, but once established they are just as likely to continue as other mothers (NICE, 2004). Delayed mother–baby contact can result in lower postnatal mood for up to 8 months (Rowe-Murray & Fisher, 2001).

Observations. Regular observations can identify any problems early. Check half-hourly for the first 2 hours then 'hourly thereafter' (NICE, 2004): usually around 2 hours if all is well. Local guidelines may apply. Obviously report any problems to an obstetrician.

- **Pulse, BP, respiratory rate**
- **Pain and sedation.** Ensure the woman is comfortable. Opioid analgesia can over-sedate some women.

Also:

- **Observe lochia and wound site.**
- **Check urine output.** Ensure the catheter is free draining and the tubing not kinked.

Analgesia. Women may vary greatly in their needs. Opioid drugs and non-steroidal anti-inflammatories (NSAIDs) (check for contraindications) give good pain relief following CS (NICE, 2004), with paracetamol for milder pain. NSAIDs reduce the need for opioids, so should be used as an adjunct to any analgesia (NICE, 2004).

Check analgesia has been prescribed and given. Advise the woman to ask for further analgesia early, as pain is easier to control before it has built up; regular analgesia is usually sensible for the first few days as pain can be debilitating for a new mother with a baby to care for.

If patient-controlled analgesia is used, check it is working properly: overdosage can be serious.

Beware of drugs written on *anaesthetic charts* but not transferred to prescription sheets: this may result in drug errors.

Thromboprophylaxis. Thromboembolism is the most common cause of direct maternal death; 80% of women who died had identifiable risk factors for pulmonary embolism (CEMACH, 2004). Thromboembolic stockings +/− low-molecular-weight heparin should be prescribed for post-CS women particularly if other risk factors are present, e.g. high body mass index (RCOG, 2004). Ensure she is wearing stockings and that any necessary thromboprophylaxis has been prescribed.

Eating and drinking can be resumed when the woman wishes if she is recovering well with no complications (NICE, 2004).

General support. Women will need lots of assistance particularly in the first few hours. Make sure that she is comfortable with plenty of supportive pillows and a drink and the call bell is accessible. Reassure her that she can ring at anytime for help with the baby. Tuck the baby in with her if she wishes, and is awake enough: ensure the baby is safe. Try to anticipate her needs as well as respond to them.

Postnatal discussion. Women who have emergency CS should be offered the opportunity afterwards to discuss the reasons for it and the implications for future pregnancies with a knowledgeable professional (NICE, 2004; Murphy *et al.*, 2005) (see Chapter 11). She may wish to tell her story endlessly at first, particularly if the CS was an emergency; give her space to do this. Referral to a support group may help.

Tell a woman that she has been very brave to undergo major abdominal surgery for the sake of her baby.

Summary

- The steep rise in CS has not improved maternal or neonatal health.
- Good midwifery care and avoiding unnecessary interventions reduces CS.
- Women requesting elective CS should have a full discussion of risks and benefits.
- Consider a birth plan for elective CS.
- Politely challenge a CS which you believe is unnecessary.
- Give maximum emotional support to the woman and birth partner.
- Ignore negativity: make the woman the centre of attention.
- Physical care:
  - ○ Site intravenous cannula; obtain FBC result
  - ○ Give antacids
  - ○ Insert catheter (usually) and shave
  - ○ Ensure warm theatre
  - ○ Check if she wants a screen in situ
  - ○ Prophylactic antibiotics are recommended
  - ○ Take cord bloods if emergency CS
  - ○ Call an advanced newborn clinician if fetal compromise suspected
- Try to enable SSC with mother: if not, suggest father.

Postnatally:

- Breastfeed in recovery room ASAP.
- Observe vital signs, lochia, wound and urine output.
- Ensure that analgesia and thromboprophylaxis prescribed, given and *recorded on drug chart* (not just anaesthetic sheet).
- She can eat and drink when she wishes.
- Give lots of support and help her get comfortable.
- Postnatal review for emergency CS is helpful.

Support groups for women following CS

Birth Trauma Association (BTA)   Website: www.birthtraumaassociation.org.uk
Caesarean birth and VBAC information   Website: www.caesarean.org.uk
National Childbirth Trust   Website: www.nct.org.uk

Further reading

Gallagher-Mundy, C. (2004) *Caesarean Recovery.* Carroll & Brown, London.

National Childbirth Trust (1999) *Caesarean Sections.* NCT, London.

NHS Institute for Innovation and Improvement website *Pathways to Success: A Self-Improvement Toolkit Guidelines to Reduce Cs.* Available at: www.institute.nhs.uk

RCOG (2007) *Green-top Guideline No. 45: Birth after Previous Caesarean Birth.* Available at: www.rcog.org.uk (accessed March 2008).

References

Alfirevic, Z., Devane, D. & Gyte, G. (2006) Continuous cardiotocography (CTG) as a form of electronic fetal monitoring (EFM) for fetal assessment in labour. *Cochrane Database of Systemic Reviews*, Issue 3.

Buckley, S., (2005) *Gentle Birth, Gentle Mothering.* One World Press, Brisbane, Queensland.

Confidential Enquiry into Maternal and Child Health (CEMACH) (2004) *Why Mothers Die 2000–2002. The Sixth Report of Confidential Enquiries into Maternal Deaths in the United Kingdom.* RCOG Press, London. Available at: www.cemach.org.uk (accessed March 2008).

Dimond, B. (1999) Is there a legal right to choose a caesarean? *British Journal of Midwifery* **7** (8), 515–8.

Dodwell, M. (2002) Should women have the right to a clinically unnecessary CS? *MIDIRS Midwifery Digest* **12** (2), 274–7.

Department of Health (DoH) (2001) *Good Practice in Consent Implementation Guide: Consent to Examination or Treatment.* DoH Publications, London.

Department of Health (DoH) (2004) *National Service Framework for Children, Young People and Maternity Services – Executive Summary* 40496. Available at: www.dh.go.uk (accessed November 2007).

Ellis, J. (2005) Neonatal hypothermia. *Journal of Neonatal Nursing* **11**, 76–82.

Erlandsson, K., Dsilna, A., Fagerberg, I. & Christensson, K. (2007) Skin-to-skin care with the father after caesarean birth and its effect on newborn crying and prefeeding behaviour. *Birth* **34** (2), 105–13.

Ghoreishi, J (2003) Indwelling urinary catheters in caesarean delivery. *International Journal of Gynaecology and Obstetrics* **83** (3), 267–70.

Henderson, J., McCandlish, R., Kumiega, L. & Petrou, S. (2001) Systematic review of economic aspects of alternative modes of delivery. *British Journal of Obstetrics and Gynaecology* **108**, 149–57.

Hodnett, E.D., Gates, S., Hofmeyr, G.J. & Sakala, C. (2004) Continuous support for women during childbirth (Cochrane Review). *The Cochrane Library*, Issue 1.

Horowitz, E., Yogev, Y. & Ben-Haroush, A. (2004) Urine culture after catheterisation. *International Journal of Gynaecology & Obstetrics* **85**, 276–8.

Kitzinger, C. & Kitzinger, S. (2007) Birth trauma: talking to women and the value of conversation analysis. *British Journal of Midwifery* **15** (5), 256–64.

Kolas, O., Saugstad, A., Dalveit, A., Nilsen, S. & Oian, P. (2006) Planned caesarean vs planned vaginal delivery at term: comparison of newborn infant outcomes. *American Journal of Obstetrics and Gynaecology* **195** (6), 1538–43.

Lowdon, D. & Chippington Derrick, D. (2007) *CS and VBAC Information.* Available at: www.caesarean.org.uk (accessed August 2007).

Murphy, D., Pope, C., Frost, J. & Liebling, R. (2005) Women's views on the impact of operative delivery in the second stage of labour: qualitative interview study. *BMJ* **327** (7427), 1132–5.

National Collaborating Centre for Women's and Children's Health (NCCWCH) (2004) *Caesarean Section: Clinical Guideline.* RCOG Press, London.

National Institute for Health and Clinical Excellence (NICE) (2001) *Clinical Guideline D – Induction of Labour.* National Institute for Health and Clinical Excellence, London. Available at: www.nice.org.uk (accessed March 2008).

National Institute for Health and Clinical Excellence (NICE) (2004) *Clinical Guideline 13 – Caesarean Section.* National Institute for Health and Clinical Excellence, London. Available at: www.nice.org.uk (accessed March 2008).

National Institute for Health and Clinical Excellence (NICE) (2007) *Clinical Guideline 55: Intrapartum Care.* National Institute for Health and Clinical Excellence, London.

NHS 2005/6 (2007) *Information Center for Health and Social Care.* NHS Maternity Statistics, England. Available at: www.ic.nhs.uk/webfiles/publications/maternity0506/NHSMaternityStatsEngland200506.pdf (accessed November 2007).

NHS Institute for Innovation and Improvement (2007) *Delivering Quality and Value. Pathways to Success Toolkit.* NHS Institute for Innovation and Improvement, London. Available at: www.institute.nhs.uk (accessed November 2007).

Odent, M. (2004) *The Caesarean.* Free Association Books, London.

Royal College of Midwives (RCM) (2007) *Campaign for Normal Birth.* Available at: www.rcmnormalbirth.org.uk (accessed November 2007).

RCOG (2004) Thromboprophylaxis during pregnancy, labour and after vaginal delivery. *RCOG Green Top Guidelines.* Available at: rcog.org.uk (accessed November 2007).

Rowe-Murray, H.J. & Fisher, J.R.W. (2001) Operative intervention in delivery is associated with compromised early mother-infant interaction. *BJOG International Journal of Obstetrics and Gynaecology* **108** (10), 1068–75.

Thomas, J. & Paranjothy, S. (2001) *National Sentinel Caesarean Section Audit Report.* RCOG Press, London.

World Health Organisation (WHO) (1985) Appropriate technology for birth. *Lancet* **2**, 436–7.

Appendix: NICE CS algorithm

Caesarean section

Pregnant women should be given evidence-based information on caesarean section (CS) – as 1 in 5 will have a CS – including indications, what the procedure involves, risks and benefits, and implications for future pregnancies.

Offer planned CS to women with:

✔ A term singleton breech (if external cephalic version is contraindicated or has failed)
✔ A twin pregnancy with breech first twin
✔ HIV
✔ Both HIV and hepatitis C
✔ Primary genital herpes in the third trimester
✔ Grade 3 and 4 placenta praevia

Do not routinely offer planned CS to women with:

✗ Twin pregnancy (first twin is cephalic at term)
✗ Preterm birth
✗ A 'small for gestational age' baby
✗ Hepatitis B virus
✗ Hepatitis C virus
✗ Recurrent genital herpes at term

Maternal request for CS

• Is not on its own an indication for CS
• Explore and discuss specific reasons
• Discuss benefits and risks of CS
• Offer counselling if fear of childbirth
• The clinician can decline a request for CS, but should offer referral for a second opinion

Planning place of birth

Inform healthy pregnant women with anticipated uncomplicated pregnancies that:
• Home birth reduces CS
• Birth in a 'midwifery-led unit' does not affect CS

Reducing CS rates

✔ Offer external cephalic version if breech at 36 weeks
✔ Facilitate continuous support during labour
✔ Offer induction of labour beyond 41 weeks
✔ Use a partogram with a 4-hour action line in labour
✔ Involve consultant obstetricians in CS decision
✔ Do fetal blood sampling before CS for abnormal cardiotograph in labour
✔ Support women who choose vaginal birth after caesarean section (VBAC)

No influence on likelihood of CS

• Walking in labour
• Non-supine position during the second stage of labour
• Immersion in water during labour
• Epidural analgesia during labour
• Active management of labour or early amniotomy to augment the progress of labour
• Raspberry leaves during labour

These measures may affect other outcomes that are outside the scope of this guideline

Summary of the effects of CS compared with vaginal birth for women and their babies

Increased with CS
- Abdominal pain
- Bladder injury
- Ureteric injury
- Need for further surgery
- Hysterectomy
- Intensive therapy/high dependency unit admission
- Thromboembolic disease
- Length of hospital stay
- Readmission to hospital
- Maternal death
- Antepartum stillbirth in future pregnancies
- Placenta praevia
- Uterine rupture
- Not having more children
- Neonatal respiratory morbidity

No difference after CS
- Haemorrhage
- Infection
- Genital tract injury
- Faecal incontinence
- Back pain
- Dyspareunia
- Postnatal depression
- Neonatal mortality (except breech)
- Intracranial haemorrhage
- Brachial plexus injuries
- Cerebral palsy

Reduced with CS
- Perineal pain
- Urinary incontinence
- Uterovaginal prolapse

This table shows the direction of the effects of CS on risk of complications, but not the size of the effects. The risks do not apply to all women in all circumstances. Appendix E of the NICE guideline has details of the absolute and relative risks.

Pregnancy and childbirth following CS

The decision about mode of birth should consider maternal preferences and priorities, general discussion of the overall risks and benefits of CS (specific risks and benefits uncertain), risk of uterine rupture and perinatal mortality and morbidity.

Women who want VBAC should be supported and:
• Be informed that uterine rupture is very rare but is increased with VBAC (about 1 per 10,000 repeat CS and 50 per 10,000 VBAC)
• Be informed that intrapartum infant death is rare (about 10 per 10,000 – the same as the risk for women in their first pregnancy), but increased compared with planned repeat CS (about 1 per 10,000)
• Be offered electronic fetal monitoring during labour
• Should labour in a unit where there is immediate access to CS and on-site blood transfusion
• If having induction of labour should be aware of the increased risk of uterine rupture (80 per 10,000 if non-prostaglandins are used, 240 per 10,000 if prostaglandins are used)
• Be informed that women with both previous CS and a previous vaginal birth are more likely to give birth vaginally

CS is the end point of a number of care pathways. This algorithm includes the common reasons for CS, but the list is not exhaustive. CS may be required for complex or rare conditions that are outside the scope of this guideline.

Making the decision for CS

✔ Communication and information should be provided in a form that is accessible
✔ Consent for CS should be requested after providing pregnant women with evidence-based information

✔ A competent pregnant woman is entitled to refuse the offer of treatment such as CS, even when the treatment would clearly benefit her or her baby's health

---

Timing of planned CS: CS should be carried out after 39 weeks' gestation to decrease the risk of respiratory morbidity.

Emergency CS: In cases of suspected or confirmed acute fetal compromise, delivery should be accomplished as soon as possible. The accepted standard is within 30 minutes.

Document the urgency of CS
1) Immediate threat to the life of the woman or fetus
2) Maternal or fetal compromise which is not immediately life-threatening
3) No maternal or fetal compromise but needs early delivery
4) Delivery timed to suit woman or staff

Procedural aspects of CS

Preoperative assessment

✔ Check haemoglobin
✔ Prescribe antibiotics (one dose of first-generation cephalosporin or ampicillin)
✔ Assess risk for thromboembolic disease (offer graduated stockings, hydration, early mobilisation and low molecular weight heparin)
✔ Site an indwelling bladder catheter

For healthy women with an uncomplicated pregnancy, don't offer:
✗ Grouping and saving of serum
✗ Cross-matching of blood
✗ Clotting screen
✗ Preoperative ultrasound to localise the placenta

Anaesthetic care

✔ Discuss post-CS analgesia options
✔ Offer antacids and H_2 receptor analogues
✔ Offer anti-emetics
✔ Offer regional anaesthesia
✔ Reduce risk of hypotension using:
– intravenous ephedrine or phenylephrine infusion

– volume preloading with crystalloid or colloid
– lateral tilt of 15°
✔ General anaesthesia for emergency CS should include preoxygenation and rapid sequence induction to reduce the risk of aspiration

Maternity units should have a drill for failed intubation

Surgical techniques (For pregnancies at term where there is a lower uterine segment. These techniques may need modification in situations such as repeat CS or placenta praevia.)

Do
✔ Wear double gloves for CS for women who are HIV-positive
✔ Use a transverse lower abdominal incision (Joel Cohen incision)
✔ Use blunt extension of the uterine incision
✔ Give oxytocin (5 IU) by slow intravenous injection
✔ Use controlled cord traction

for removal of the placenta
✔ Close the uterine incision with two suture layers
✔ Check umbilical artery pH if CS performed for fetal compromise
✔ Consider women's preferences for birth (such as music playing in theatre)
✔ Facilitate early skin-to-skin contact for mother and baby

Don't
✗ Close subcutaneous space (unless > 2 cm fat)
✗ Use superficial wound drains
✗ Use separate surgical knives for skin and deeper tissues
✗ Use forceps routinely to deliver baby's head
✗ Suture either the visceral or the parietal peritoneum
✗ Exteriorise the uterus
✗ Manually remove the placenta

The effects of different suture materials or methods of skin closure are uncertain

A practitioner skilled in the resuscitation of the newborn should be present at CS with a general anaesthetic or with presumed fetal compromise

Postoperative monitoring

✔ Recovery area – one-to-one observations until the woman has airway control and cardiorespiratory stability and can communicate
✔ In the ward – half-hourly observations (respiratory rate, heart rate, blood pressure, pain and sedation) for 2 hours, then hourly if stable

✔ Intrathecal opioids – hourly observation of respiratory rate, sedation and pain scores for 12 hours for diamorphine and 24 hours for morphine
✔ For epidural opioids and patient-controlled analgesia with opioids – hourly monitoring during the CS, plus 2 hours after discontinuation

Care of the woman and her baby after CS

✔ Provide additional support to help women to start breastfeeding as soon as possible
✔ Offer diamorphine (0.3–0.4 mg intrathecally) or epidural diamorphine (2.5–5 mg) to reduce the need for supplemental analgesia
✔ Offer non-steroidal anti-inflamatory analgesics to reduce the need for opioid analgesics
✔ Women who are feeling well and have no complications can eat or drink when they feel hungry or thirsty

✔ After regional anaesthesia remove catheter when woman is mobile (> 12 hours after top-up)
✔ Remove wound dressing after 24 hours; keep wound clean and dry
✔ Discuss the reasons for the CS and implications before discharge from hospital
✔ Offer earlier discharge (after 24 hours) to women who are recovering, are apyrexial and have no complications

Recovery following CS

• Offer postnatal care, plus specific post-CS care, and management of pregnancy complications
• Prescribe regular analgesia
• Monitor wound healing
• Inform women that they can resume activities (such as driving, exercise) when pain not distracting or restricting

Consider CS complications:
• Endometritis if excessive vaginal bleeding
• Thromboembolism if cough or swollen calf
• Urinary tract infection if urinary symptoms
• Urinary tract trauma (fistula) if leaking urine

This algorithm should, where necessary, be interpreted with reference to the full guideline.

Reproduced with kind permission from the National Institute of Clinical Excellence.

11 Vaginal birth after caesarean section

Vicky Chapman

Introduction

'An evaluation of differences between maternity units that had low CS and those that had higher rates revealed an important attitudinal factor was a belief and pride in a low CSR and culture of birth as a normal physiological process' (Royal College of Obstetricians and Gynaecologists (RCOG), 2001).

Women who have had a previous caesarean section (CS) may decide to try for a vaginal birth in subsequent pregnancies. This is commonly referred to as *vaginal birth after caesarean* (VBAC). The National Caesarean Section Audit, 2001, recommended 'A trial of labour should be considered in women who have had a previous CS' (RCOG, 2001).

Women choose VBAC because they are influenced by the shorter recovery time after birth, want the experience of a natural birth or fear another CS (Emmett *et al.*, 2006). However, fear of repeating past negative labour experiences and the unpredictability of the outcome is a daunting prospect for these women (Lowdon & Chippington Derrick, 2007).

Incidence

- The caesarean section rate (CSR) was 23.5% in England in 2005–2006 (NHS Maternity Statistics England, 2007).
- 14% of these caesareans are women undergoing repeat elective CS.
- The VBAC success rate is 72–76% (RCOG, 2007).
- Successful VBAC is more common following one previous vaginal birth (success rate 87–90%), or if previous CS was for breech.
- VBAC is marginally less successful if previous CS was for perceived cephalopelvic disproportion, oxytocin had been used (National Institute for Health and Clinical Excellence (NICE), 2004), or the previous baby was >4000 g (RCOG, 2007).

- Uterine rupture is very rare, but is increased in women attempting VBAC at 0.35% (35 per 10 000) compared with 0.12% (12 per 10 000) for women having planned repeat CS (NICE, 2004).
- Just over half of the cases of true uterine rupture are in women who have not had a previous CS (Enkin, 2000).

Facts

- In 1985 the World Health Organisation issued a consensus statement suggesting there were no additional health benefits associated with a CSR above 10–15%.
- Surveys suggest that around 25% obstetricians would choose elective CS over vaginal birth in a straightforward pregnancy (RCOG, 2001). Fewer female obstetricians than male would choose a CS (Groom *et al.*, 2002; MacDonald *et al.*, 2002). These rates are higher than reported in other women surveyed (RCOG, 2001), and in contrast to personal preferences of midwives, 96% of whom would prefer a vaginal delivery (Dickson & Willett, 1999). This may have implications for obstetric advice on VBAC.
- Obstetricians have a strong influence over women's CS/VBAC decision which they may be unaware of (RCOG, 2001).
- Most obstetricians surveyed believed that elective CS was not the safest option for the mother, although 50% thought it was the safest option for the baby (RCOG, 2001).
- CS is more costly than vaginal birth. For approximately every 800 births without complications conducted as normal deliveries as opposed to CS, the NHS would save £1 million (OHE, 2007).

VBAC or elective CS

Women's perception of risk varies according to personal circumstances and previous delivery experiences. While many women describe feeling supported by their obstetrician, many describe uncertainty regarding mode of delivery which may continue even after the birth (Emmett *et al.*, 2006).

Obstetricians advising women often describe the process of CS rather than debating the risks and benefits. CS is recommended more frequently by obstetricians who are male and/or less experienced and/or working in private health care (RCOG, 2001). A large national study found that only 44% of women undergoing CS were offered a trial of labour in subsequent pregnancies. This varied from 8 to 90% in individual hospitals (RCOG, 2001). Most women opted for a repeat elective CS and only 33% chose VBAC. Most obstetricians failed to recognise the degree of their influence over women's CS/VBAC decision (RCOG, 2001).

Some factors increase the likelihood of CS, including advanced maternal age, body mass index >30, non-white ethnicity, short stature and previous preterm CS delivery (RCOG, 2007). However, there are very few situations where VBAC is not a reasonable option. There are accounts of supportive obstetricians and midwives have enabling 'higher risk' women to achieve a safe and satisfying VBAC birth, e.g. twins, breech or two or more previous CS (Lowdon & Chippington Derrick, 2007).

CS and vaginal birth have similar rates of haemorrhage, infection, faecal incontinence, dyspareunia, neonatal mortality (except in breech) intracranial haemorrhage, brachial plexus injuries and cerebral palsy (NICE, 2004). However other risks differ as follows.

Risks associated with VBAC

- The intrapartum infant death risk is small (about 10 per 10 000); however, this is higher than for planned repeat CS (about 1 per 10 000) and is the same as for a primigravida (NICE, 2004).
- Vaginal delivery is associated with postnatal perineal pain, increased risk of urinary incontinence and uterovaginal prolapse (NICE, 2004).
- Uterine rupture is rare but is marginally increased following induction/ augmentation of labour particularly if prostaglandins are used (RCOG, 2007), possibly following previous 'single-suture closure technique' CS (RCOG, 2007) and if conception occurred less than a year following previous CS (Lowdon & Chippington Derrick, 2007).

Risks associated with CS

- Operative risks include bladder/ureter injury, hysterectomy, need for high dependency/intensive therapy and postnatal readmission (NICE, 2004).
- Postnatal effects include abdominal pain, slower recovery, longer hospital stay and higher risk of thromboembolic disease (NICE, 2004).
- Neonatal risks include neonatal respiratory morbidity, especially pre-39 weeks (Morrison *et al.*, 1995).
- Long-term effects of CS include serious risk for subsequent pregnancies: increased risk of placenta praevia, placenta accreta (Langdana *et al.*, 2001) antepartum stillbirth and reduced future fertility (NICE, 2004).

Induction of labour for VBAC

Induction of labour increases the risk of uterine rupture to 80:10 000 if non-prostaglandins are used and to 240:10 000 if prostaglandins are used (NICE, 2004). The rate of vaginal delivery in this group of women is thought to be similar to that quoted for spontaneous labour after a previous CS at about 75% (Vause & Macintosh, 1999).

- Only attempt to induce labour when there is valid indication to do so.
- Induction of labour should take place on the labour ward (NICE, 2001).
- Artificial rupture of the membranes and/or oxytocin should be used cautiously and selectively (Enkin, 2000).
- Also refer to Chapter 18.

Midwifery care for VBAC labour

A woman who has had a previous CS is considered 'high risk' and NICE (2004) advises that labour should take place in a unit with access to immediate CS and on-site blood transfusion services. Women should not be pressured to consent to any particular aspect of care. Since a ruptured uterus is rare, many women undergo 'routine' interventions which involve iatrogenic risk and subsequent morbidity.

First stage

One-to-one midwifery care. Continuous intrapartum care is important for recognition and management of uterine scar rupture (NICE, 2004). However emotional support is equally important. Women may approach a VBAC labour with great trepidation. They may have strong memories of a previous long stressful labour perhaps ending in a frightening emergency situation (Horn, 2007). Particular reassurance may be required at the point in labour when the previous CS occurred (Wainer Cohen, 1991). Knowing the reason for the previous CS may even help prevent a recurrence.

Monitoring the fetal heart rate (FHR). RCOG (2007) and NICE (2004) recommend continuous fetal monitoring (CTG) in labour for women aiming for VBAC. Where is no specific FHR or uterine activity pattern that indicates the onset of a uterine rupture, 55–87% cases of ruptured uterus have an abnormal CTG (Guise *et al.*, 2004); often variable and/or late decelerations followed by fetal bradycardia (Menihan, 1999).

Some VBAC support groups challenge this, supporting a woman's right to choose intermittent auscultation over CTG to increase the likelihood of a normal birth (Beech Lawrence, 2001). A CTG in high-risk women increases labour interventions, including CS, and has not been shown to affect the perinatal mortality rate (Alfirevic *et al.*, 2007). Unfortunately NCT and AIMS receive regular reports of staff acting unprofessionally or threateningly, exaggerating risks and coercing women into CTG monitoring. Any woman who has weighed up her personal risks and declines CTG still needs to be supported in labour as any other and her choices respected. Intermittent auscultation is a valid alternative to electronic fetal monitoring and the FHR should be auscultated particularly scrupulously, especially if there is any suspicion of a problem.

Epidural. Some clinicians recommend epidurals 'just in case' a CS is needed and others suggest it could mask the pain of uterine rupture. The RCOG (2007) states that VBAC should not be a contraindication to an epidural. However, women should be aware that epidurals do carry a risk of additional complications and associated interventions (RCOG, 2007) which may complicate an otherwise straightforward labour.

Slow labour. Enkin (2000) suggests that slow progress should not always result in CS: careful oxytocin use following consultant opinion and maternal discussion (RCOG, 2007) may be effective.

- Oxytocin must be titrated to avoid uterine hyperstimulation: contractions should not exceed 3–4 in 10 minutes (RCOG, 2007).
- Serial vaginal examination, preferably by the same person, may help assess progress (RCOG, 2007).
- Chapter 8 also deals with other methods to stimulate uterine contractions.

Possible precautions

- **Intravenous cannula and bloods** for full blood count analysis/cross-matching (these can be kept and only tested in an emergency). If the woman declines a cannula, it is quite possible to site one quickly in an emergency, just as for any other emergency CS.

- **Fasting.** Gastric aspiration is associated with poor general anaesthetic technique, not directly due to food in the stomach. Conversely, NICE suggests that the effect of eating in labour on the risk of aspiration under anaesthesia is uncertain. It suggests that women should be informed that having isotonic drinks during labour prevents ketosis without a concomitant increase in gastric volume (NICE, 2004).
- **Regular antacids** (e.g. ranitidine, cimetidine). VBAC women are considered higher risk, and are likely to be offered 4-hourly antacids, although there is no strong evidence to support the use of routine antacids in normal labour to prevent gastric aspiration (Gyte & Richens, 2006).

Second stage of labour

Some suggest too many VBACs are forceps or ventouse assisted as obstetric fear of uterine rupture and lack of confidence in the birth process leads to a desire to conclude VBAC as quickly as possible.

> 'If, however, the only reason a speedy delivery is being considered is that the sand in the egg timer has run out, and mother and baby are coping just fine, there is little justification for mending what is not broken' (Lowdon & Chippington Derrick, 2002).

- Care should be as per a normal second stage of labour (see Chapter 1).
- Restricting the duration of the second stage is not evidence based and is associated with increased iatrogenic morbidity for the mother.
- Active pushing (valsalva) is potentially dangerous for VBAC women as it includes prolonged breath holding and forced bearing down which carries multiple risks including raised intrauterine pressures.

Third stage

- There are no special precautions if all has gone well.
- A scar on the uterus is not a contraindication to a physiological third stage.
- If there are difficulties delivering the placenta, consider it may have adhered to the myometrium of the previous scar (placenta accreta). Placenta accreta is only diagnosable and deliverable surgically, sometimes requiring hysterectomy to control haemorrhage (Langdana *et al.*, 2001). Inform the doctor early if the placenta appears retained as bleeding may be concealed. Observe the woman for shock.

Uterine scar rupture

Although uncommon, the uterus can rupture in the antenatal period, at induction, during labour/birth, and even during the third stage of labour.

Be vigilant and listen to the woman. While there is no clinical feature indicative of uterine rupture (RCOG, 2007), many women and midwives report a woman's *unease* or *distress* as a common feature (Lowdon & Chippington Derrick, 2002). If in doubt, contact a senior obstetrician immediately. If at home or a birthing centre, then arrange immediate ambulance transfer to hospital.

For signs and symptoms of uterine rupture and treatment of shock see Chapter 16.

Preparing for birth at home/birthing centre

Each woman has a right to unemotive, unbiased information about the potential risks and benefits within her own individual circumstances. Women who feel pressured, obstructed or unsupported sometimes opt out of the acute hospital system. Most birthing centres do not encourage VBAC, although women may still choose to give birth there. Some NHS midwives are uncomfortable to support home birth VBAC. Women may turn to independent midwives (Lowdon & Chippington Derrick, 2007). However, as discussed in Chapter 6 (Home birth), all midwives have a responsibility to provide care and support at home, even if the pregnancy is not considered low risk. Some suggest that birthing at home can reduce women's risk of encountering problems since labour and birth at home is physiologically spontaneous and not 'interfered with'. Conversely, any emergency transfer to an acute unit will obviously involve some delay. So while unlikely, a ruptured uterus is a potentially life-threatening emergency.

VBAC labour care at home

See also Chapter 6.

- **Care as per normal labour.** The midwife must instil confidence in the woman and strike a balance between maintaining a warm, reassuring persona while also being unobtrusively vigilant for signs of possible rupture.
- **Ruptured uterus.** While there are no reported cases of this occurring at a home birth (Lowdon & Chippington Derrick, 2007), the midwife should be well supported by colleagues and aware of VBAC issues (for signs and symptoms of rupture see Box 16.1, p. 225).
- **Transfer.** The transfer rate for a woman attempting a VBAC at home is thought to be higher than the national average, possibly as midwives and mothers tend to be cautious and transfer at the first sign of trouble. One small study reported a 28% VBAC transfer rate although none was for a ruptured uterus (Chamberlain *et al.*, 1994).

Summary

In hospital

- Extra reassurance and one-to-one midwifery care.
- Possible precautions:
  - Cannula and bloods (test only in an emergency)
  - Eating and drinking is not contraindicated but be cautious
  - CTG
- Observe unobtrusively for signs of uterine rupture: listen to the woman.
- Prostaglandin/artificial rupture of the membranes/oxytocics should be used with caution.
- Epidural is not contraindicated.

At home/birthing centre

- Offer reassurance and positive care with unobtrusive vigilance for signs of uterine rupture.
- Be prepared for transfer, if necessary.

Useful contacts

Association for Improvements in the Maternity Services (AIMS)   AIMS Helpline: 0870 765 1433. Website: www.aims.org.uk

CS and **VBAC**   information. Website: www.caesarean.org.uk

References

Alfirevic, Z., Devane, D. & Gyte, G.M. (2007) Continuous cardiotocography (CTG) as a form of electronic fetal monitoring (EFM) for fetal assessment during labour (Review). *The Cochrane Library*, Issue 3, Art. No. CD006066.

Beech Lawrence, B. (2001) Electronic fetal monitoring: do NICE's new guidelines owe too much to the medical model of childbirth? *The Practising Midwife* **4** (7), 31–3.

Chamberlain, G., Wraight, A. & Crowley, P. (1994) *National Birthday Trust Report – Report of the Confidential Enquiry into Home Births.* Parthenon Publishing Group, London.

Dickson, M.J. & Willett, M. (1999) Midwives would prefer a vaginal delivery. *BMJ* **319**, 1008.

Emmett, C., Shaw, A., Montgomery, A. & Murphy, D. (DiAMOND study group) (2006) Women's experience of decision making about mode of delivery after a previous caesarean section: the role of health professionals and information about health risks. *An International Journal of Obstetrics and Gynaecology* **113** (12), 1438–45.

Enkin, M. (2000) Labour and birth after a previous caesarean section. In *A Guide to Effective Care in Pregnancy and Childbirth*, 3rd edn (Enkin, M., Keirse, M.J.N.C., Neilson, J., *et al.*, eds), pp. 359–71. Oxford University Press, Oxford.

Groom, K.M., Patterson-Brown, S. & Fisk, N.M. (2002) Temporal and geographical variation in UK obstetricians' personal preference regarding mode of delivery. *European Journal of Obstetrics, Gynecology, and Reproductive Biology* **100**, 185–8.

Guise, J.M., McDonagh, M.S., Osterweil, P., Nygren, P., Chan, B.K. & Helfand, M. (2004) Systematic review of the incidence and consequences of uterine rupture in women with previous caesarean section. *BMJ* **329**, 19–25.

Gyte, G.M.L. & Richens, Y. (2006) Routine prophylactic drugs in normal labour for reducing gastric aspiration and its effects. *Cochrane Database of Systematic Reviews*, 2006, Issue 3, Art. No. CD005298.

Horn, A. (2007) *VBAC at Home*. Available at: www.homebirth.org.uk (accessed August 2007).

Langdana, F., Geary, M., Haw, W. & Keane, D. (2001) Peripartum hysterectomy in the 1990s: any new lessons? *Journal of Obstetrics and Gynaecology* **21**, 121–3.

Lowdon, D. & Chippington Derrick, D. (2002) VBAC on whose terms. *AIMS Journal* **14**, 1.

Lowdon, D. & Chippington Derrick, D. (2007) *CS and VBAC Information*. Available at: www.caesarean.org.uk (accessed August 2007).

MacDonald, C., Pinion, S. & McCLeod, U. (2002) Scottish female obstetricians views on elective caesarean section and personal choice for delivery. *Journal of Obstetrics & Gynaecology* **22**, 586–9.

Menihan, C.A. (1999) The effect of uterine rupture on fetal heart rate patterns. *Journal of Nurse-Midwifery* **44** (1), 40–46.

Morrison, J.J., Rennie, J.M. & Milton, P.J. (1995) Neonatal respiratory morbidity and mode of delivery at term: influence of timing of elective caesarean section. *British Journal of Obstetrics and Gynaecology* **102**, 101–6.

National Institute for Health and Clinical Excellence (NICE) (2001) *Clinical Guideline D – Induction of Labour.* National Institute for Health and Clinical Excellence, London.

National Institute for Health and Clinical Excellence (NICE) (2004) *Clinical Guideline 13 – Caesarean Section.* National Institute for Health and Clinical Excellence, London.

NHS Maternity Statistics England 2005/6 (2007) *Information Center for Health and Social Care.* Available at: www.ic.nhs.uk/webfiles/publications/maternity0506/NHSMaternityStatsEngland200506.pdf (accessed March 2008).

OHE Compendium Health Statistics (2007) *How UK NHS Expenditure and Staffing Has Changed: Rising UK Birth Rates and Causes of Increasing Numbers of Caesarean Deliveries.* Press release 26 February 2007.

Royal College of Obstetricians and Gynaecologists (RCOG) (2001) Royal College of Obstetricians and Gynaecologists Clinical Effectiveness Support Unit. *National Sentinel Caesarean Section Audit Report* (Thomas, J. & Paranjothy, S., eds). RCOG Press, London.

Royal College of Obstetricians and Gynaecologists (RCOG) (2007) *Green-top Guideline No. 45: Birth After Previous Caesarean Birth.* Available at: www.rcog.org.uk (accessed March 2008).

Silverton, L. (1993) *The Art and Science of Midwifery.* Prentice Hall International, London.

Vause, S. & Macintosh, M. (1999) Evidence based case report: use of prostaglandins to induce labour in women with a caesarean section scar. *BMJ* **318**, 1056–8.

Wainer Cohen, N. (1991) *Open Season: Survival Guide for Natural Childbirth and VBAC in the 90s.* Bergin and Gavery, New York.

12 Preterm birth

Vicky Chapman

Introduction

'The birth of a baby should be one of the most special and joyful experiences a family can have and yet every year thousands of families experience the pain of losing a baby or seeing a tiny child fight for life' (Briley *et al.*, 2002).

Preterm birth is defined as the delivery of a baby before 37 completed weeks gestation (Tucker & McGuire, 2004) and is often associated with pre-existing conditions such as:

- Infection
- Pre-eclampsia
- Antepartum haemorrhage
- Placenta praevia
- Inadequate fetal growth
- Maternal disease

Preterm births are more prevalent in multiple pregnancies and among babies with congenital malformations (Keirse, 2000).

Incidence

- The UK preterm birth rate of 5–7% has remained static over the past 30 years. 1–2% of all births are <32 weeks gestation. Most neonatal mortality and morbidity associated with prematurity occurs in infants born before this time (Tucker & McGuire, 2004).
- Survival rates for babies born between 27 and 28 weeks gestation have improved, with 88% surviving for 28 days after delivery. Survival rates have more than doubled in recent years (Royal College of Obstetricians and Gynaecologists (RCOG), 2001).

Facts

- Identifying women at risk of preterm labour is imprecise; also prediction does not yet mean prevention. Several prediction methods are available, e.g. cervical scanning and biochemical markers (fetal fibronectin, salivary oestriols and interleukins), but no single reliable method of predicting preterm delivery exists (Briley *et al.*, 2002).
- The most important predictors of spontaneous preterm delivery are a history of preterm birth and poor socioeconomic background of the mother (Tucker & McGuire, 2004).
- Preterm babies are more prone to hypothermia, hypoglycaemia, jaundice, infection and respiratory distress. More serious risks are intraventricular haemorrhage, deafness, retinopathy of prematurity, blindness, necrotising enterocolitis, cerebral palsy and death (Kenyon *et al.*, 2001b).
- Higher survival rates in preterm infants are attributed to the following:
  ○ Cephalic vaginal birth
  ○ Singleton birth
  ○ Babies with a higher weight for gestation
  ○ Gender: girls have a greater survival rate than boys

Place of delivery

This will depend on gestation due to the specialist facilities needed for extremely premature births. Babies <35 weeks may benefit from specialist neonatal facilities with those born at 24–28 weeks requiring intensive care.

Some preterm babies are born unplanned at home or in a hospital with limited facilities and will need prompt transfer to appropriate neonatal services. Transfer is advisable for women with threatened preterm labour; however, it is usually unsafe to transfer if:

- The birth is imminent
- Her condition is unstable, e.g. bleeding or severe pre-eclampsia.

If transfer is required, decide whether a midwife is needed to accompany the woman. Any escorting staff must be trained to assist in transfer (CESDI, 2003).

Preterm, prelabour rupture of membranes

Preterm, prelabour rupture of membranes (PPROM) is associated with 40% of preterm births and can cause significant neonatal mortality and morbidity, with one-third of women testing positive to infection (RCOG, 2006).

- If PPROM occurs at 24–34 weeks gestation, 50% of women will deliver within 4 days and 70–80% within 1 week (Walkinshaw, 2001).
- The three causes of neonatal death associated with PPROM are prematurity, sepsis and pulmonary hypoplasia (RCOG, 2006).
- Antibiotics following PPROM significantly reduce chorioamnionitis, neonatal infection, abnormal cerebral ultrasound and can extend the pregnancy (RCOG, 2006).

- Erythromycin (250 mg orally 6 hourly) should be given for 10 days following the diagnosis of PPROM (Co-amoxiclav is not recommended) (RCOG, 2006).

Infection

Infection is a major cause of preterm labour, and infants born with sepsis have a mortality rate four times higher than those without sepsis (RCOG, 2006).

The ORACLE trial (Kenyon *et al.*, 2001a) suggests that:

- If infection is suspected/diagnosed or PPROM confirmed, commence antibiotics as quickly as possible.
- If there is no sign of infection or PPROM then antibiotics are of no benefit.

Signs and symptoms of maternal infection

Early signs of infection:

- Slight maternal pyrexia
- Fetal tachycardia
- General malaise

Advanced signs of infection:

- Feeling very unwell
- High pyrexia
- Maternal and/or fetal tachycardia
- Uterine tenderness and an offensive smelling vaginal discharge/liquor
- Baby ill at birth
- Intrauterine death

Screening and assessment:

- Obstetric referral
- Maternal temperature, pulse rate and urinalysis
- Fetal heart rate (FHR) auscultation
- Two sets of blood cultures
- Depending on history and clinical picture, send urgent and repeated bacterial specimens (Department of Health (DOH) 2001) e.g. vaginal/cervical swabs, urine specimen and maybe throat swab, sputum sample and faeces for culture

Midwifery care during uncomplicated preterm labour and birth

Diagnosing preterm labour

It can be difficult to distinguish *threatened* from *actual preterm labour* at the outset. Every area should have clear guidelines for the diagnosis and management of preterm labour. Any woman reporting preterm *regular* painful contractions or suspected ruptured membranes should be assessed in a consultant unit.

A careful history should be taken. Abdominal palpation and FHR auscultation should be performed. Perform a speculum rather than digital vaginal examination (VE) to take swabs and attempt to visualise the cervix (RCOG, 2006). Avoid digital VE if possible, or keep to a minimum, as it can introduce infection, cause prostaglandin release and augment labour (Atalla *et al.*, 2000).

Digital VE is *contraindicated* in cases of suspected infection or PPROM (CESDI, 2003; RCOG, 2006).

Tocolysis

Tocolytic drugs are sometimes used to delay preterm delivery. RCOG (2002) suggests that there is no clear evidence that they improve the outcome, but a few days may be gained if necessary to complete a course of corticosteroids, or transfer in utero.

Tocolytic drugs have serious side effects, and if used, nifedipine (not licensed for this use in the UK) or atosiban is effective and has fewer adverse effects than ritodrine.

The use of tocolytics should be avoided in the following:

- Fetal death or fetal abnormality incompatible with life
- Fetal or maternal condition requiring urgent delivery
- Active vaginal bleeding (as tocolytics relax the uterus)
- Preterm rupture of the membranes and/or infection

Use of corticosteroids

A single course of corticosteroids should be administered ≤34 weeks to women at risk of preterm birth. Antenatal corticosteroids encourage the release of pulmonary surfactant in fetal lungs, reducing the risk of respiratory distress syndrome, cerebroventricular haemorrhage, systemic infection <48 hours of age, necrotising enterocolitis and death (Roberts & Dalziel, 2007).

Fetal heart rate monitoring

National Institute for Health and Clinical Excellence (NICE) (2007) lists preterm labour as one indication for continuous electronic fetal monitoring (EFM). However, Cochrane review found that EFM in preterm labour appears to have no advantage over intermittent auscultation (IA) and increases maternal morbidity, caesarean section (CS) and possibly cerebral palsy (Alfirevic *et al.*, 2007).

Preterm EFM is an unreliable tool for predicting future neurodevelopmental impairment of premature infants of very low birth weight (Nisenblat *et al.*, 2006). Very premature, small babies can be difficult to monitor continuously, and preterm fetal heart rates may be difficult to interpret as they differ from those at term (Atalla *et al.*, 2000). So if continuous cardiotocography (CTG) monitoring is performed, it is likely to be more easily interpretable in older preterm babies than very early ones. Preterm (particularly very preterm) CTGs tend to have a higher baseline (sometimes 170 bpm) and decelerations which are not necessarily truly pathological, and Atalla *et al.* (2000) suggests that most preterm babies with unsatisfactory CTG traces will not be acidotic. However, once a CTG is performed it is natural that clinicians will have a low threshold for action in a preterm labour. If it is decided to perform IA, it should be carried out scrupulously (see Chapter 3).

First stage of labour

Most care and support will be the same as for any labour (see Chapter 1):

- **Continuous, supportive, one-to-one midwifery care** is proved to reduce interventions and improves maternal and fetal outcomes (Hodnett *et al.*, 2007).
- **Discuss with the parents** what may occur at the birth and immediately afterwards: who will be present, what type of resuscitation is anticipated and the likelihood of their baby needing special care.
- **Minimise environmental stress.** Try to reduce external stressful stimuli of bright lights, noise, interruptions and lack of privacy.
- **Liaise with colleagues.** Ensure that neonatal intensive care units (NICU) are well briefed. Ideally the delivery suite coordinator will keep the relevant clinicians updated so the midwife can remain with the mother.
- **Encourage mobility and upright position** to aid optimal fetal positioning, progress and descent. As with any labour, avoid the supine position as it may cause FHR abnormalities, increased duration of second stage, episiotomy and instrumental delivery (Gupta *et al.*, 2004). A non-supine position also improves outcomes in women with epidurals (Roberts *et al.*, 2005).
- **Monitor the FHR.**
- **Minimise digital VEs.** Always consider what is to be gained by them. They may lead to ascending vaginal infection, especially if the membranes have ruptured.
- **Eating and drinking is not contraindicated**, although it may be wise to administer regular antacids/hydrogen ion inhibitors, e.g. ranitidine or cimetidine, in case an emergency anaesthetic is required (Johnson *et al.*, 2000).
- **Avoid narcotic analgesia**, e.g. pethidine: it can cause neonatal respiratory depression, drowsiness and depressed reflexes, including the suck reflex (NICE, 2007) which is more of a problem for a preterm baby.
- **Artificial rupture of the membranes (ARM) is not recommended** since any potential cord compression may be particularly serious for a preterm baby and there is a risk of exacerbating ascending infection/chorioamnionitis.
- **Fetal blood sampling is contraindicated** <34 weeks (NICE, 2007) and has not been shown to hold an advantage over CTG without fetal blood sampling (Alfirevic *et al.*, 2007).
- **Prepare the resuscitaire.** Check equipment. Provide baby clothes, hat and warm towels. Preterm labours can progress rapidly, so be prepared.

Second stage of labour

- **Keep the room warm.** Shut windows and switch off fans when birth is close.
- **Avoid forced pushing.** Prolonged breath holding and closed glottis pushing is associated with fetal compromise, forceps delivery and lower Apgars (Keirse, 2000) which can have more serious consequences for a preterm infant. Let the woman push at her own pace.
- **Avoid episiotomy.** The only indications for an episiotomy are acute fetal compromise and, if absolutely necessary, an unyielding perineum (Keirse, 2000). This procedure does not protect the fetal head.

- **Ventouse delivery is not recommended** in gestations <34 weeks due to the baby's soft skull (Keirse, 2000).
- **Forceps delivery may damage the fetal head** (Keirse, 2000) and the old practice of preterm elective forceps delivery has been abandoned.

Mode of delivery

Mode of delivery for preterm infants remains controversial. Almost 50% preterm infants are delivered by CS (RCOG, 2001) despite no clear evidence of advantages of a CS over a vaginal birth (Keirse, 2000).

Care immediately after birth

Skin-to-skin contact in preterm infants

Conventional care involves early cutting of the cord and immediate maternal–infant separation possibly including the use of a space blanket or placing the baby in a plastic bag (Vohra *et al.*, 1999) for heat conservation despite evidence of the clinical superiority of a more humane approach.

However, there is good evidence that skin-to-skin contact (SSC) should be considered the 'gold standard' of care for most preterm infants as there appear to be many physiological, and possibly psychological, benefits for the mother and baby (see Box 12.1). It must be remembered, however, that there may be times when the urgent clinical needs of the baby outweigh the benefits of SSC, particularly if the baby has significant respiratory difficulty and/or is very preterm.

Aim to deliver the baby onto the mother's chest immediately or as soon as possible if born by CS. Cover the outer part of the baby with a pre-warmed blanket or space

Box 12.1   Skin-to-skin contact (SSC) at birth in preterm infants.

Skin-to-skin contact at birth
- **Improves clinical outcomes** in both term and preterm infants (Moore *et al.*, 2007) stabilising the heart rate, respiratory response/rate and oxygen requirements (Christensson *et al.*, 1992; Bergman *et al.*, 2004).
- **Provides better warmth** compared to radiant overhead heaters or incubators (Bergman *et al.*, 2004) protecting even infants <1500 g (Christensson *et al.*, 1998) against hypothermia.
- **Reduces cardiorespiratory instability.** Separated preterm infants weighing 1200–2200 g demonstrate hyperarousal and separation anxiety response patterns (Bergman *et al.*, 2004) many hours following birth, affecting heart rate and respiration. SSC relaxes the baby and normalises breathing and heart rate.
- **Promotes maternal–infant attachment and pleasure** of the mother and her baby, and also significantly improves breastfeeding uptake and duration (De Chateau & Wilbert, 1997; Moore *et al.*, 2007) which is particularly beneficial for preterm infants.
- **Promotes earlier positive feelings in fathers** (Sullivan, 1999).
- **Seems to have no side effects** making it the most obvious and sensitive form of care for preterm infants.

SSC should not be pursued however if the baby is born in poor condition requiring intensive intervention, e.g. urgent need for intubation and ventilation.

blanket (but do not put it between baby and mother) and put on a hat (Moore *et al.*, 2007).

Delayed cord clamping

NICE (2007) recommends early cord clamping for all actively managed third stages, but this advice might be challenged, particularly for preterm babies. NICE suggests that even though limited evidence shows benefit to anaemic babies, there is some risk of hyperbilirubinaemia. Other meta-analyses however suggest there is no increase in symptomatic polycythaemia or jaundice treatment following delayed cord clamping (DCC) (Mercer, 2001; Hutton & Hassan, 2007), and NICE accepts the evidence base is incomplete.

Keirse (2000) states that there is no justification for clamping and cutting the cord unless active and immediate resuscitation is required. A Cochrane review shows that DCC, even for a short time, ensures that extra blood from the placenta passes to the baby. This improves blood flow to the baby's lungs and brain particularly in the first 24 hours of birth (Baenziger *et al.*, 2007) reducing the need for supplemental oxygen. DCC also reduces serious complications including anaemia requiring blood transfusion, intraventricular haemorrhage and late-onset sepsis (Rabe *et al.*, 2004; Mercer *et al.*, 2006). DCC even during CS is effective at transfusing extra blood (Cernadas *et al.*, 2006).

For most babies 1 minute of DCC may be enough, especially if they breathe quickly after birth. However, Philip (2006) suggests that only when the baby cries does a significant amount of blood transfer from the placenta to the large vascular bed created by lung expansion. Hence, in babies requiring assistance to breathe, it may be helpful to delay cord clamping, if possible, until the baby has breathed/the lungs have been expanded and adapt to administer initial, simple resuscitation at the woman's side (Philip, 2006). This may mean DCC for several minutes.

It may be difficult, in practice, to challenge NICE recommendations for normal labour, but many studies of preterm infants as a sub-group show significant evidence of benefit from DCC.

Whenever the cord is cut, leave the baby's end long in case umbilical catheterisation is required later.

All studies on DCC involve active management of the third stage. If a physiological third stage occurs, the cord is normally not clamped until the delivery of the placenta, so that transfer of blood should occur as part of the physiological process.

Resuscitation of the preterm newborn

Neonatal resuscitation is covered fully in Chapter 17. Remember the following:

- Keep the baby *warm and dry* during resuscitation: the importance of this cannot be overstressed for preterm babies. *It is not an optional extra but a vital step in the resuscitation process.*
- If NICU transfer is necessary, try to let the mother see and touch her baby first. Encourage her partner to accompany if possible.
- Ensure that the baby is labelled and up-to-date notes provided for NICU staff as soon as it is practical.

Care related to specific types of preterm labour

Very preterm infants (22–26 weeks)

The increasingly high survival rates of very preterm infants are compounded by an increasing level of disability (CESDI, 2001). The EPICure study in 1995 found that of those babies born at 25–26 weeks gestation half of those who survived had either mental and psychomotor development disabilities, neuromotor function disabilities or sensory and communication function disabilities (Costeloe *et al.*, 2000).

In 10–15% preterm births, the baby has died before labour starts or has lethal malformations incompatible with life. These very sad situations will come as a shock to the parents and this can be an extremely distressing time. Care should be directed towards the needs of the mother and family:

- Prior to the birth the parents should be able to discuss with an experienced paediatrician the prognosis for their baby, the likely events following the birth and whether or not to commence treatment or resuscitation in a very preterm or extremely malformed baby. This discussion should be documented.
- Due to heightened emotions and anxiety, many parents find it difficult to process information. Carers must be prepared to repeat explanations and talk in sensitive, understandable terms about the possible outcome, however bleak, for the baby.
- An ultrasound scan should be available to exclude serious abnormalities and confirm fetal presentation (Keirse, 2000).
- Staff trained in neonatal resuscitation and thermal care of neonates and at least one clinician experienced in tracheal intubation should attend the delivery of any infant <28 weeks (CESDI, 2003).

Breech presentation

Breech presentation is more common in preterm infants and is associated with increased incidence of congenital abnormalities, antepartum stillbirth and neonatal mortality than cephalic preterm infants (Keirse, 2000). Preterm breech infants are also more likely to present as incomplete presentations such as footling, with associated increased risk of umbilical cord prolapse and a premature urge to push (see Chapter 13 for more information on breech birth).

Multiple pregnancies

Multiple pregnancies are more likely to deliver preterm, and women expecting multiples are usually aware of this possibility (see Chapter 14 for more detail on multiple births).

Preterm birth at home

Unplanned, quick birth at home is usually very straightforward, but it can occasionally present the midwife with a compromised preterm baby. Sometimes the mother too is unwell; indeed this may have caused her preterm labour.

The main risks of unattended births are maternal haemorrhage, retained placenta and neonatal heat loss. Risks may be reduced by training ambulance staff not to clamp and cut the cord when an oxytocic has not been given (Loughney *et al.*, 2006) and to promote SSC after birth:

- Hypothermia is extremely serious in preterm babies (CESDI, 2003) and the primary risk for babies 'born before arrival' (BBA) (Loughney *et al.*, 2006). Dry the baby thoroughly at birth, and give SSC promptly with the mother (see Box 12.1 for benefits). In addition, put a hat on the baby and cover well. Keep the room warm.
- Hospital transfer is advisable for any baby <35–36 weeks; many preterm babies appear well at delivery but can develop respiratory and other difficulties in the hours following birth.
- Unless the baby requires active resuscitation, consider SSC for transfer. Ambulance staff may be reluctant to transfer an 'unsecured' baby but common sense should prevail.

Summary

- Identifying women at risk of preterm delivery remains imprecise. Previous preterm delivery and the woman's socioeconomic status are the single best predictors.
- Parents should receive clear sensitive information and be involved in decisions on their baby's care. Be prepared to repeat information.
- Experienced staff should provide neonatal resuscitation.
- The room should be warm and draught free.
- Dry the baby following birth, and keep warm even during resuscitation.
- Encourage SSC unless the baby needs immediate and intensive attention.

Evidence supports:

- Corticosteroid administration if <34 weeks
- Antibiotic administration if PPROM or suspected maternal infection

Evidence supports *avoiding*:

- ARM or 'routine' VE
- Narcotic analgesia
- Active pushing
- Supine maternal position
- Ventouse
- Non-indicated episiotomy/forceps
- Early clamping of the umbilical cord

Useful contacts

BLISS the Premature Baby Charity   Telephone: 0870 7700337. Helpline: 0500 618 140. Website: www.bliss.org.uk

Confidential Enquiry into Maternal and Child Health (CEMACH)   CEMACH changed from Confidential Enquiry into Stillbirths and Deaths in Infancy (CESDI) in April 2003. Website: www.cemach.org.uk

Tommy's the Baby Charity Information Telephone: 0870 777 3060. Website: www.tommys-campaign.org Research, education and information for parents and professionals.

References

Alfirevic, Z., Devane, D. & Gyte, G.M. (2007) Continuous cardiotocography (CTG) as a form of electronic fetal monitoring (EFM) for fetal assessment during labour (Review). *The Cochrane Library*, Issue 3, Art. No. CD006066.

Atalla, R., Kean, L. & McParland, P. (2000) In *Best Practice in Labor Ward Management* (Kean, L., Baker, P. & Edelstone, D., eds). WB Saunders, Edinburgh.

Baenziger, O., Stolkin, F., Keel, M., von Siebenthal, K., Fauchere, J.C., Das Kundu, S., Dietz, V., Bucher, H.U. & Wolf, M. (2007) The influence of the timing of cord clamping on postnatal cerebral oxygenation in preterm neonates: a randomized, controlled trial. *Pediatrics* **119** (3), 455–9.

Bergman, N.J., Liney, L.L. & Fawcus, S.R. (2004) Randomized controlled trial of skin-to-skin contact from birth versus conventional incubator for physiological stabilization in 1200- to 2199-gram newborns. *Acta Paediatrica* **93** (6), 779–85.

Briley, A., Crawshaw, S. & Hughes, J. (2002) *Premature Labour – Information for Parents.* Tommy's the Baby Charity, London.

Cernadas, J.M.C., Carroli, G. & Lardizabal, J. (2006) Effect of timing of cord clamping on neonatal venous hematocrit values and clinical outcome at term: a randomized, controlled trial: in reply. *Pediatrics* **118** (3), 1318–9.

CESDI (2001) *Confidential Enquiry into Stillbirths and Deaths in Infancy, 8th Annual Report.* Maternal and Child Health Consortium, London.

CESDI (2003) *Project 27/28: An Enquiry into Quality and Care and Its Effect on Survival of Babies Born at 27/28 Weeks.* Stationary Office, London.

Christensson, K., Bhat, G.J., Amadi, B.C., Eriksson, B. & Hojer, B. (1998) A randomised study of skin-to-skin versus incubator care for rewarming low risk hypothermic neonates. *The Lancet* **352**, 1115.

Christensson, K., Siles, C., Moreno, L., Belaustequi, A., De La Fuente, P., Lagercrantz, H., Puyol, P. & Winberg, J. (1992) Temperature, metabolic adaption and crying in healthy full-term newborns cared for skin-to-skin or in a cot. *Acta Paediatrica* **91**, 488–93.

Costeloe, K., Hennessy, E. & Gibson, A. (2000) EPICure study: outcomes to discharge from hospitals for infants born at the threshold of viability. *Pediatrics* **106**, 659–71.

De Chateau, P. & Wilbert, B. (1997) Long-term effect on mother infant behaviour of extra contact during the first hour postpartum. II. A follow up at 3 months. *Acta Paediatrica* **66**, 145–51.

Department of Health (DOH) (2001) *Why Mothers Die, 1997–1999. The Fifth Report of the Confidential Enquiries into Maternal Deaths in the United Kingdom.* Department of Health, RCOG Press, London.

Gupta, J.K., Hofmeyr, G.J. & Smyth, R. (2004) Position in the second stage of labour for women without epidural anaesthesia. *Cochrane Database of Systematic Reviews*, 2004, Issue 1, Art. No. CD002006.

Hodnett, E.D., Gates, S., Hofmeyr, G.J. & Sakala, C. (2007) Continuous support for women during childbirth. *Cochrane Database of Systematic Reviews*, 2007, Issue 3, Art. No. CD003766.

Hutton, E.K. & Hassan, E.S. (2007) Late vs early clamping of the umbilical cord in full-term neonates: systematic review and meta-analysis of controlled trials. *JAMA* **297**, 1241–52.

Johnson, C., Keirse, M.J.N.C., Enkin, M. & Chalmers, I. (2000) Hospital practices – nutrition and hydration in labour. In *A Guide to Effective Care in Pregnancy and Childbirth*, 3rd edn (Enkin, M., Keirse, M.J.N.C., Neilson, J., *et al.*, eds), pp. 255–66. Oxford University Press, Oxford.

Keirse, M. (2000) *A Guide to Effective Care in Pregnancy and Childbirth*, 3rd edn (Enkin, M., Keirse, M. & Neilson, J., eds). Oxford University Press, Oxford.

Kenyon, S., Taylor, D. & Tarnow-Mordi, W. (2001a) Broad spectrum antibiotics for spontaneous preterm labour: the ORACLE I randomised trial. *The Lancet* **375**, 979–88.

Kenyon, S., Taylor, D. & Tarnow-Mordi, W. (2001b) Broad spectrum antibiotics for spontaneous preterm labour: the ORACLE II randomised trial. *The Lancet* **375**, 989–94.

Loughney, A., Collis, R. & Dastgir, S. (2006) Birth before arrival at delivery suite: associations and consequences. *British Journal of Midwifery* **14** (4), 204–208.

Mercer, J. (2001) Current best evidence: a review of the literature on umbilical cord clamping. *Journal of Midwifery and Women's Health* **46** (6), 404–14.

Mercer, J., Vohr, B.R., McGrath, M.M., Padbury, J.F., Wallach, M. & Oh, W. (2006) Delayed cord clamping in very preterm infants reduces the incidence of intraventricular hemorrhage and late-onset sepsis: a randomized, controlled trial. *Pediatrics* **117** (4), 1235–42.

Moore, E.R., Anderson, G.C. & Bergman, N. (2007) Early skin-to-skin contact for mothers and their healthy newborn infants (review). *The Cochrane Library*, Issue 3, Art. No. CD003519.

National Institute for Health and Clinical Excellence (NICE) (2007) *Clinical Guideline 55: Intrapartum Care*. National Institute for Health and Clinical Excellence, London.

Nisenblat, V., Alon, E., Barak, S., Gonen, R., Bader, D. & Ohel, G. (2006) Fetal heart rate patterns and neurodevelopmental outcome in very low birth weight infants. *Acta Obstetricia et Gynecologica Scandinavica* **85** (7), 792–6.

Philip, A. (2006) Delayed cord clamping in preterm infants. *Pediatrics* **117** (4), 1434–5.

Rabe, H., Reynolds, G. & Diaz-Rossello, J. (2004) Early versus delayed umbilical cord clamping in preterm infants. *Cochrane Database of Systematic Reviews*, 2004, Issue 4, Art. No. CD003248.

Roberts, C.L., Algert, C.S., Cameron, C.A. & Tovaldsen, S. (2005) A meta-analysis of upright positions in the second stage to reduce instrumental deliveries in women with epidural analgesia. *Acta Obstetricia et Gynecologica Scandinavica* **84** (8), 794–8.

Roberts, D. & Dalziel, S. (2007) Antenatal corticosteroids for accelerating fetal lung maturation for women at risk of preterm birth. *Cochrane Database of Systemic Reviews*. Issue 4, Update software, Oxford.

Royal College of Obstetricians and Gynaecologists (RCOG) (2001) Clinical effectiveness support unit. In *National Sentinel Caesarean Section Audit Report* (Thomas, J. & Paranjothy, S., eds). RCOG Press, London.

Royal College of Obstetricians and Gynaecologists (RCOG) (2002) *Tocolytic Drugs for Women in Preterm Labour*. RCOG Clinical Guideline No. 1(b).

Royal College of Obstetricians and Gynaecologists (RCOG) (2006) *Preterm Pre Labour Rupture of Membranes*. Green-top guideline No 44, London.

Sullivan, J.R. (1999) Development of father-infant attachment in fathers of preterm infants. *Neonatal Network* **18** (7), 33–9.

Tucker, J. & McGuire, W. (2004) Epidemiology of preterm birth. *British Medical Journal* **329**, 675–8.

Vohra, S., Frent, G., Campbell, V., *et al.* (1999) Effect of polythene occlusive skin wrapping on heat loss in very low birth weight infants at delivery: a randomised controlled trial. *Journal of Paediatrics* **134**, 547–51.

Walkinshaw, S. (2001) *Turnbull's Obstetrics*, 3rd edn (Chamberlin, G. & Steer, P., eds). Churchill Livingstone, London.

13 Breech birth

Lesley Shuttler

Introduction

Breech presentation is where the lie of the baby is longitudinal and the baby's buttocks are in the lower segment of the mother's uterus.

Following the term breech trial (TBT) (Hannah *et al.*, 2000), midwives today may have limited experience of seeing or being involved in caring for a woman having a vaginal breech birth. They may approach a vaginal breech birth with the same lack of confidence and fear observed in inexperienced obstetricians. However, midwives need to remember that in carefully selected/assessed women, vaginal breech birth can be a safe and fulfilling birth option (Alarab *et al.*, 2004; Royal College of Obstetricians and Gynaecologists (RCOG), 2006b).

Incidence

- 25% of babies adopt a breech position at some time in pregnancy, and 3–4% remain breech at term (RCOG, 2006b).
- The TBT (Hannah *et al.*, 2000) has increased breech caesarean section (CS) rates. The UK CS rate for breech presentation rose from 69% in 1993 to 88% in 2001 (RCOG, 2001), and is rising still. Breech now accounts for 11% of all caesareans (RCOG, 2007).
- Other countries have had similar increases: the Netherlands CS rate for breech has risen from 57 to 81% (Schutte *et al.*, 2007), whilst in France it rose from 43% in 1998 to 75% in 2003 (Carayol *et al.*, 2007).

Facts

- Many babies appear to adopt a breech presentation for no particular reason. However, a minority will adopt a breech position because of 'problems' such as short or entangled cord, prematurity, placenta praevia or fetal abnormalities.

- Irrespective of mode of delivery, breech presentation is associated with increased subsequent disability; in a few cases failure to adopt a cephalic presentation may be a marker for fetal impairment (RCOG, 2006b).
- For a woman with predisposing factors, such as diabetes, fetopelvic disproportion, a previous macrosomic baby, or a suspected large baby and poor labour progress, a CS is usually advisable (RCOG, 2006b).
- Evidence suggests that external cephalic version (ECV) should be offered to all women with an uncomplicated breech baby at term (37–42 weeks) (National Institute for Health and Clinical Excellence (NICE), 2003; RCOG, 2006a).
- Following TBT the RCOG (2006b) advises, 'Women should be advised that planned (breech) CS carries a reduced perinatal mortality and early neonatal morbidity . . . compared with planned vaginal birth', but the TBT trial has been criticised for clinical and methodological flaws. Later follow-up of TBT babies shows fewer perinatal deaths with planned CS were balanced by more babies with neurodevelopmental delay (Whyte et al., 2003).
- Women should be facilitated to make an informed choice about their birth options and should not be coerced into one particular mode of delivery. These discussions should include the possible differences between a 'managed' vaginal breech birth and one 'facilitated' by a skilled practitioner.
- Midwives working in all environments should be prepared for the possibility of being the only professional around when faced with an unexpected or undiagnosed breech baby. It is, therefore, important that they are prepared to deal with this eventuality and that they have the training, knowledge and skills to assist the woman and her baby at this time (CESDI, 2000; Robinson, 2000).
- Whilst having a good heart rate, breech babies may be slower to breathe spontaneously than cephalic babies, and may require bag-and-mask resuscitation to establish breathing.

Types of breech presentation

The baby in a breech presentation will adopt a variety of positions, similar to a cephalic baby, with the sacrum being the denominator. Table 13.1 describes different breech presentations.

Women's options and the provision of care

The midwife needs to explore his/her own feelings and prejudices and remain unbiased and non-judgemental, acting in a manner that will facilitate both informed choice and decision making as well as enabling the woman to access appropriate care.

- Explore the options – ECV, vaginal breech birth, and CS; home or hospital.
- Women can choose who assists at the birth: an NHS midwife, an independent midwife or an obstetrician.
- Discuss the possible difference between a vaginal breech birth that is 'managed' and one that is 'facilitated' by a skilled practitioner/midwife. Managed/medicalised breech birth tends to include a package of epidural anaesthesia, routine episiotomy and lithotomy position for the delivery. A facilitated birth encourages the breech

Table 13.1 Types of breech presentation.

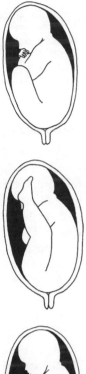

Complete (flexed or full breech)
Incidence: 10% of term and preterm breeches (Frye, 2004)

The baby sits cross-legged with flexed knees and hips: feet are tucked up against its bottom

This position is most common in multigravidae

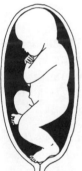

Extended (incomplete or frank breech)
Incidence: 45–50% (AAFP, 2004) or 60–70% (Frye, 2004) of term breeches

The baby's legs are flexed at the hip but with straight knees: the legs lie alongside the trunk

This position is most common in primigravidae near term as knee flexion is restricted by firm uterine and abdominal muscles

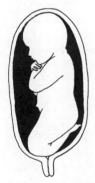

Footling
Incidence: 20–25% of preterm breeches and 10–20% (Frye, 2004) or 35–45% (AAFP, 2004) of term breeches

One or both knees and/or hips are extended with one or more feet below the buttocks

Knee/kneeling
Incidence: <5% of term breeches (Frye, 2004)

One or both hips are extended and the knees are flexed: the knees are at the height of or below the buttocks

This is the rarest presentation

Others
Occasionally a presentation may be compound, e.g. one leg footling, the other extended

baby to birth through supporting the woman in upright postures and only inter-vening should a direct indication arise.

- Choice may be restricted due to 'local policy' or a lack of suitably skilled practition-ers.
- Where a hospital is unable to safely offer the woman the option of a vaginal breech birth, she should be referred to another hospital where this choice is available (RCOG, 2006b).

Self-help measures

A woman may wish to try self-help measures to turn a breech antenatally, thus pro-moting a feeling of active involvement and enabling her to retain a feeling of active participation in her situation. Methods include postural management, e.g. knee-chest position and pelvic rocking, visualisation, swimming, massage, talking to her baby as well as complementary therapies such as hypnotherapy, homeopathy, acupuncture, acupressure, moxibustion, chiropractic or osteopathic intervention. There is little hard evidence for any of these methods. Only acupuncture and moxibustion have under-gone randomised controlled trials (Neri *et al.*, 2004; Coyle *et al.*, 2005). Whilst these results look promising, the evidence base is still incomplete for these and all self-help/complementary measures.

External cephalic version

All women should be offered information about the safety and benefits of ECV at term. When it is undertaken by a trained operator, the success rate will be around 50%; however, this rate may vary from 30 to 80% and depend on a number of factors includ-ing engagement of the breech, liquor volume, uterine tone, race and parity (RCOG, 2006a).

- The success rate of ECV may be increased by the use of tocolysis (RCOG, 2006a).
- Following successful ECV, spontaneous reversion to breech presentation is said to be less than 5% (Impey & Lissoni, 1999).
- Hofmeyr (2000) suggests that even when a breech presentation is encountered in labour and the membranes remain intact, the limited data available indicates that ECV performed with tocolysis has a reasonable success rate.
- Rhesus negative women who have ECV performed should be offered anti-D pro-phylaxis (NICE, 2002).

Caesarean section

Many obstetricians now recommend CS for breech presentation regardless of individ-ual circumstances. This is primarily due to the TBT (Hannah *et al.*, 2000), which reported an increased 1% mortality risk and 2.4% early neonatal morbidity risk in breech vagi-nal delivery over CS. Hannah *et al.* concluded: 'planned caesarean section is better than planned vaginal birth for the term fetus in the breech presentation'. Whilst this recom-mendation has been largely accepted and implemented by obstetricians, others have challenged it (Robinson, 2000/2001; Banks, 2001; Gyte, 2001; Lancet Correspondence, 2001). One criticism is that the 'vaginal' breech deliveries in the TBT were dorsal 'managed' breech extractions, and women were not allowed to labour in upright positions. Some women also moved from their randomised groups, potentially confounding the result. Glezerman (2006) concludes that in the light of serious methodological and clinical flaws 'the original term breech trial recommendations should be withdrawn'. Alarab *et al.* (2004) state that with strict selection criteria, adherence to a careful intrapartum protocol and an experienced obstetrician in attendance a vaginal breech delivery at term can be achieved safely.

In a 2-year follow-up study to the TBT (Whyte *et al.*, 2003), an unexpectedly high number of babies born by breech CS showed later neurodevelopmental delay, which balanced the smaller numbers of perinatal deaths in that group. Another observational prospective study with an intent-to-treat analysis demonstrated a lower mortality and morbidity than the TBT (Goffinet *et al.*, 2006).

The practice of CS for breech babies in the belief that it is safer may become a self-fulfilling prophecy as attendants become less skilled in vaginal breech birth. With a rising breech CS rate too, few clinicians have vaginal breech experience (RCOG, 1999, 2006b). It is to be hoped that in the next few years, the debate following the TBT will lead to a better understanding of breech issues, and that women will not be pressured into CS without proper consideration of the relative risks.

Extracts from RCOG (2006b) Guidelines for the Management of Breech Presentation state that:

- Women should be fully informed on all aspects relating to breech birth both for current and future pregnancies and have careful assessment before selection for vaginal breech birth.
- Induction of labour may be considered if individual circumstances are favourable.
- Augmentation in labour is not advisable. Slow progress at any stage should be considered as possible fetopelvic disproportion, and a CS may then be indicated.
- Routine CS for a preterm breech baby should not be advised.
- Diagnosis of breech presentation during labour should not be a contraindication for vaginal breech birth.
- In a twin pregnancy where the first baby is breech, it is suggested that the data relating to a singleton breech can be used to aid decision making. Where the second twin is breech, the RCOG (2006b) states that routine CS should not be performed. (For more information on twins see Chapter 14.)

Midwives are strongly advised to read and evaluate all the literature for themselves. It may also fall to them to inform colleagues, managers and obstetricians of current national guidelines.

Concerns and possible complications with a breech birth

Hypoxia

Hypoxia has been identified as the commonest cause of death in breech babies. CESDI (2000) suggests that lack of recognition and inaction are major factors.

Umbilical cord prolapse

Incidence: 3.7% in breech (Confino *et al.*, 1985).
  Umbilical cord prolapse is

- More frequent in primigravidae than multigravidae (6% and 3%, respectively).
- More common in premature labour and incomplete presentations (e.g. footling).
- More common where artificial rupture of membranes (ARM) is performed, which increases the incidence of cord compression.

Prolapse does not always cause cord compression. Where the cervix is fully dilated, a vaginal birth may still be possible (see Chapter 16).

Entrapment of aftercoming head

Incidence: 0–8.5% at term (Cheng & Hannah, 1993).
  It is thought that if the diameters of a baby's bottom are smaller than those of its head it is more likely to pass through a cervix that is not fully dilated. This may result in the entrapment of the aftercoming head behind a partially open cervix.
  However, the specific presentation of the breech baby appears significant. It is now suggested that the diameters of the term breech baby's bottom will be the same size as the head (Stevenson, 1993), with the bitrochanteric diameter measuring around 9 cm, similar to the average biparietal diameter of 9.5 cm (Frye, 2004).

- 'If the frank or complete breech passes easily through the pelvis, the head can be expected to follow without difficulty' (Hofmeyr, 2000).
- In a term baby, if the head is not going to pass through the cervix and pelvis, the buttocks would also be obstructed and labour will not progress (Hofmeyr, 2001 citing Gebbie, 1982).
- Entrapment is more common in a preterm baby (Stevenson, 1993) and may be related to maternal pushing being encouraged prior to, or following, misdiagnosis of full dilatation.

Hyperextension of the baby's head (star gazing)

Incidence: 5% (Confino *et al.*, 1985).
  If hyperextension of the head is detected by ultrasound scan (USS) at term, a CS will be advised.
  Hyperextension may occur due to:

- Cord around baby's neck
- Placental location
- Muscle spasm in baby
- Abnormalities in either the uterus or the baby
- May be caused in labour by unnecessary intervention of the carer. Spontaneous pushing, not traction, should be encouraged; traction may cause extension of the baby's arms and head (Hofmeyr, 2000).

Head and neck trauma

Forceful traction by the carer may cause iatrogenic brain and spinal injuries (Banks, 1998).

Premature placental separation

This may be linked to maternal position in the second stage of labour, especially where the woman adopts a fully upright position. This is due to the centre of gravity being higher in a breech than in a cephalic birth, resulting in more traction being placed on the cord and placenta by gravity (Cronk, 1998).

Labour and birth

Preparation/birth planning

Frank and open discussion between the midwife, the woman and her partner, where all options available are explored, will help the woman reach a decision about whether or not to have a vaginal breech birth. It may also clarify issues for the woman and enable her to develop an appropriate and individual birth plan.

Points to consider include the following:

- The baby is in a good position and not considered too large.
- A skilled and competent midwife will support the woman in a breech birth.
- The woman, her partner and the midwife are informed regarding the anticipated process and progress of a breech labour and birth.
- The woman has confidence in her body and her midwife.
- Good communication between the woman and the midwife at all times.

The midwife's role

- To support the woman in her innate ability to birth her baby.
- To have confidence in the woman's ability to birth her baby.
- Not to 'manage' the woman's care or labour process, encourage and enable the woman to respond intuitively and to express her own needs and wishes.
- To ensure and maintain a sound knowledge of skills and techniques to assist a breech birth, should it become necessary.
- To recognise, assess and respond to problems, should they occur.
- To act as advocate for the woman at all times.

It is important that midwives ensure they have appropriate support for themselves. Having a colleague present who is experienced in non-medicalised breech birth will provide support for the midwife.

Mechanisms of a breech birth

Midwives should refer to a suitable textbook to familiarise themselves with the various mechanisms. A very detailed and comprehensive description, supported by diagrams, can be found in the book by Anne Frye (2004).

Onset of labour

Midwifery care and support is the same as for any labour.

- With maternal consent, palpate the abdomen to check that the presentation and position of the baby has not changed.
- Banks (1998) suggests that a vaginal assessment in early breech labour is important to determine the presenting part and to exclude cord, foot, knee or compound presentation. This should be carried out with the woman's consent and awareness of the purpose of the examination. She should be advised that it is expected that cervical dilatation may be minimal at this stage to avoid her feeling demotivated.
- Cooper (1992) suggests that the presenting part is often higher in the pelvis than the midwife would expect with a cephalic presentation, and that the station is likely to go up and down more during labour.
- If the woman is examined in a semi-recumbent position, assist her into an upright position immediately afterwards to avoid problems such as postural hypotension, fetal heart rate (FHR) irregularities and slowing of labour progress (Sleep *et al.*, 2000; Gupta *et al.*, 2004).

Pain management

Encourage the woman to apply skills she may have learnt antenatally such as relaxation, visualisation, vocalisation and mobility. Use massage, TENS, support and so on.

The use of a birthing pool is controversial and needs to be explored on an individual basis according to the wishes of the woman, the experience of the individual midwife and the place of the birth. The benefits of water are well documented (see Chapter 3), and those benefits, it could be argued, would be of use to a woman having a spontaneous vaginal breech birth, especially in the first stage of labour. This may prove challenging for both the woman and her carer where local guidelines on the use of a birthing pool exclude any presentation other than cephalic.

Midwives interested in exploring the use of water in breech presentation (and other unusual situations) may find work by Dr Herman Ponette in Belgium and Cornelia Enning in Germany helpful (see 'Useful contacts').

There is no evidence that the routine use of an epidural is appropriate in a vaginal breech birth; women should have a choice of analgesia (RCOG, 2006b). However, obstetricians may recommend it believing that it may prevent the premature urge to push and also enable them to carry out obstetric manoeuvres. This may be acceptable to the woman and be part of her decision-making process. Women need to be fully informed of the risks and benefits of an epidural including the restrictions it may place on them in terms of mobility and the inability to adopt upright positions to facilitate a breech birth.

First stage

- Care and observations are the same as for a cephalic birth:
  - Avoid unnecessary vaginal examinations (VEs)
  - Food and drink as desired by the individual woman
  - Encourage regular emptying of the bladder

Also use midwifery skills to monitor alternative signs of progress (see Chapter 1).

- There may be a long latent phase due to a lack of application of the presenting part to the cervix, but progress may escalate rapidly once an active first stage is reached.
- The woman may feel breathless during or after contractions due to the pressure of the baby's head against her diaphragm. She may experience the pain more in her back than the front.
- Multigravidae may experience little or no discomfort in early labour; it is not unusual for the cervix to be 4 cm dilated before they become aware they are in labour (El Halta, 1989).
- No ARM. If membranes rupture spontaneously, do a vaginal examination to exclude cord prolapse, foot or knee presentation, and check the fetal heart for any effects of cord compression.
- No augmentation of labour.
- The RCOG (2006b) states that continuous electronic fetal monitoring (EFM) should be offered to women with a breech presentation in labour, and local guidelines/policy may reflect this. Advancements in fetal monitoring equipment and the provision of systems that can provide continuous waterproof EFM have already been developed and are available (Price, 2001).
- A woman may choose or decline to comply with unit policy EFM. If used, do so in a way to encourage mobility rather than restrict it.
- Fetal blood sampling from the buttocks is not advised (RCOG, 2006b).
- A premature urge to push is unlikely in the term breech baby. The hip size in an extended or flexed breech baby is likely to equal the head size (Stevenson, 1993).

Second stage

A latent phase may occur, as with cephalic birth, between full dilatation and the spontaneous urge to push. The woman will often doze during this period. Second-stage contractions are often less frequent, shorter and less powerful. Maternal anal dilatation and pressure may 'diagnose' the second stage, or a VE may be used to confirm full dilatation. In principle, remember 'hands off the breech'. Just watch, wait and support. If a baby requires assistance, refer to Table 13.2 for assisted breech delivery techniques.

- Multigravidae may experience the sensation and 'feel' the descent of the baby as being different to a previous cephalic baby.
- Meconium is to be expected due to the pressure on the baby's buttocks. Its presence does not necessarily indicate that the baby is, or has been, distressed (Hulme, 1992). However, Frye (2004) suggests that if is evident prior to 6 cm dilatation, it should be considered as a possible sign of fetal compromise.
- When the buttocks reach the perineum, it may be necessary to do an episiotomy if it is tight or rigid and not stretching despite good contractions and maternal effort, or to expedite the birth for fetal compromise. The RCOG (2006b) supports the use of selective rather than routine episiotomy in breech birth.
- Banks (1998) suggests that if the membranes are intact, they should be broken when the buttocks reach the perineum to allow any meconium to drain from the vagina. However, the close fit of the baby's bottom in the vagina usually prevents meconium from getting to the liquor around the baby's head.

- A rocking or up-and-down motion during the descent of the baby's bottom ('rumping') is the same process as that of 'crowning' (Stevenson, 1993).

The birth

- No touching unless absolutely necessary or there is a complication (see Table 13.2 for techniques to assist a breech birth).
- Extended legs look never-ending but usually flop out on their own, shortly followed by the arms (Cronk, 1998).
- When born to the umbilicus, the cord may be compressed between the baby's head and maternal pelvis (both bony). Wharton's jelly affords some protection but expect the FHR to be slower. The lower heart rate is also due to the reduction in the placental site and thought to be an automatic reflex to conserve oxygen in the baby (Stevenson, 1993).
- If there is tension, a loop of cord may be brought down, but handle gently to avoid stimulating constriction and thus reducing oxygen to the baby.
- Allow the baby's body to take some of the weight. This will bring the chin on to the perineum, followed by the birth of the head.
- The midwife can give gentle support either by placing her hand under the buttocks, the baby 'sitting' in her hand, or by supporting the baby by the hips. This may be necessary, in some situations, to slow the birth of the head, prevent sudden decompression and thus avoid a tentorial tear or perineal trauma.
- When born to the nape of the neck, the heart rate can be felt or observed over the baby's chest.
- Flexion (chin-to-chest) of the baby's head may be assisted by gently placing a finger on the back of the baby's head (occiput) and with the other hand gently placing two fingers on the baby's cheekbones. Inserting a finger in the baby's mouth is no longer recommended as traction on the jaw may cause dislocation (American Academy of Family Physicians (AAFP), 2004).

There is divided opinion over optimal positions for vaginal breech birth, as the subject has been under-researched. Midwives should encourage and enable the woman to adopt whatever position is best for her. Box 13.1 summarises the basic positions.

Assisted breech birth

Many midwives used to be taught that assisted breech manoeuvres were the only way to deliver a breech, and they are still favoured by many obstetricians, although even the RCOG (2006b) does not now recommend them routinely over spontaneous birth. However, these techniques may be used to assist the birth of the baby's head if descent is very slow/arrested, or where legs, arms or head have become extended (Table 13.2).

The baby at birth

It is important to remember, and discuss with parents, that the mechanism of a breech birth is different from that of a cephalic baby and their appearance and response are

Box 13.1 Maternal positions for labour and birth.

In the absence of conclusive research in breech birth positions, the following are suggested:

Squatting
- Expands the pelvic outlet.
- Advocated by Odent (1984) as being mechanically efficient, gravity reduces the delay between delivery of the baby's umbilicus and its head. Less likely to need intervention to assist birth.
- Squatting (even supported) is tiring and may need to be practised during pregnancy.
- Squatting may increase blood loss (but this may be due to ease of measuring it).

Standing
- Believed by some to be more natural physiological position as gravity aids descent.
- Cronk (1998) speculates that standing:
  - Causes a quicker birth which may cause rapid head decompression.
  - May encourage the babies' arms to be swept over its head, complicating their delivery and risking Erb's palsy.
  - May increase traction on cord and placenta risking early separation and/or hypoxia.
- As the baby's body hangs straight down, this may encourage a deflexed head.
- May increase perineal tearing and blood loss.

Hands and knees (all fours)
- Complements the attitude and angle of the uterus.
- Allows the baby's body and arms to manoeuvre naturally.
- Gravity helps the baby descend.
- Prevents undue traction or pressure on the placenta or cord.
- Facilitates the birth of the baby's head.

likely to be different. This may be reflected in a lower 1-min Apgar score in breech babies born vaginally (Thorpe-Beeston *et al.*, 1992).

Cephalic babies often 'rest' between the birth of the head and the body allowing adjustment from compression to decompression of the head. This does not occur with a breech birth, and this may be a factor in the occasional need for resuscitation. Breech babies may be slower than cephalic babies to breathe spontaneously and may initially have lax muscle tone and poor reflexes whilst having a good heart rate. A bag and mask or a resuscitaire should be on hand and ready to use if necessary. Whilst the baby is still on the pulsating cord, it is receiving oxygen from the mother if the placenta remains attached to the uterine wall.

The best place to give supportive measures, if required, is in the mother's arms to enable her to stimulate the baby by voice and touch. If more extensive measures are required, they should be carried out close to the mother (for more detail see Chapter 17).

Third stage

This should be conducted according to the woman's wishes, subject to events and discussion (see Chapter 1). Oxytocics should be withheld until the birth of the baby's head is completed.

Table 13.2 Techniques for an assisted breech birth.

Burns Marshall manoeuvre
- Baby 'hangs' by its own weight to encourage descent and flexion of the head. Avoid the head delivering too quickly.
- When the nape of the neck and hairline are visible, grasp the baby's ankles in one hand and lift the body in an arc over the mother's abdomen.
- Use the other hand to support the perineum and avoid sudden delivery of the head.
- Once the mouth is clear, the baby will be able to breathe. Allow the rest of the head to deliver slowly.

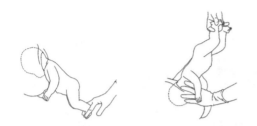

Mauriceau–Smellie–Veit manoeuvre
- This is useful if the hairline does not become visible after the baby has been allowed to support its weight briefly, i.e. the head may have become extended.
- Straddle the baby on one arm – usually the left in a right-handed individual.
- Gently place a finger on the back of the baby's head (occiput) and with the other hand gently place two fingers on the baby's cheekbones to assist flexion if necessary. Putting a finger in the baby's mouth is no longer recommended as it can cause jaw fracture (AAFP, 2004).
- A second person can apply suprapubic pressure if necessary.
- Now place two outer fingers of the other hand over the baby's shoulders with the middle finger on the occiput to assist and maintain flexion.

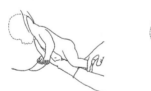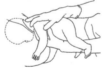

Extended legs
- If the legs appear to be splinting the body, preventing lateral flexion of the trunk, place a finger in each of the baby's groins and apply gentle traction until the backs of the knees are visible.
- Apply popliteal pressure to abduct and flex the knees.

Extended arms: Lovset's manoeuvre
- The arms are swept up alongside the head. This may occur when the head delivers rapidly or when traction has been applied to deliver the trunk.
- Grasp the baby's thighs with your thumbs over the sacrum.
- Keep the back uppermost and pull the baby gently downwards.
- At the same time rotate the baby through 180° to bring the posterior shoulder anteriorly, beneath the symphysis pubis.
- Friction of the arm against the pelvic wall will bring the arm down to be released.
- Release the other arm by repeating the manoeuvre in the opposite direction.

Summary

- *Hands off the breech* – damage is often a result of too much force being used.
- No unnecessary VEs.
- No 'routine' ARM; if spontaneous rupture of membranes, check no cord/foot is presenting.
- Avoid epidurals.
- Enable women to adopt positions spontaneously.
- No augmentation: if there is poor progress, consider CS.
- Check FHR regularly and act appropriately.
- Enable women to push spontaneously; give guidance if necessary.
- Meconium is to be expected.
- Episiotomy only if felt necessary.
- Breech babies may be slower to breathe spontaneously than cephalic – be prepared.
- Conduct third stage as the woman wishes, unless contraindicated.
- Ensure that you are well supported by like-minded people.
- Enjoy and celebrate the birth!

Useful contacts

Association for Improvements in the Maternity Services (AIMS)   Helpline: 0870 765 1433. Website: www.aims.org.uk.

Birthspirit Ltd.   Website: www.birthspirit.co.nz

Cornelia Enning   (a German midwife who has championed water birth) Website: www.hebinfo.de/ (website in German but good pictures).

Dr Herman Ponette   (a Belgian obstetrician with a medicalised approach to water birth, but still very interesting) Website: www.helsinki.fi/~lauhakan/whale/waterbaby/p0.html

Henry Serruys Hospital, Oostende, Belgium   Telephone: 058 51 15 58. Hospital that specialises in water birth including expertise in breech birth in water.

Independent Midwives Association   Telephone: 01483 821104. Website: www.independentmidwives.org.uk

National Childbirth Trust (NCT)   Enquiry line: 0870 444 8707. Website: www.nct-online.org

References

American Academy of Family Physicians (AAFP) (2004) *Advanced Life Support in Obstetrics (ALSO)*. Course Syllabus Manual, 4th edn. American Academy of Family Physicians, Leawood, Kansas.

Alarab, M., Regan, C., O'Connell, M.P., Keane, D.P., O'Herlihy, M.D. & Foley, M. (2004) Singleton vaginal breech delivery at term: still a safe option. *Obstetrics & Gynecology* **103**, 407–12.

Banks, M. (1998) *Breech Birth Woman Wise*. Birthspirit Books, Hamilton, New Zealand.

Banks, M. (2001) *Breech Birth Beyond the Term Breech Trial*. Birthspirit. Available at: www.birthspirit.co.nz (accessed March 2008).

Carayol, M., Blondel, B., Zeitlin, J., Breart, G. & Goffinet, F. (2007) Changes in the rates of caesarean delivery before labour for breech presentational term in France:

1972–2003. *European Journal of Obstetrics and Gynaecology and Reproductive Biology* **132** (1), 20–26.

CESDI (2000) *Confidential Enquiry into Stillbirths and Deaths in Infancy*, 7th Annual Report. Maternal and Child Health Research Consortium, London.

Cheng, M. & Hannah, M. (1993) Breech delivery at term: a critical review of the literature. *Obstetrics and Gynaecology* **82** (4), 605–18.

Confino, E., Gleicher, N., Elrad, H., Isajovich, B. & David, M.P. (1985) The breech dilemma – a review. *Obstetrical and Gynaecological Survey* **40** (6), 330–37.

Cooper, M. (1992) *Twins, Breech and VBAC (Audiotape)*. Midwifery Today, Eugene, Oregon.

Coyle, M.E., Smith, C.A. & Peat, B. (2005) Cephalic version by moxibustion for breech presentation (Cochrane Review). *The Cochrane Database of Systematic Reviews*, Issue 2.

Cronk, M. (1998) Birthing a baby by the breech. *AIMS Journal* **10** (3), 6–8.

El Halta, V. (1989) Advanced midwifery seminar: moving midwifery forward: essays and outlines, workshop manual. Garden of Life, Dearborn MI. Care during labor and birth. In *Holistic Midwifery. A Comprehensive Textbook for Midwives in Home Birth Practice*, Vol. 11 (Frye, A., ed.), p. 937. Labrys Press, Portland, Oregon.

Frye, A. (2004) Care during labor and birth. In *Holistic Midwifery. A Comprehensive Textbook for Midwives in Home Birth Practice*, Vol. 11. Labrys Press, Portland, Oregon.

Glezerman, M. (2006) Five years to the term breech trial: the rise and fall of a randomized controlled trial. *American Journal of Obstetrics and Gynaecology* **194**, 20–25.

Goffinet, F., Caroyal, M., Foidart, J.M., Alexander, S., Uzan, S., Subtil, D. & Breart, G. (2006) PREMODA Study Group. Is planned vaginal delivery for breech presentation at term still an option? Results of an observational prospective study in France and Belgium. *American Journal of Obstetrics and Gynaecology* **194**, 1002–11.

Gupta, J., Hofmeyr, G. & Smyth, R. (2004) Position in the second stage of labour for women without epidural anaesthesia. *The Cochrane Database of Systematic Reviews*, Issue 1.

Gyte, G. (2001) Planned caesarean section versus planned vaginal birth for breech presentation at term: a randomised multicentre trial. *MIDIRS Midwifery Digest* **11** (1), 80–83.

Hannah, M.E., Hannah, W.J., Hewson, S.A., Hodnett, E.D., Saigal, S. & Willan, A.R. (2000) Planned caesarean section versus vaginal birth for breech presentation at term: a randomised multicentre trial. *The Lancet* **356**, 1375–83.

Hofmeyr, G.J. (2000) Suspected fetalpelvic disproportion and abnormal lie. In *A Guide to Effective Care in Pregnancy and Childbirth* (Enkin, M., Keirse, M.J.N.C., Neilson, J., Crowther, C., Duley L., Hodnett, E. & Hofmeyr, J., eds), pp. 185–95. Oxford University Press, Oxford.

Hofmeyr, G.J. (2001) Abnormal fetal presentation and position. In *Turnbull's Obstetrics* (Chamberlain, G. & Steer, P., eds), p. 557. Churchill Livingstone, Edinburgh.

Hulme, H. (1992) Meconium aspiration syndrome: reflections on a midwifery subject. *MIDIRS Midwifery Digest* **2** (2), 177.

Impey, L. & Lissoni, D. (1999) Outcome of external cephalic version after 36 weeks gestation without tocolysis. *Journal of Maternal and Fetal Medicine* **8**, 203–207.

Lancet Correspondence (2001) Term breech trial. *The Lancet* **357** (9251), 225–8.

National Institute for Health and Clinical Excellence (NICE) (2002) *Technology Appraisal Guidance No 41: Guidance on the Use of Routine Anti-D Prophylaxis for RhD-negative Women*. National Institute for Health and Clinical Excellence, London.

National Institute for Health and Clinical Excellence (NICE) (2003) *Clinical Guideline 6. Antenatal Care: Routine Care for the Healthy Pregnant Woman*, p. 22. National Institute for Health and Clinical Excellence, London.

Neri, I., Airola, G., Contu, G., Allais, F., Fachinetti, F. & Benedettoo, C. (2004) Acupuncture plus moxibustion to resolve breech presentation: a randomised controlled study. *Journal of Maternal, Fetal and Neonatal Medicine* **15** (4), 247–52.

Odent, M. (1984) *Birth Reborn*. Souvenir Press, London.

Price, S. (2001) Electronic fetal monitoring equipment. *British Journal of Midwifery* **9** (9), 579–82.

Robinson, J. (2000) Midwives need training in the lost art of breech birth. *British Journal of Midwifery* **8** (7), 447.

Robinson, J. (2000/2001) Breech babies – caesarean or vaginal birth? *AIMS Journal* **12** (4), 12–13.

Royal College of Obstetricians and Gynaecologists (RCOG) (1999) *Effective Procedures in Maternity Care Suitable for Audit. 4.7 Breech Presentation at Term*. Royal College of Obstetricians and Gynaecologists: Clinical Audit Unit, RCOG Press, London.

Royal College of Obstetricians and Gynaecologists (RCOG) (2001) Clinical Effectiveness Support Unit. *National Sentinel Caesarean Section Audit Report*. RCOG, London.

Royal College of Obstetricians and Gynaecologists (RCOG) (2006a) *External Cephalic Version and Reducing the Incidence of Breech Presentation. Guideline No. 20a*. RCOG, London.

Royal College of Obstetricians and Gynaecologists (RCOG) (2006b) *The Management of Breech Presentation. Guideline No. 20b*. RCOG, London.

Royal College of Obstetricians and Gynaecologists (RCOG) (2007) TOG release: planned vaginal breech delivery births – choice or safety? *The Obstetrician & Gynaecologist*. RCOG, London.

Schutte, J.M., Steegers, A.P., Santema, J., Schuitemaker, N. & Van Roosemalen, J. (2007) Maternal deaths after elective caesarean section for breech presentation in the Netherlands. *Acta Ocstetricia et Gynecologica Scandinavica* **86** (2), 240–43.

Sleep, J., Roberts, J. & Chalmers, I. (2000) The second stage of labor. In *A Guide to Effective Care in Pregnancy and Childbirth*, 3rd edn (Enkin, M., Keirse, M.J.N.C., Neilson, J., Crowther, C., Duley L., Hodnett, E. & Hofmeyr, J., eds), pp. 289–99. Oxford University Press, Oxford.

Stevenson, J. (1993) More thoughts on breech. *Midwifery Today*, **26**, 24–5.

Thorpe-Beeston, J.G., Blanfield, P.J. & Saunders, N.J.S. (1992) Outcome of breech delivery at term. *British Medical Journal* **305**, 746–7.

Whyte, H., Hannah, M. & Saigal, S. (2003) Term Breech Trial Collaborative Group. Outcomes of children at 2 years of age in the term breech trial. *American Journal of Obstetrics and Gynaecology* **189**, 857.

14   Twins and higher-order births

Jo Coggins

Introduction

The news of a multiple pregnancy is often met with delight by both mothers and mid-wives. The rarity of twins and higher-order births ensures that they remain a somewhat special phenomenon. However, it can be a daunting time for women as they may feel their choices are swept away by a plethora of obstetric concerns and interventions. Midwives have a key role in limiting this by advocating women's choices and ensuring that medical intervention is reserved only for those who need it.

Incidence and facts

- In the UK approximately 1 in 67 pregnancies results in a multiple birth (ONS, 2004).
- Twin birth rates have increased in recent years due to advances in fertility treatment.
- In the UK one-third of twins are monozygotic (identical) and two-thirds are dizygotic (non-identical).
- Monoygotic twins occur when one fertilised ovum splits during the early stages of pregnancy. There are no known causal factors.
- Dizygotic twins occur when the mother produces two ova during her menstrual cycle, which are fertilised separately. Rates are influenced by age, parity, race and family history (Blickstein, 2005).
- The presence of one placenta (for monozygotic twins) or two (for dizygotic twins) may be inaccurate for determining zygosity as one-third of monozygotic twins develop with separate placentae. Usually monozygotic twins have one chorion and two amnions, but DNA testing is the only accurate test for zygosity (Twins and Multiple Births Association (TAMBA), 2006a).

- The incidence of triplets and higher-order births is comparatively low (159 triplet births throughout the UK in 2005 and just 2 quadruplet births) (ONS, 2004).
- The average gestation at birth is 37 weeks for twins, 33 weeks for triplets and 31 weeks for quads.
- Multiple pregnancies are associated with increased risks for both mothers and babies. For mothers, these include pre-eclampsia, antepartum haemorrhage, preterm delivery and caesarean section (CS) amongst others. Babies are more likely to be of low birth weight and require admission to neonatal intensive care unit (NICU)/special care baby unit (SCBU) (Jolly *et al.*, 2000).

Place of delivery

The risks associated with multiple pregnancies are generally accepted to be greater than those of singletons. Stillbirth risk for twins is more than twice that of a singleton, and greater still for triplets (TAMBA, 2007). Neonatal morbidity and mortality is also higher. However, as obstetric litigation increases, obstetricians can place disproportionate emphasis on these risks when counselling women. Consequently, most women choose consultant-led units for delivery (Kalish & Skupski, 2002). For some though the idea of a hospital birth and the interventions likely to accompany, it contradicts the ethos of 'normal birth', and they choose homebirth. Women considering this option may benefit from the care of an independent midwife, who may have more experience in caring for women with multiple births at home.

Mode of delivery

Many women carrying twins can enjoy safe vaginal births (El Halta (1996) cited by Evans (2000)). However, a lack of research into higher-order births results in practice varying worldwide. In the UK, where obstetricians are the lead caregiver, 59% of all twins and almost all triplets and higher-order births deliver by elective CS (Kalish & Skupski, 2002). This begs the question: 'Are women offered true choice or are their decisions swayed by obstetricians who lean towards a more medical view of birth?'

A woman's choice regarding twin birth is usually influenced by the presentation of the babies. Most commonly, they present vertex/vertex (~40%), followed by vertex/non-vertex (~30%), non-vertex/vertex (~20%) and non-vertex/non-vertex (~10%) (Blickstein, 2005). Historically, obstetricians have recommended CS for any woman whose leading twin is non-vertex. However, evidence suggests that other factors are of greater or equal importance in determining a safe vaginal delivery, such as predicted birth weights (Blickstein, 2005).

Triplet and quadruplet birth

In the UK, almost all triplets and quadruplets are delivered operatively (Kalish & Skupski, 2002). It is unclear whether this is due to lack of an evidence base or because of rising litigation. Interestingly, evidence from studies in other countries, including USA, concludes outcomes for mothers and babies are improved by vaginal delivery, providing it is in a hospital and attended by appropriately skilled clinicians (Grobman *et al.*, 1998). This is mainly due to a reduction in post-operative complications for mothers and a lower incidence of respiratory distress syndrome in babies. Sheppard *et al.* (1999) support this, highlighting the fact that mothers recover more quickly following vaginal birth, and are therefore better placed to begin caring for their babies. It seems UK women may be currently disadvantaged as obstetricians continue to routinely advocate elective CS for triplets and higher-order births.

Twin birth

Care in labour

Midwives' knowledge and understanding of normal birth is invaluable when caring for a mother of twins in labour. This is sometimes a difficult role, as the midwife must act as an advocate for the mother whilst working alongside obstetric colleagues. The key is to remember that women's choice is the priority and that those who feel empowered to make informed decisions are more likely to feel at ease and have a positive outcome.

If the birth is in hospital, women may wish to look around the unit at some stage during their pregnancy. A tour of NICU/SCBU may be appreciated as around 50% of twins and almost all triplets will require admission (TAMBA, 2006b). This is mainly due to low birth weight resulting from prematurity. Prematurity is one of the most significant risks associated with multiple pregnancies, and midwives must be aware of the implications when caring for women in labour (see Chapter 12).

In hospital, when the woman is in labour the midwife should inform the relevant professionals. The birthing room should be prepared adequately with equipment checked and accessible. Instrumental delivery or theatre preparation equipment should be nearby but not visible as this may disturb the birthing environment and concern the woman unnecessarily. Likewise, in the absence of complications, there is little need for anyone other than the attending midwife to be in the room, usually joined by a second midwife during the second stage.

Care during the first stage of labour should be similar to that offered to any woman. A calm, kind midwife who offers appropriate explanations and plenty of praise and reassurance will help ensure the woman feels safe and confident. There are some special considerations for twin mothers:

- **Positioning.** The woman should be comfortable and able to mobilise freely, maintaining an upright position to aid labour progress. The increased uterine size in a multiple pregnancy can cause considerable discomfort, and frequent changes of position may be needed.
- **Intravenous (IV) cannulation.** In many hospitals it is routine practice to site an IV cannula to administer emergency drugs if complications arise. However, this is ultimately the woman's choice and should be based on her potential risk or the condition of her veins, rather than being a blanket policy.
- **Fasting.** Some obstetricians advocate fasting or fluids only to prevent gastric aspiration if a general anaesthetic is required. Johnson *et al.* (2000) contest this, as gastric aspiration is associated with poor anaesthetic technique and happens even when women have fasted. Limiting a woman's intake during labour can inhibit progress and lead to a cascade of intervention so midwives should avoid this practice. However, offering a hydrogen ion inhibitor (e.g. ranitidine, cimetidine) to encourage

rapid emptying of stomach contents may confer benefits, should an emergency CS be required (Johnson *et al.*, 2000).

- **Epidural Analgesia.** Women may feel pressured into having an epidural in case of the need for emergency procedures, e.g. cephalic version or CS. However, epidurals slow labour by reducing oxytocin levels and restricting mobility. This leads to interventions, e.g. IV oxytocin and instrumental delivery (Dickersin, 2000). The midwife should ensure that the woman is appropriately informed and support her decisions. This includes discussion regarding other suitable forms of analgesia.

Monitoring the fetal heart rates

There is much debate as to whether continuous or intermittent auscultation is the best option during a twin labour. NICE guidelines advocate continuous electronic fetal monitoring (National Institute for Health and Clinical Excellence (NICE), 2007), although the evidence underpinning this is debatable (Beech Lawrence, 2001). It is often restrictive and uncomfortable for women and is associated with increased intervention (Grant, 2000; NICE, 2007). Intermittent auscultation may be preferable although the difficulties in locating two or more heartbeats can make it impractical. In practice, midwives are usually under pressure to perform continuous cardiotocograph (CTG) although this is not always practicable either. Ultimately, women have the right to choose and may decline electronic monitoring or prefer to have only periodic CTG traces. The following points offer some guidance for both methods:

- **Intermittent auscultation**
  - ○ Both heartbeats must be heard simultaneously to ensure they are separate.
  - ○ A second midwife can help using a second pinards or another doppler device.
  - ○ Midwives should 'listen in' for up to 1 min following a contraction approximately every 15 min in the first stage and every 5 min in the second stage (NICE, 2007).
- **Electronic monitoring**
  - ○ The benefits of CTG are unproved although it is often advocated for twins and higher-order births. Midwives should ensure that women are well informed and that they have the right to decline.
  - ○ CTG should only be used in active labour as it restricts mobility and may cause unnecessary anxiety.
  - ○ Poor contact via abdominal transducers can be a problem during twin labours and may distract care away from the mother. In high-risk labours a fetal scalp electrode may be indicated (see Chapter 3).
  - ○ Electronic fetal monitoring does not require the woman to recline on the bed. Consider using a birthing ball or chair.

Second stage of labour

As the woman approaches the second stage, inform the second midwife. Unless there is concern about the mother or babies, the birthing environment should remain calm and quiet with as few people present as possible. Low lighting, relaxing music and speaking in a whispered voice will convey an atmosphere of confidence and calm to anyone entering the room. On sensing this, they are likely to adopt similar behaviour, causing minimal disturbance to the woman at this pivotal moment.

Birth of the first twin

The birth of the first baby should take place as any other, and providing this goes well, it should be placed skin-to-skin with the mother, leaving the umbilical cord unclamped and able to pulsate. It is now important to auscultate the second baby's heartbeat intermittently or by CTG as appropriate.

Birth of the second twin

The mother's contractions usually resume in due course and the presenting part of the second twin begins its descent into the pelvis. Evans (2000) postulates this interval between births is nature's way of giving the mother time to greet her first baby before the second is born. In the absence of complications, midwives should protect this special time between the woman and baby by ensuring that unnecessary interventions are avoided.

The interval between the birth of the first and second twin is when emergency procedures are most often required (Levin & Levy, 2005). Complications at this stage usually derive from malpresentation or cord damage/prolapse. One study reported an emergency CS rate of 9.25% for the second twin, due mainly to malpresentation followed by fetal distress (Wen *et al.*, 2004). Another study found that with a cephalic presentation the main complications were cord prolapse and fetal distress, increasing the risk of CS and instrumental delivery rates to 6.3 and 8.3%, respectively (Yang *et al.*, 2005). It is arguable that this is often due to unnecessary intervention, e.g. clamping/cutting the first twin's cord or artificially rupturing the membranes (ARM) of the second twin.

Midwives should consider proactive measures to aid normality:

- **Upright positioning/avoiding lithotomy.** Helping the woman into an upright position may aid the natural descent of the second twin and reduce malpresentations and positional fetal heart rate (FHR) anomalies.
- **Listening to the fetal heart.** As the second twin descends, the usual second-stage FHR changes may occur, e.g. early decelerations. However, persistent late decelerations or bradycardia may indicate malpresentation or cord prolapse. A vaginal examination (VE) may help determine this.
- **Determining the lie/presentation of the second twin.** Palpation and/or VE are commonly performed at this stage although the benefits are unclear if the FHR is normal and labour is progressing normally. Both procedures are uncomfortable and some clinicians will reserve them for situations in which there are concerns regarding the presentation or FHR of the second twin.
- **Time interval between the births.** Research is inconclusive, but if the FHR of the second twin is normal, evidence suggests 30 min is a safe cut-off due to the gradual deterioration in the arterial cord pH, although one study showed babies still had good outcomes up to an hour (McGrail & Bryant, 2005). Another study found that birth interval was only a significant predictor of Apgar score for breech second twins >1900 g, and that gestational age was the single most important predictive factor overall (Evrim *et al.*, 2003).

- **Avoid ARM.** ARM for the second twin is often practised by obstetricians but carries multiple risks, e.g. cord compression and/or prolapse (Prabulos & Philipson, 1998), FHR anomalies (Goffinet *et al.*, 1997), rupture of the first twin's cord and malpresentation/malposition of the second twin caused by balloting the presenting part away from the pelvic rim. As the risks outweigh the benefits, this practice should be avoided.

  After birth each baby and their cord should be labelled 'twin 1 or twin 2' in case anomalies are detected when examining the placentae and membranes or if cord pHs were taken. Cord clamps can be used (i.e. one for twin 1, and two for twin 2); however, an alternative method is necessary for a physiological third stage where cord clamping is contraindicated. Following this the mother can be helped into a comfortable position in which she can greet her babies and initiate their first feed.

Third stage of labour

Twin mothers are often encouraged to have an actively managed third stage due to the increased risk of postpartum haemorrhage resulting from a larger placental site (Levin & Levy, 2005). Ultimately, it is woman's right to choose, and as long as she is well informed, midwives should support her decision. Support for a physiological third stage includes helping her into an upright position and ensuring she is relaxed and unhurried. The immediate postpartum period is a precious time and should not be unnecessarily disturbed. If there is no heavy vaginal bleeding, there is no indication to augment this stage, although helping the woman into a comfortable position to breastfeed her babies is helpful. If there is sudden and continuous heavy vaginal bleeding, proceed with active management: administer an oxytocic and then apply controlled cord traction to both cords simultaneously, whilst guarding the uterus with the other hand.

Care after the birth

Care immediately following the birth should allow for the mother's private time with her new family. Inspection for perineal trauma and any necessary repair can wait if she is not bleeding. If breastfeeding, she may require help and extra pillows to achieve a comfortable position in which the babies can root and find the breast. If she wishes to have private time alone with her family, the midwife can continue the documentation outside the room. Equally, if she prefers the midwife to stay for further support or simply for reassurance, this should be respected.

Examination of the placentae and membranes is crucial to ensure none is retained by the mother. Many women are intrigued by their babies placentae; therefore, this may be done in her presence. Finally, when the mother is ready and has had refreshments, she can be helped to bathe and change into fresh clothing.

Documentation

The midwife is responsible for contemporaneous record keeping throughout the woman's labour and delivery. In the event of an emergency or circumstances preventing documentation in real time, it is important to record events in retrospect.

Summary

- Women with multiple pregnancies often need extra emotional/psychological support and should not feel their choices are swept away by obstetric concerns.
- In the UK, CS is advocated for triplets and higher-order births, yet studies in other countries conclude better maternal/neonatal outcomes with vaginal delivery.
- Multiple births carry increased risks for mothers and babies. The second twin has a small increased mortality rate due to potential second-stage complications, i.e. hypoxia, cord prolapse and malpresentation.
- Give special consideration to positioning, analgesia and fetal monitoring and labour.
- Avoid ARM of second twin
- NICE recommends CTG in active labour although the evidence base is poor.
- A physiological third stage is not always contraindicated. If no complications, the woman's choice should prevail.
- Twin mothers may require extra support to find a comfortable position for skin-to-skin and breastfeeding.

Useful contacts

The Association of Independent Midwives Telephone: 0870 850 7539. Website: www. information@independentmidwives.org.uk

The Association of Radical Midwives Telephone: 01695 572776. Website: www.radmid. demon.co.uk

The Multiple Births Association Telephone: 0208 383 3519. Website: www.multiplebirths. co.uk

The Twins and Multiple Births Association Telephone: 0800 138 0509. Website: www. tamba.org.uk

Twins UK Telephone 01670 354463. Website: www.twinsuk.co.uk

References

Beech Lawrence, B. (2001) Electronic fetal monitoring: do NICE's new guidelines owe too much to the medical model of childbirth? *The Practising Midwife* **4** (7), 31–3.

Blickstein, I. (2005) Definition of multiple pregnancy. In *Multiple Pregnancy: Epidemiology, Gestation and Perinatal Outcome*, 2nd edn (Blickstein, I. & Keith, L., eds). Taylor & Francis, London.

Dickersin, K. (2000) Control of pain in labour. In *A Guide to Effective Care in Pregnancy and Childbirth*, 3rd edn (Enkin, M., Keirse, M.J.N.C., Neilson, J., Crowther, C., Duley L., Hodnett, E. & Hofmeyr, J., eds), pp. 313–31. Oxford University Press, Oxford.

El Halta, V. (1996) A study outline of twin pregnancy, labor and delivery. *Midwifery Today* **39**, 18–19; cited by Evans, J. (2000) [updated online version] 'Can a Twin Birth be a Positive Experience?' Available at: http://www.radmid.demon.co.uk (accessed 12 January 2007).

Evans, J. (2000) *Can a Twin Birth be a Positive Experience?* [updated online version]. Available at: http://www.radmid.demon.co.uk (accessed 28 March 2007).

Evrim, E., Tamer, M., Tapisiz, O.L., Ustunyurt, E. & Caglar, E. (2003) Effect of inter-twin delivery time on Apgar score of the second twin. *Australian and New Zealand Journal of Obstetrics and Gynaecology* **43** (3), 203–206.

Goffinet, F., Fraser, W., Marcoux, S., Breart, G., Moutquin, J. & Darvis, M. (1997) Early amniotomy increases the frequency of fetal heart rate abnormalities. *British Journal of Obstetrics
and Gynaecology* **104**, 548–53.

Grant, A. (2000) Care of the fetus during labour. In *A Guide to Effective Care in Pregnancy
and Childbirth*, 3rd edn (Enkin, M., Keirse, M.J.N.C., Neilson, J., Crowther, C., Duley, L.,
Hodnett, E. & Hofmeyr, J., eds), pp. 267–80. Oxford University Press, Oxford.

Grobman, W.A., Peaceman, A.M., Haney, E., Silver, R. & MacGregor S. (1998) Neonatal
outcomes in triplet gestations after a trial of labour. *American Journal of Obstetrics and
Gynecology* **179** (4), 942–5.

Johnson, C., Keirse, M., Enkin, M. & Chalmers, I. (2000) Hospital practices – nutrition and
hydration in labour. In *A Guide to Effective Care in Pregnancy and Childbirth*, 3rd edn (Enkin,
M., Keirse, M.J.N.C., Neilson, J., Crowther, C., Duley L., Hodnett, E. & Hofmeyr, J., eds),
pp. 255–66. Oxford University Press.

Jolly, M., Sebire, N., Harris, J., Robinson, S. & Regal, L. (2000) The risks associated with
pregnancy in women over 35. *Human Reproduction* **15 (11)**, 2433–7.

Kalish, R.B. & Skupski, D.W. (2002) Delivery route in triplets. In *Triplet Pregnancies and Their
Consequences* (Keith, L. & Blickstein, I., eds). Parthenon Publishing Group, New York.

Levin, D. & levy, R. (2005) Epidemiology of bleeding and haemorrhage in multiple gestations.
In *Multiple Pregnancy: Epidemiology, Gestation and Perinatal Outcome*, 2nd edn (Blickstein,
I. & Keith, L., eds). Taylor & Francis, London.

McGrail, C.D. & Bryant, D.R. (2005) Intertwin time interval: how it affects the immediate
neonatal outcome of the second twin. *American Journal of Obstetrics and Gynecology* **192** (5),
1420–22.

National Institute for Health and Clinical Excellence (NICE) (2007) *Clinical Guideline 55:
Intrapartum Care.* National Institute for Health and Clinical Excellence, London. Available
at: www.nice.org (accessed March 2008).

Office for National Statistics (ONS) (2004) *Incidence of Multiple Births in the UK.* cited by
TAMBA (2007) [online]. *Multiple Births Fact Sheet.* Available at: http://www.tamba.org.uk
(accessed 14 September 2007).

Prabulos, A.M. & Philipson, E.H. (1998) Umbilical cord prolapse-is time from diagnosis to
delivery critical. *Journal of Reproductive Medicine* **43** (2), 129–32.

Sheppard, C., Malinow, A. & Alger, L. (1999) Vaginal delivery versus caesarean section
for triplets and quadruplets: no difference in immediate measures of neonatal outcome.
American Journal of Obstetrics and Gynecology **180** (1S–II) Supplement.

Twins and Multiple Births Association (TAMBA) (2006a) *Multiple Births Fact Sheet* [online].
Available at: http://www.tamba.org.uk (accessed 2 January 2007).

Twins and Multiple Births Association (TAMBA) (2006b) *A Midwife's Guide to Twins, Triplets
and More* [online]. Available at: http://www.tamba.org.uk (accessed 2 January 2007).

Twins and Multiple Births Association (TAMBA) (2007) *Multiple Births Factsheet* [online].
Available at: http://www.tamba.org.uk (accessed 8 January 2007).

Wen, S., Fung, K., Oppenheimer, L., Demissie, K., Yang, Q. & Walker, M. (2004) Occurrence
and predictors of caesarean delivery for the second twin following vaginal delivery of the
first. *The American Journal of Obstetrics and Gynecology* **103** (3), 413–9.

Yang, Q., Wen, S.W., Chen, Y., Krewski, D., Fung Kee Fung, K. & Walker, M. (2005) Occurrence
and clinical predictors of operative delivery for the vertex second twin after normal vaginal
delivery of the first twin. *American Journal Obstetric Gynecology* **192** (1), 178–84.

15 Haemorrhage

Sheila Miskelly

Introduction

Haemorrhage may be defined as blood loss sufficient to cause haemodynamic instability (American Academy of Family Physicians (AAFP), 2004).

Heavy bleeding in the antenatal, intrapartum or immediate post-delivery period can become a serious emergency requiring rapid action. It is a comparatively common occurrence, and every midwife will face at least one serious haemorrhage at some time in his/her career. It can be terrifying for a woman and her partner (Mapp & Hudson, 2005). Timely and methodical management usually resolves the situation, but occasionally the haemorrhage can be catastrophic, even leading to death (CEMACH, 2004).

Incidence and facts

- The death rate from haemorrhage is approximately 6.5/million materni- ties (CEMACH, 2004). The 2004 Confidential Enquiries into Maternal Deaths (CEMACH) report cites 17 deaths directly due to haemorrhage.
- Haemorrhage can occur prior to, during or following birth; it can be dramatic and sudden or slow and incipient. Slow, continuous bleeding often goes unnoticed, but may still lead to maternal death (AAFP, 2004).
- Accurate visual estimation of blood loss is known to facilitate timely resuscitation (Bose *et al.*, 2006). Blood loss >300 ml is often underestimated, with greater inaccu- racy as volume increases (World Health Organization (WHO), 2006).
- Higher-risk groups include women with placenta praevia (especially those with a previous caesarean or myomectomy scar), uterine fibroids, placental abruption or previous third-stage complications (CEMACH, 2004). A woman's risk of haemor- rhage should be assessed antenatally by the midwife. Women with increased risk should be advised to have their babies in a consultant unit with an on-site blood bank (CEMACH, 2004).

- Each unit should have a multidisciplinary massive haemorrhage protocol and regularly rehearsed drills (CEMACH, 2004; Clinical Negligence Scheme for Trusts (CNST), 2006). Practical sessions with real blood spillages may improve blood loss estimation (Bose *et al.*, 2006).
- The principles of haemorrhage management are the same whatever the setting, but *early intervention* is particularly important at home or birthing centres (see Chapter 6). On transfer give concise information to receiving clinicians as to the emergency encountered.

Placenta praevia

Placenta praevia is the abnormal implantation of the placenta in the lower uterine segment, with partial or complete coverage of the cervical os. Haemorrhage is a significant risk. Incidence rises in the third trimester with the development of the lower segment and uterine contractions.

Incidence and facts

- 0.5% of pregnancies (AAFP, 2004) of which 15% of placenta praevia are complicated by placenta accreta (McDonald, 1999).
- Four maternal deaths were cited as due to placenta praevia in the 2004 CEMACH report.
- The only safe mode of delivery for complete placenta praevia is by caesarean section (CS) as the os will be obstructed (Royal College of Obstetricians and Gynaecologists (RCOG), 2005).
- All women with placenta praevia and their partners should have antenatal discussions regarding delivery, haemorrhage and possible blood transfusion, even hysterectomy (RCOG, 2005), and their views sensitively managed.
- Placenta praevia is more common in women with a uterine scar (RCOG, 2005), previous uterine surgery (AAFP, 2004) and in multiparity (McDonald, 1999).
- Both an obstetric and an anaesthetic consultant should be available as a CS hysterectomy may become necessary due to uncontrollable haemorrhage (CEMACH, 2004). Admission is advisable when repeated bleeding occurs (CEMACH, 2002; RCOG, 2005).
- Autologous blood donation (Dinsmoor & Hogg, 1995) or intra-operative blood cell salvage if available (National Institute for Health and Clinical Excellence (NICE), 2005) may be options for women declining transfusion. Alternative arrangements should preferably be discussed antenatally (CEMACH, 2004).

For diagnosis of placenta praevia see Table 15.1 and for care of a woman with placenta praevia see p. 208.

Placental abruption

Placental abruption is the partial or total separation of the placenta from the uterus during pregnancy or labour. It is a major cause of perinatal mortality (McGeown, 2001).

Incidence and facts

- 1–2% of pregnancies (AAFP, 2004).
- 10% of stillbirths have been attributed to antepartum haemorrhage (CEMACH, 2006). The risk of stillbirth is proportionate to the degree of placental separation (AAFP, 2004).
- Three maternal deaths were attributed to placental abruption in the 2004 CEMACH report (CEMACH, 2004).
- Many cases are mild and the pregnancy uneventful. Severe cases require the co-ordinated care of obstetricians, midwives, anaesthetists and haematologists (McGeown, 2001).
- Abruption should be considered in any woman with abdominal pain, with or without bleeding (AAFP, 2004).
- For smaller bleeds facilitating vaginal delivery (with continuous electronic fetal monitoring (EFM)) and if necessary inducing/augmenting with intravenous (IV) oxytocin) may reduce the CS rate by 50% without effecting perinatal mortality (Fraser & Watson, 2000).
- Symptoms of shock are a late sign and represent a blood loss of ≥30% of blood volume (AAFP, 2004).
- One-third of women with abruption and fetal demise will develop coagulopathy as thromboplastins from the placental site are released, potentially activating the clotting cascade (AAFP, 2004). Consumptive coagulopathy and disseminated intravascular coagulopathy may follow (AAFP, 2004).

Risk factors for placental abruption

- Hypertension in 25–50% of cases (Lockwood, 1996).
- Abdominal trauma, e.g. domestic violence and road traffic incidents (AAFP, 2004).
- High parity and advanced maternal age (AAFP, 2004).
- Growth restriction (Ananth & Wilcox, 2001).
- Uterine overdistension: polyhydramnios and multiple gestation (AAFP, 2004).
- Smoking (AAFP, 2004) and some substance abuse (Miller *et al.*, 1995).
- Some thrombophilias (McGeown, 2001).

Care of a woman with placenta praevia/placental abruption

For diagnosis see Table 15.1.

With severe placenta praevia, CS delivery is likely. Abruption/low-grade placenta praevia may be managed expectantly if bleeding is mild to moderate, is settling (AAFP, 2004) and/or the baby is very preterm and the mother is stable (Fraser & Watson, 2000).

- **Assess and record blood loss**.
- **Note location of abdominal tenderness.** It may relate to placental site, back pain associated with posterior placenta (AAFP, 2004).
- **Monitor vital signs.** Tachycardia >90 bpm with systolic BP <100 mm Hg and/or diastolic <50 mm Hg may indicate impending hypovolaemic shock (WHO, 2003).

Table 15.1   Diagnosis of placenta praevia and placental abruption.

	Placenta praevia	Placental abruption
Pain	Usually painless	Varies from mild to severe
		Uterine pain or back pain if placenta posterior or concealed abruption (AAFP, 2004)
Uterus	Soft/usually relaxed	Tense/tender
	25% experience variable strength contractions (Lockwood, 1996)	Hypertonus generally seen in severe cases when the baby has died and with concealed abruption (AAFP, 2004)
Bleeding	Usually visible (AAFP, 2004)	Usually visible but 20% present with concealed bleeding (Frazer & Watson, 2000; AAFP, 2004)
Symptoms of shock (see p. 235)	May be present	May be present
Baby	Commonly non-engaged, ballotable presenting part 35% present as unstable lie (Lockwood, 1996)	Usually normal lie and presentation
Vaginal examination	Contraindicated: may exacerbate bleeding (Frazer & Watson, 2000)	Not contraindicated
Ultrasound scan (US)	Review US reports for placental location and fetal gestation. Transvaginal US may confirm placental edge (AAFP, 2004). Magnetic resonance imaging may enhance placental image quality (RCOG, 2005)	Ultrasound scan to exclude placenta praevia. Differentiation between fresh bleeding and placental tissue can be difficult as haematomas become hypoechoic after a week (Nyberg, 1987)

- **Perform EFM** (AAFP, 2004). A non-reassuring fetal heart rate may indicate the need to expedite delivery due to the significant risk of fetal demise (AAFP, 2004) (see the Appendix in Chapter 3).
- **Palpate/monitor contractions.** Abruption may cause a high resting tone and super-imposed small frequent contractions (AAFP, 2004).
- **Site large gauge IV cannula.** Check full blood count and blood group. If bleeding persists give IV fluids. Maintain a fluid balance chart.
- Ensure **cross-matched blood** (4 units) is ordered.
- **Consider clotting studies** as disseminated intravascular coagulopathy may develop (AAFP, 2004) fibrinogen levels, prothrombin time/international normalised ratio/activated partial thromboplastin time.
- **Consider Kleihauer testing** if woman is rhesus negative (Crowther & Keirse, 2002) to detect fetal cells in the maternal circulation.
- **Inform team:** obstetrician, anaesthetist, paediatrician, neonatal intensive care unit and theatres. If condition serious inform the intensive care unit.

In labour

- **Analgesia and support.** Placental abruption can be very painful. Support, reassurance and analgesia are essential. Assist the woman to get comfortable, use bean bags/pillows, massage, touch and pharmacological analgesia.
- **Monitor labour progress.** Continue EFM throughout (AAFP, 2004), monitor contractions and document fluid balance, blood loss and maternal vital signs. Rapid intervention may be required.
- **Give regular antacids**/hydrogen ion inhibitors in anticipation of possible anaesthetic (RCOG, 2004).
- **Expedite delivery** if bleeding is heavy, ongoing or greater than infusion ability (AAFP, 2004). There is evidence of compromise to mother or baby (Hayashi, 2000) or labour is not progressing (AAFP, 2004).
- **If haemorrhage continues**
  - Site a **second large gauge cannula**.
  - A **central venous pressure** line may be sited to accurately monitor fluid volume.
  - **Record hourly urine volume** via catheter. Output should be ≥30 ml/hour (AAFP, 2004).
  - **Order blood** urgently: platelet and fresh frozen plasma infusion may be required prior to operative delivery if coagulopathy is present (AAFP, 2004).

See also basic care for shock, Box 16.4, p. 235.

Third-stage management

- **Delay cord clamping** by ≥30 seconds if possible as the baby is at risk of anaemia (Mercer, 2001). Delayed clamping increases blood volume to the baby increasing the haemoglobin and haematocrit (Prendiville & Elbourne, 2000).
- **Leave a long cord** to enable umbilical cord catheterisation if required.
- **Take paired cord blood samples** for pH testing. If the mother is rhesus negative, a **direct Coombs' test** from umbilical cord blood may indicate antibody presence; consequent haemolysis may cause neonatal hyperbilirubinaemia.
- **Active management is recommended** to reduce risk of postpartum haemorrhage (PPH).
- Have a **syntocinon infusion** ready in case of PPH.
- **Remember** that blood loss is frequently underestimated (WHO, 2006).

Postpartum haemorrhage

The World Health Organization defines PPH as 500 ml blood loss in first 24 hours post-delivery (WHO, 2003). However, any blood loss that causes the woman's condition to deteriorate is considered a PPH (WHO, 2006). Early summoning of quality and senior help by the midwife can save valuable time and prevent a situation getting out of control.

Women who suffer a PPH usually find the experience frightening and traumatic. Remembering fear and pain may increase their anxiety in any subsequent birth. The woman's birth partner may experience feelings of helplessness and concern manifested as quiet anxiety, asking many questions or occasionally showing panic or aggression.

Incidence and facts

- PPH occurs in 4% of vaginal deliveries (AAFP, 2004) and 4–8% of CS (RCOG, 2004).
- PPH has four causes, the 4Ts: Tone (uterine atony), Tissue, Trauma and, rarely, Thrombophilias (clotting problems). Incidence: 70% tone, 20% trauma, 10% tissue and 1% thrombin (AAFP, 2004).
- Life-threatening haemorrhage is estimated at 6.7 per 1000 deliveries (CEMACH, 2004), and it remains a major cause of death globally (AAFP, 2004).
- Ten maternal deaths occurred due to PPH in the 2004 CEMACH report, with two deaths of women who refused blood transfusion (CEMACH, 2004).
- Clinicians should be aware of predisposing risk factors for haemorrhage, and those considered 'high risk' should be encouraged to deliver in a consultant unit (CEMACH, 2004). However, PPH is unpredictable and can occur in women with no identifiable risk factors (AAFP, 2004).
- Insidious blood loss can occur, causing maternal fatality if not recognised early (AAFP, 2004).

The 4Ts

Tone (uterine atony)

Around 70% of PPHs are caused by uterine atony. Predisposing risk factors include polyhydramnios, multiple pregnancy, high parity, prolonged/induced/augmented labours, instrumental delivery, pregnancy-induced hypertension, placental abruption, placenta praevia and PPH (AAFP, 2004). The aim of care is to deliver the placenta, if in situ, and ensure the uterus is well contracted by rubbing up a contraction and administering oxytocics (Fig. 15.1).

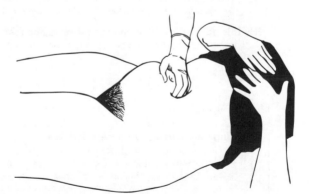

Fig. 15.1 Rubbing up a contraction.

For management see Box 15.1.

Tissue

Retained tissue in the uterus can consist of either placental fragments or an adherent placenta (AAFP, 2004). The uterus cannot contract efficiently due to retained tissue, resulting in haemorrhage. The placenta must be delivered to allow uterine contraction.

Always check the placenta and membranes after delivery for completeness.

Box 15.1   Management of PPH.

Women considered at high risk of PPH should be advised to have a large gauge IV cannula sited (CEMACH, 2004). An up-to-date haemoglobin result should be available and blood cross-matched (CEMACH, 2004).

Call for help
- At a home birth, call for a paramedic ambulance and follow guidelines given in Chapter 6. In hospital summon more midwives and an obstetrician.

Deliver the placenta if in situ
- If the placenta is completely adhered, there is usually no bleeding.
- If separation is partial, the bleeding can be copious and delivery of an incomplete placenta may occur.
- Always check the placenta for completeness.

Rub up a contraction
- Rub the fundus in a firm circular motion – keep rubbing as required for up to a minute. The uterus should feel hard, not 'boggy' or soft.
- Regularly re-assess and re-rub if the uterus starts to relax under the fingers.

Give oxytocics/site IV
- Administer a second oxytocic agent (see Chapter 24) either:
  - IM Syntometrine
  - IV oxytocin (Syntocinon) bolus
  - IM (or cautiously IV) ergometrine
- Be wary of oxytocic overload and antidiuretic effects (AAFP, 2004).
- Warn the woman; she may feel sick/vomit.
- Site a large gauge cannula and take routine emergency bloods: full blood count, clotting, group and cross-match.
- Commence IV Syntocinon 5–30 IU in 500 ml fluids (Hartmann's or normal saline) as per protocol.

Catheterisation
- Ensures no impediment to uterine contractility and enables renal function assessment. Satisfactory urine output is at least 100 ml in 4 hours (WHO, 2006).

By this point, most bleeding is controlled and responding to oxytocics; if not, summon the senior obstetrician and anaesthetist immediately.

Re-assess
- If bleeding settling, continue to observe.
- If not settling do not delay, perform a detailed examination of the genital tract (Campbell & Lees, 2000).

Ongoing haemorrhage/replace blood loss
- Site a second large gauge cannula.
- Commence IV fluids: infuse 3 ml for every ml of blood loss (WHO, 2003). Options are
  (a) crystalloid infusion, e.g. Ringer's Lactate
  (b) colloid infusion, e.g. Gelofusine. This will remain within the circulatory vessels for longer; beware of potential fluid overload.
- Infuse blood products as necessary.
- Carboprost/Hemabate (kept in the fridge) injected intramuscularly (IM) (warn the woman that the drug will make her feel unwell).

Continued severe haemorrhage
- In hospital conduct bimanual compression (Box 15.2); prepare the woman for theatre to undergo exploration of the uterine cavity and surgical management of the haemorrhage.
- At home conduct bimanual compression until surgical intervention. In extreme maternal collapse with a retained placenta, the midwife may perform urgent manual removal of the placenta (NMC, 2004) (see Box 15.2).
- In severe loss, IV fluids of a balanced electrolyte solution should be continued at 1 litre 6-hourly for the following 48 hours, although individual cases will vary (WHO, 2003).

Trauma

Trauma may consist of lacerations of the cervix, vagina, perineum, anus or episiotomy, pelvic haematomas and uterine inversion/rupture (AAFP, 2004). Occasionally large blood vessels are involved. Predisposing risk factors include enforced expulsive pushing, macrosomia, instrumental delivery (AAFP, 2004), also malpositions; persistent occipitoposterior, brow, compound presentations. An episiotomy if large or performed too early before the perineum has thinned can cut through blood vessels resulting in uncontrolled bleeding. Episiotomy also increases the risk of third- and fourth-degree tears (Sleep *et al.*, 2000).

Despite heavy blood loss, the uterus usually feels well contracted and does not gush blood when pressed. Many midwives choose to give a precautionary dose of an oxytocic if they remain unsure of the source of the bleeding.

Treatment of trauma

External bleeding:

- Locating the source of the bleeding can be very painful – entonox can be offered. The midwife should talk through what she is doing and suggest the woman says if she needs the midwife to stop at any time.
- A bleeding vessel can be hidden behind clots or oozing blood loss. Methodically check the area – the clitoris, labia and perineum – dabbing firmly with gauze.
- Once located, a bleeding vessel is obvious as when dabbed clear it instantly oozes or pumps blood, obscuring the view. Apply pressure to the bleeding point using some sterile gauze, or similar material, and hold firmly for approximately 5 min. This may be sufficient but keep checking the area in the following hours.
- If still oozing, the bleeding vessel should be clamped and will require tying off (see Fig. 15.2). The midwife should do this promptly.
- If the bleeding is internal, or excessive, contact a senior obstetrician (CEMACH, 2004).

Internal bleeding:

- An experienced obstetrician should be contacted to carry out further examination.
- If at a home birth or birthing centre, the midwife must undertake this examination as prompt arrest of the bleeding is essential.
- Bleeding from the cervix or deep in the vagina requires a speculum examination using a good light source and plenty of gauze. Use a clamp or sponge holder forceps wrapped in gauze for dabbing the blood away allowing a view of the bleeding point.
- If the bleeding is high up, apply direct pressure or pack with gauze; the woman will require suturing under anaesthesia. Sutures should not be placed blindly deep in the vaginal fornix as they can cause uterine injury. Occasionally, very high tears need repairing via the abdomen (Kean, 2000).
- Compression of the abdominal aorta, just above and to the left of the umbilicus, may be necessary in extreme cases (AAFP, 2004).
- Keep a count of gauze swabs used before and after, as one could easily become lost.

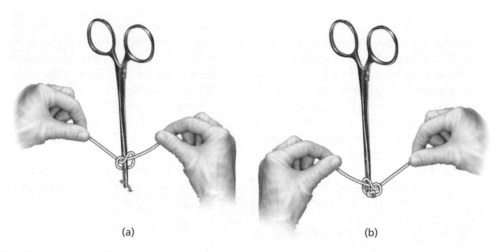

(a)   (b)

Fig. 15.2   Tying off a bleeding vessel. Bleeding vessels can be awkward to reach and tying them off may be painful for the woman. Grasp the vessel with a pair of forceps, then loop some thread around the forceps (this may require the aid of an assistant). Tie one throw of a knot – left thread over right (a) and slip the knot down past the end of the forceps to encircle the vessel. Pull the knot right and then tie a second throw – right thread over left (b). The knot should be square and not slip. Trim the thread and then release the forceps carefully.

Haematoma

This is a solid swelling formed by blood in the tissues. An acute haematoma is rare, approximately 1 per 1000 births. The volume of blood is often underestimated (Kean, 2000). Episiotomy is usually a related factor in 85–90% of haematomas (Kean, 2000).

Signs and symptoms of haematoma

- Visible discoloured swelling and blood-filled oedematous tissues; the mass may appear to distort the vagina and rectum (AAFP, 2004). The bleeding is usually concealed and may lie beneath sutures.
- There may be no external signs, and internal examination may be intolerable due to severe vaginal/vulval/rectal pain/back pain or unrelenting vulval/rectal pressure.
- Signs of hypovolaemic shock.

Treatment

- For small haematomas <3 cm, offer analgesia and observe (Kean, 2000; AAFP, 2004).
- Most large haematomas require not only analgesia but prompt surgical intervention (AAFP, 2004), i.e. incision, drainage and stemming of any bleeding vessel(s), followed by packing or suturing depending on tissue friability (Kean, 2000).
- Treat any hypovolaemia promptly (see basic treatment for shock, p. 235).

Thrombophilias/clotting problems

Thrombophilias and clotting problems are directly accountable for only 1% of PPHs as most are identified and treated antenatally (AAFP, 2004).

Some pregnancy-related conditions result in clotting problems: e.g. large placental abruption (classically accompanied by fetal demise), severe pre-eclampsia/eclampsia, intrauterine death, amniotic fluid embolism and sepsis (AAFP, 2004). Some uncommon conditions, e.g. thrombocytopenia and von Willebrand's disease, can also affect clotting. The clotting cascade once triggered can lead to disseminated intravascular coagulation (AAFP, 2004).

Signs and symptoms

- Continued bleeding and lost blood does not clot.
- Oozing from puncture sites.

Treatment

- Care should involve senior anaesthetic, obstetric, midwifery and haematology staff.
- Treat the underlying disorder (AAFP, 2004). Admission to ICU may be required. Blood testing for immediate full blood count and clotting studies (AAFP, 2004) and cross-matching.
- Urgent fluid and blood product replacement, depending on the diagnosed coagulopathy (AAFP, 2004) (see basic treatment for shock, p. 235).

Snapped cord

A short or friable cord can snap at, or following, birth. It occurs in 3% of vaginal births (Prendiville & Elbourne, 2000). If the cord snaps, or can be felt tearing away on applying traction, then providing there is no haemorrhage encourage delivery of the placenta by maternal effort. Pushing in an upright position is usually successful unless the placenta is truly adhered. Ensure the bladder is empty. If the placenta does not deliver after an hour (AAFP, 2004), see retained placenta.

Retained placenta

A retained placenta and manual removal can have a negative effect on the quality of contact the woman has with her newborn, reducing time spent feeding and getting to know the new baby, and can leave the woman anaemic, tender and sore. Rarely, the placenta is truly adherent and imbedded due to scanty or absent decidua, resulting in placenta accreta/increta or percreta. In more severe cases it can result in acute haemorrhage, infection, secondary postpartum haemorrhage, hysterectomy and even maternal death (AAFP, 2004).

Incidence and facts

- A retained placenta occurs in 3% of vaginal births (AAFP, 2004).
- 15% of retained placentas recur in women who have had a previous retained placenta (AAFP, 2004).
- There is a moderate level of evidence that an actively managed third stage of ≥ 30 minutes is associated with an increased incidence of PPH (NICE, 2007). NICE also

cites one study suggesting PPH risk rises after 30 minutes and peaks at 75 minutes with both active and physiological management (Combs & Laros, 1991), but this old US data (from 1976 to 1985) may not be applicable to current UK physiological management.

- A physiological third stage lasts <60 minutes in 95% of women (NICE, 2007).
- NICE (2007) therefore defines a *prolonged third stage* (not necessarily a retained placenta) if the placenta is not delivered within 30 minutes of active management or 60 minutes of expectant management.
- Active management is recommended if physiological management has been unsuccessful after 60 minutes (NICE, 2007). Only if active management has been unsuccessful would more interventionist procedures be used, and the term 'retained placenta' be appropriate.
- For suspected placenta accreta/percreta urgent manual removal is indicated in theatre since both are responsible for adverse outcomes including maternal death (CEMACH, 2004). This high-risk situation should be managed by the consultant obstetrician, consultant anaesthetist and involve the haematologist to ensure the best outcome (RCOG, 2005).
- Minimal bleeding can be evident with a totally adherent placenta, but increased volumes with partial adherence (AAFP, 2004).
- In the absence of medical aid and in an extreme emergency, manual removal of the placenta can be undertaken by a midwife (Nursing and Midwifery Council (NMC), 2004) (see Box 15.2).

Box 15.2   Manual removal of the placenta and bimanual compression.

Manual removal (only conducted by a midwife in an extreme emergency)

Manual removal is likely to be very painful for the woman and risks infection and uterine rupture if performed too roughly. The woman should be offered entonox or alternative analgesia. The procedure should be explained to her and her birth partner, who may wish to stay and give support, or leave the room (Crafter, 2002).

- Wear sterile gloves.
- Place the external hand on the fundus to prevent it moving away.
- Insert the fingers, then the hand into the vagina, through the os and trace the cord to locate the placenta.
- Locate the edge of the placenta (cleavage plane), and using a side-to-side movement gently coax the placenta away from the uterus (Crafter, 2002), cupping the separated cotyledons in the palm of the hand (AAFP, 2004).
- Aim to deliver the placenta intact (AAFP, 2004).
- Once separated deliver the placenta by cord traction.
- Keep the hand inside the uterus to 'brush' gently over the placental site and dislodge any possible fragments left behind (Crafter, 2002).

Bimanual compression

This is extremely painful and should only be performed if bleeding continues and medical assistance is not available.

Rub up a contraction with the external hand on the fundus. Insert the other hand and make a clenched fist shape, pushing up against the anterior fornix of the vagina, thereby pressing the walls of the uterus together (Crafter, 2002).

Role of the midwife in delivering a retained placenta

Provided blood loss is normal, the midwife can try the following:

- **Observation of pulse and blood pressure** is recommended (WHO, 2003).
- **Breastfeeding and nipple stimulation.** This stimulates natural oxytocin, which helps the uterus contract.
- **Proceed to active management** of third stage if the placenta does not deliver with physiological management. NICE (2007) recommends active management after 60 minutes; however, some midwives may doubt the quality of the evidence and wait for longer if the woman is not bleeding and is happy to continue.
- **Controlled cord traction.** If an oxytocic has been administered, attempt to deliver the placenta by applying cord traction and guarding the uterus. If any heavy bleeding occurs, stop cord traction.
- **Maternal position.** Assist the mother to remain upright, e.g. squatting/kneeling or sitting on the toilet/bedpan.
- **Encourage active pushing.** The woman may experience contractions as period-type pains and they may be infrequent. Encourage her to push with these pains. Anecdotally, midwives who recommend this suggest that pushing may take a while and require many attempts but that it is often successful.
- **Palpable bladder.** A full bladder may displace the uterus. Offer a bedpan/toilet, however urination is often unachievable, and if the bladder is palpable discuss passing a catheter. Offer entonox during any catheterisation.
- **Establish IV access.** Oxytocin infusion should not be used to facilitate delivery of the placenta (NICE, 2007); however, it should be commenced promptly with any active bleeding.

If the placenta remains undelivered, inform the obstetrician who may:

- Perform a vaginal examination to determine degree of separation, if any, as sometimes the placenta has separated and is lying in the vagina/cervix.
- Attempt removal by fundal pressure and/or cord traction.
- Inject 20 IU oxytocin in 20 ml saline directly into the umbilical vein of the clamped and cut cord (NICE, 2007). *Caution*: ensure that the baby is separated from the mother's cord before attempting this.
- If unsuccessful, proceed to digital manual removal of the placenta (MROP) in theatre under regional (occasionally general) anaesthesia. Attempted manual removal of an adherent placenta may cause catastrophic bleeding requiring hysterectomy (AAFP, 2004).
- IV oxytocin infusion, prophylactic antibiotics and close observation for signs of PPH or infection are recommended post-procedure (AAFP, 2004).

Summary

Placenta praevia and placental abruption

- Monitor vital signs, pain, uterine tone and FH
- Take blood and treat hypovolaemia

- If severe, prepare for emergency delivery, possibly CS
- Remember the risk of PPH

Postpartum haemorrhage
Tone (uterine atony) (see Box 15.1)
Tissue (partial or complete retention of placenta):

- Try to deliver placenta
- Check placental completeness
- Control haemorrhage

Trauma:

- Apply pressure over bleeding point
- Clamp and tie off bleeding vessel
- Serious trauma/haematomas will go to theatre

Thrombophilias/clotting disorders:

- A rare cause of haemorrhage
- Bleeding from puncture sites; blood does not clot
- Treat underlying causes

Retained placenta

- Bleeding worse if partial rather than full adherence
- Give IV fluids and oxytocics as per local protocol
- Injecting cord with oxytocic may help but MROP usually required

References

American Academy of Family Physicians (AAFP) (2004) *Advanced Life Support in Obstetrics (ALSO) Course Syllabus Manual, Revised*, 4th edn. American Academy of Family Physicians, Leawood, Kansas.

Ananth, C. & Wilcox, A. (2001) Placental abruption and perinatal mortality in the U.S. *American Journal of Epidemiology* **153** (4), 332–7.

Bose, P., Regan, F. & Paterson-Brown, N. (2006) Improving the accuracy of estimated blood loss at obstetric haemorrhage, using clinical reconstruction. *British Journal of Obstetrics and Gynaecology* **113** (8), 919–24.

Campbell, S. & Lees, C. (2000) Obstetric emergencies. In *Obstetrics by Ten Teachers*, 17th edn (Campbell, S. & Lees, C., eds), pp. 303–17. Edward Arnold, London.

CEMACH (2004) *Why Mothers Die 2000–2002. The Sixth Report of Confidential Enquiries into Maternal Deaths in the United Kingdom*. RCOG Press, London.

CEMACH (2006) *Perinatal Mortality Surveillance Report. England, Wales & N. Ireland*. CEMACH, London.

Clinical Negligence Scheme for Trusts (CNST) (2006) *Maternity Clinical Risk Management Standards*. NHS Litigation Authority.

Combs, C. & Laros, R., Jr (1991) Prolonged third stage of labor: morbidity and risk factors. *Obstetrics and Gynaecology* **77** (6), 863–7.

Crafter, H. (2002) Intrapartum and primary postpartum haemorrhage. In *Emergencies around Childbirth: A Handbook for Midwives* (Boyle, M., ed.), pp. 11–26. Radcliffe Medical Press, Oxford.

Crowther, C. & Keirse, M.J.N.C. (2002) Anti D Administration in pregnancy. *The Cochrane Library*, Issue 4. Update Software, Oxford.

Dinsmoor, M.J. & Hogg, B. (1995) Autologous blood transfusion with placenta praevia – is it feasible? *American Journal of Perinatology* **12**, 382–4.

Fraser, R. & Watson, R. (2000) Bleeding in the latter half of pregnancy. In *A Guide to Effective Care in Pregnancy and Childbirth*, 3rd edn (Enkin, M., Keirse, M.J.N.C., Neilson, J., Crowther, C., Duley, L., Hodnett, E. & Hofmeyr, J., eds), pp. 178–84. Oxford University Press, Oxford.

Hayashi, R. (2000) Obstetric collapse. In *Best Practice in Labor Ward Management* (Kean, L.H., Baker, P.N. & Edelstone, D.I., eds), pp. 415–33. WB Saunders, Edinburgh.

Kean, L. (2000) Other problems of the third stage. In *Best Practice in Labour Ward Management* (Kean, L.H., Baker, P.N. & Edelstone, D.I., eds), pp. 435–50. WB Saunders, London.

Lockwood, C. (1996) Third trimester bleeding. In *Protocols for High Risk Pregnancies*, 3rd edn (Queenan, J.T. & Hobbins, J.C., eds), pp. 568–72. Blackwell Science, Oxford.

Mapp, T. & Hudson, K. (2005) Feelings and fears during obstetric emergencies. *British Journal of Midwifery* **13** (1), 30–35.

McDonald, S. (1999) Physiology and management of the third stage of labour. In *Myles Textbook for Midwives* 13th edn (Bennet, V.R. & Brown, L.K., eds), pp. 465–88. Churchill Livingstone, Edinburgh.

McGeown, P. (2001) Practice recommendations for obstetric emergencies. *British Journal of Midwifery* **9** (2), 71–3.

Mercer, J.C. (2001) Current best evidence: a review of the literature on umbilical cord clamping. *Journal of Midwifery and Women's Health* **46** (6), 402–14.

Miller, J.M., Boudreaux, M.C. & Regan, F.A. (1995) A case control study of cocaine use in pregnancy. *American Journal of Obstetrics and Gynaecology* **172**, 180–85.

National Institute for Health and Clinical Excellence (NICE) (2005) *Intra-operative Blood Cell Salvage in Obstetrics: Interventional Procedure Guidance 144*. National Institute for Health and Clinical Excellence, London.

National Institute for Health and Clinical Excellence (NICE) (2007) *Clinical Guideline 55: Intrapartum Care*. National Institute for Health and Clinical Excellence, London.

Nursing and Midwifery Council (NMC) (2004) *Midwives Rules*. Available at: www.nmc-uk.org (accessed March 2008).

Nyberg, D.A. (1987) Ultrasound scanning and placental abruption. *American Journal of Roentgenology* **148** (1), 161–4 .

Prendiville, W. & Elbourne, D. (2000) The third stage of labor. In *A Guide to Effective Care in Pregnancy and Childbirth*, 3rd edn (Enkin, M., Keirse, M.J.N.C., Neilson, J., Crowther, C., Duley L., Hodnett, E. & Hofmeyr, J., eds), pp. 300–309. Oxford University Press, Oxford.

Royal College of Obstetricians and Gynaecologists (RCOG) (2004) *Caesarean Section Guideline. No. 13*. RCOG, London.

Royal College of Obstetricians and Gynaecologists (RCOG) (2005) *Placenta Praevia and Placental Accreta: Diagnosis and Management: Revised Green Top Guideline No. 27*. RCOG, London.

Sleep, J., Roberts, J. & Chalmers, L. (2000) The second stage of labor. In *A Guide to Effective Care in Pregnancy and Childbirth*, 3rd edn (Enkin, M., Keirse, M.J.N.C., Neilson, J., Crowther, C., Duley L., Hodnett, E. & Hofmeyr, J., eds) pp. 289–99. Oxford University Press, Oxford.

World Health Organization (WHO) (2003) *Integrated Management of Pregnancy & Childbirth: Managing Complications in Pregnancy & Childbirth: A Guide for Midwives & Doctors*. WHO, Geneva.

World Health Organization (WHO) (2006) Managing postpartum haemorrhage. In *Midwifery Education Modules*, 2nd edn. WHO, Geneva.

16 Emergencies in labour and birth

Sheila Miskelly

Introduction

A small but significant proportion of women develop complications which may threaten their lives or those of their babies. Emergency situations can be very disturbing and provoke a range of emotional responses and consequences for all involved (World Health Organization (WHO), 2003). Acute units must have comprehensive multidisciplinary facilities for rapid response to obstetric emergencies. In birth centres and at home births the midwife is responsible for emergency measures and prompt transfer (Department of Health (DoH), 2004). Regular skills drills have been shown to improve outcomes (Paxton *et al.*, 2005).

Clear, calm explanations of the emergency procedure and the risks involved will help to reduce anxiety for the woman and her partner. Be respectful of the woman's dignity, be aware that her choices may be reduced, acknowledge her fears and give sensitive responses to her needs (WHO, 2003).

> 'Even when serious emergencies occur, midwives can do much to create an environment which respects the woman as a person with feelings and emotions rather than an object to be rushed to theatre.' (Weston, 2001).

Cord prolapse and cord presentation

Cord presentation means that a loop of umbilical cord lies below the presenting part of the fetus, with intact membranes. If the membranes rupture this is known as a cord prolapse. The prolapse can be occult, i.e. alongside the presenting part, or frank, where the cord escapes through the cervix and may even be visible outside the vagina.

Incidence and facts

- Cord prolapse is reported as 0.4% in vertex presentations, 0.5% in frank breeches, 4–6% in complete breeches and 15–18% in footling breeches (American Academy of Family Physicians (AAFP), 2004).
- 50% of cord prolapse cases occur following artificial rupture of membranes (ARM) (Prabulos & Philipson, 1998).
- Umbilical cord prolapse is associated with poor perinatal outcomes, even when emergency delivery facilities are available (Prabulos & Philipson, 1998).
- Squire (2002) suggests that mortality is predominantly associated with congenital abnormities and prematurity rather than birth asphyxia per se.
- Occult cord prolapse is associated with less perinatal morbidity than frank prolapse (Prabulos & Philipson, 1998).
- In only 41% of cases, electronic fetal monitoring aided the diagnosis of cord prolapse (Murphy & MacKenzie, 1995).

Associated risk factors

- Any situation where the presenting part may not engage well in the pelvis, e.g. high presenting part, high parity, multiple birth, polyhydramnios, small/preterm baby, malpresentation (e.g. breech) (McGeown, 2001), ARM with a high presenting part (AAFP, 2004).
- Long umbilical cord (AAFP, 2004).

Signs and symptoms of cord prolapse

- Visible cord may protrude from vagina.
- Cord felt (often pulsating) on vaginal examination.
- Fetal bradycardia/prolonged late decelerations following rupture of membranes, possibly with fresh meconium liquor.

Practice recommendations/manoeuvres

- **Call for help.** If at home/birthing centre, call paramedic ambulance even if delivery appears imminent; if in second stage, also call midwife ventouse/forceps practitioner (if available). Give accurate and concise information when communicating with the receiving obstetric unit.
- **Maintain pressure on presenting part.** Keep the fingers in the vagina firmly pushing on the presenting part, particularly during contractions, to relieve cord compression until urgent delivery is achieved (AAFP, 2004). If achievable maintain pressure during ambulance transfer or while the woman is wheeled to a birth room/theatre (AAFP, 2004). This can be uncomfortable and stressful for whoever is performing the pressure.
- **Remain calm** and briefly explain to the woman and her partner what is happening and what is required of them. The clinician conducting internal pressure cannot

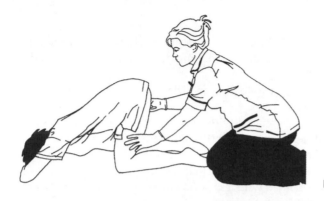

Fig. 16.1 Knee-chest position.

participate in other activities and is ideally situated to offer supportive reassurance and explanations to the woman and her partner during this frightening situation.

- **Position the mother.** The *all fours/knee-chest* position reduces pressure caused by the presenting part (see Fig. 16.1). It is possibly the most effective position, but can be uncomfortable and undignified for the woman. Cover her lower half for modesty.
- **Alternative positions:**
  - **Trendelenburg.** The woman lies on her back with a 30° tilt using a wedge to prevent aortocaval compression with a head down tilt, if possible, to relieve pressure.
  - **Exaggerated Sims.** The woman lies on her left side with her upper leg flexed and the knee resting on the bed.
- **Gently replace** the cord into the vagina if it is protruding, but do not attempt to replace into the uterus (AAFP, 2004). Keep the cord warm and wet using sterile gauze or a cloth and polythene bag if replacement is impossible (Davis, 1997) as cold air or excessive handling can cause spasm and resultant reduced oxygen delivery.
- **Fill the bladder.** Some success is reported from instilling 500–700 ml of saline into the bladder (AAFP, 2004). This may relieve cord compression and inhibit uterine activity, in cases where theatre is not immediately available. Prolonged overdistension of the bladder should be avoided.
- **Deliver urgently.** In the first stage of labour, caesarean section (CS) is normally performed. However if in advanced second stage, encourage the woman to push. Most primigravidae are unlikely to be able to deliver quickly, and an episiotomy and instrumental delivery are probable. Multigravid women may also require such intervention, but quick spontaneous birth may be achieved if they push hard: consider an upright position, as the risk of cord compression may be offset by the improved pushing. Close fetal heart monitoring is vital.
- **Assistance with resuscitation.** A baby with a frank cord prolapse is likely to require intensive resuscitation; therefore, paediatric support should be summoned. Appropriate help should be summoned at a birthing centre or at home.

Amniotic fluid embolism

Amniotic fluid embolism (AFE) is a rare but catastrophic condition, which is usually fatal (AAFP, 2004). A woman may collapse rapidly with no clear diagnosis at the time. AFE is an anaphylactic type reaction to amniotic fluid that has entered the woman's circulation (AAFP, 2004). This results in left ventricular failure and pulmonary vasospasm resulting in acute lung injury. Clotting factors are also activated with disseminated intravascular coagulation (DIC) commonly resulting (Davis, 1999; Fahy, 2001; AAFP, 2004). The rapidly deteriorating situation can be extremely stressful for staff and birth partners, particularly as death so often results.

Incidence and facts

- Incidence of AFE is reported as 1:20 000 deliveries (AAFP, 2004), with a 26.4–61% mortality rate (AAFP, 2004; Confidential Enquiry into Maternal and Child Health (CEMACH), 2004). The perinatal mortality rate is 40%.
- CEMACH (2004) reports 5 deaths from AFE, with 19 cases reported to the National AFE Register.
- Risk factors include multiparity, abruption, intrauterine fetal demise, tumultuous labour and oxytocic hyperstimulation (AAFP, 2004). AFE remains unpredictable, rapidly progressive and unpreventable (CEMACH, 2004).
- Diagnosis may be confirmed by the presence of fetal squames and lanugo hair in the pulmonary vasculature at post-mortem (CEMACH, 2004), or reliant on clinical observations if autopsy is unavailable (AAFP, 2004). Fahy (2001) suggests that the more knowledgeable clinicians become about AFE, the more frequently it is diagnosed.

Signs and symptoms of AFE

(See Table 16.1.)

Table 16.1 Signs and symptoms of AFE (Fahy, 2001).

Sign/symptom	% of women
Hypotension (shock)	100
Fetal distress (if undelivered)	100
Pulmonary oedema or adult respiratory distress syndrome	93
Cardiopulmonary arrest	86
Cyanosis	83
Coagulopathy	83
Dyspnoea (difficult or laboured breathing)	49
Seizure	48

- AFE manifests itself with the woman gasping for breath, developing rapid hypotension and shock symptoms, and usually going into cardiac arrest (AAFP, 2004). A behavioural change may precede collapse, as hypoxia and toxic confusional state develops (CEMACH, 2004).
- Sometimes haemorrhage due to DIC is the initial presentation (Davis, 1999).

Practice recommendations

- **Call for help/transfer to hospital.**
- **Think ABC.** Airway, Breathing and Circulation (see Box 16.4 and Chapter 17).

- **Early input** of co-ordinated care from the resuscitation team and consultant anaesthetist, obstetrician and haematologist (CEMACH, 2004). Rapid intensive therapy unit transfer is recommended and may increase survival (CEMACH, 2004).
- **Deliver baby** by CS as rapidly as possible in the event of maternal cardiac arrest (Managing Obstetric Emergencies and Trauma (MOET), 2003). Obstetricians do not need to prepare a sterile field and should go for the quickest incision possible (Bobrowski, 1994).
- **Aftercare.** The woman will require intensive care with supportive treatment (AAFP, 2004).

Uterine rupture

Uterine dehiscence is defined as disruption of the uterine muscle with intact serosa (Royal College of Paediatrics and Child Health (RCOG), 2007). The more serious condition of *uterine rupture* is defined as disruption of the uterine muscle extending to and involving the uterine serosa or disruption of the uterine muscle with extension to the bladder or broad ligament (RGOG, 2007). Occasionally these events occur antenatally, but more often during labour, birth or prior to delivery of the placenta (RCOG, 2007).

For additional information see Box 16.1.

Incidence and facts

- Uterine rupture is rare. Incidence in women with an unscarred uterus is reported as 2 per 10 000 and with a scarred uterus 0.5 to 2 per 10 000 deliveries (RCOG, 2007).
- 50% of cases occur in women with no uterine scar, mainly multiparous women (Enkin, 2000).
- 13% uterine ruptures occur outside the hospital setting (AAFP, 2004).
- There is no single clinical feature indicative of uterine rupture: diagnosis is ultimately confirmed at CS or postpartum laparotomy (RCOG, 2007).
- Early recognition and diagnosis may improve outcomes (AAFP, 2004).

Associated risk factors

- 50% cases associated with previous uterine surgery including CS (AAFP, 2004).
- Other associated causes: inappropriate use of prostaglandins/oxytocin to induce/augment labour (National Institute for Health and Clinical Excellence (NICE), 2004, AAFP, 2004), trauma caused by high-cavity forceps, manual manipulation for unstable lie, manual removal of placenta, road traffic incident or other blunt trauma including physical assault (Kroll & Lyne, 2002).

Signs and symptoms of uterine rupture are given in Box 16.1.

Practice recommendations

- Midwifery care: call for help/transfer to hospital.
- Discontinue intravenous (IV) oxytocin if in progress (AAFP, 2004).
- Administer oxygen and IV fluids rapidly.

Box 16.1   Signs and symptoms of uterine rupture.

Pain
- Sudden uterine or scar pain (AAFP, 2004).
- Chest or shoulder tip pain (RCOG, 2007).
- A feeling of 'giving way' (Silverton, 1993).
- Lower abdominal pain may come with a contraction, or be constant and unrelenting (AAFP, 2004).
- The woman may find it too painful to have her uterus touched or palpated.
- Pain may decrease after the rupture (WHO, 2003).

Uterus/contractions
- Solid, tonic uterus or abnormal uterine shape (WHO, 2003).
- Contractions may stop or dwindle (AAFP, 2004).

Fetus
- Abnormal cardiotocograph may occur (RCOG, 2007) culminating in prolonged fetal bradycardia (AAFP, 2004).
- Recession of the presenting part (RCOG, 2007) or suprapubic bulging (AAFP, 2004).
- Easily palpable fetal parts (WHO, 2003).

Shock
- Tachycardia (AAFP, 2004).
- Hypotension (RCOG, 2007).
- Sudden onset of shortness of breath (RCOG, 2007).

The woman may:
- Look cold and clammy.
- Appear restless, agitated or withdrawn.
- Say she is frightened and that something is wrong.
- Vomit.

Bleeding
- Fresh vaginal bleeding or blood-stained amniotic fluid may be seen.
- Haematuria may develop (RCOG, 2007).
- Following delivery a ruptured uterus may rise as it fills with blood.

Obstetricians are likely to:

- Deliver the baby by instrumental means or proceed to immediate CS (AAFP, 2004).
- Repair the uterus immediately in theatre. Haemorrhage is likely. If bleeding is uncontrollable, hysterectomy may be necessary (Bakshi & Meyer, 2000).

Aftercare

- Closely monitor the woman following surgery as she is at risk of postpartum haemorrhage (RCOG, 2007). An IV oxytocin infusion is advisable post-delivery. In severe cases the mother and baby may require intensive care. Perinatal morbidity is more common in cases of complete displacement of the baby into the abdominal cavity due to uterine rupture (AAFP, 2004).

Shoulder dystocia

Shoulder dystocia is one of the most serious birth emergencies. It is caused by the impaction of the anterior shoulder of the fetus against the maternal symphysis pubis, or less commonly the posterior fetal shoulder on the sacral promontory, after delivery of the head (RCOG, 2005), requiring additional obstetric manoeuvres to release the shoulders (RCOG, 2005). Unless the baby is born within a few minutes of its head emerging, it is likely to die. Shoulder dystocia cannot be predicted (WHO, 2003); all midwives must be able to recognise and manage this emergency promptly (Brown, 2002).

Incidence and facts

- Shoulder dystocia occurs in 0.3–1% of babies weighing 2.5–4 kg and 5–7% of babies weighing 4–4.5 kg (AAFP, 2004).
- Over 50% of shoulder dystocias occur in normal sized babies with no identifiable risk factors (AAFP, 2004).
- Preconception and prenatal risk factors have extremely poor predictive value and therefore in clinical practice do not facilitate accurate, reliable prediction of shoulder dystocia (Gherman, 2002).
- Morbidity for the baby includes obstetric brachial plexus palsy (OBPP) injuries in 7–20% following dystocia, with 1–2% of those sustaining permanent injury (AAFP, 2004). Hypoxia, fractures of the clavicle/humerus, bruising and soft tissue damage may occur, and in severe cases, fetal death may result.
- Litigation may result from OBPP: 40–60 births from 1993 to 1997 resulted in claims (NHSLA, 2003).
- Morbidity for the woman includes trauma, blood loss, bruising to the perineum/ genital tract and surrounding tissues, episiotomy/serious tears, psychological trauma, as well as, in severe cases, grief at the death of her baby.
- Simulated training sessions have been found to improve performance in shoulder dystocia management (Deering *et al.*, 2004).

Associated risk factors

All shoulder dystocia-associated risk factors have poor predictive value in clinical practice (WHO, 2003).

Antenatal associated risks:

- Macrosomia (AAFP, 2004) and previous baby >4.0 kg (CEMACH, 2004).
- Maternal diabetes, short stature and abnormal pelvic anatomy (AAFP, 2004).
- Previous instrumental delivery (AAFP, 2004).
- Post-dates pregnancy (AAFP, 2004).
- Previous shoulder dystocia (AAFP, 2004).

Intrapartum-associated risks:

- Prolonged first or second stage of labour (RCOG, 2005).

- Birthing semi-recumbent on a bed can restrict the movement of the coccyx and sacrum contributing to 'bed-birth dystocia' (Mortimore & McNabb, 1998; McGeown, 2001).
- Oxytocin augmentation (RCOG, 2005).
- Instrumental delivery (AAFP, 2004).

Recognising shoulder dystocia

Shoulder dystocia is usually preceded by a slow 'bobbing' delivery of the baby's head; the baby's chin then retracts against the perineum and 'turtlenecks' (AAFP, 2004). With the next contraction the baby will not deliver as its anterior shoulder is impacted against the symphysis pubis bone, due to the shoulder (bisacromial) diameter exceeding the diameter of the pelvic inlet (AAFP, 2004).

Beware of overdiagnosing shoulder dystocia. Sometimes anxious clinicians start to worry after only 1 or 2 minutes. Think: 'has there been a contraction yet?' Two minutes can seem like a long time, but no baby will be compromised at this point: this is quite normal. Spontaneous restitution of the shoulders may take one or two contractions. Premature traction without a contraction may give the false impression that dystocia is occurring.

Practice recommendations

Upright birthing positions improve the alignment of the mobile pelvic bones and improve the shape and capacity of the pelvis, optimising the chances of a 'good fit' between baby and pelvis (Simpkin & Ancheta, 2005). Common sense suggests that any woman at risk of shoulder dystocia should be discouraged from birthing in the semi-recumbent position.

Changing the woman's position in itself can be beneficial in preventing/shifting impacted shoulders.

Do not clamp and cut a nuchal cord. This will cut off the only oxygen supply the baby has, and hypoxia will rapidly follow.

Avoid excessive traction. Once shoulder dystocia is diagnosed, do not put any further traction on the head. A previously healthy fetus will withstand up to 10 minutes of complete anoxia before there is a significant risk of brain damage (Pasternak, 1993). Whilst a fetus who has experienced prior fetal distress may not endure more than 5 minutes of anoxia (Confidential Enquiry into Stillbirths and Deaths in Infancy (CESDI), 1998) and it may be justifiable to resume traction if other manoeuvres have repeatedly failed, any OBPP injury following a head-to-body delivery of, say, 2–3 minutes will probably be judged in court to have been due to excessive traction (Johnson, 2005). Performing the manoeuvres correctly will certainly take more than 2–3 minutes.

Avoid fundal pressure which could increase shoulder impaction and cause serious injuries, including uterine rupture, haemorrhage and even maternal death.

Use of systematic manoeuvres. Most shoulder dystocias will resolve with these manoeuvres. Prophylactic use of McRoberts or other manoeuvres prior to clinical diagnosis of shoulder dystocia requires further evaluation (Poggi, 2004). Many midwives might respond however that prevention happens all the time: optimal positioning in the second stage, e.g. squatting/all fours (which might be described as physiological

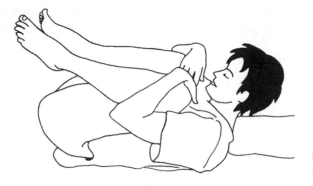

Fig. 16.2 McRoberts manoeuvre (side view).

McRoberts positions) widens the pelvic diameters (see Chapter 1) therefore logically must reduce the chances of shoulder dystocia. Indeed the all fours position appears so successful in managing shoulder dystocia (Kovavisarach, 2006) that Walsh (2007) has even suggested that it should be the first mnemonic option for shoulder dystocia.

The HELPERR drill

The AAFP (2004) states that HELPERR manoeuvres serve to:

- Increase the functional size of the bony pelvis.
- Decrease the bisacromial (fetal shoulder) diameter.
- Change the relationship of the bisacromial diameter within the bony pelvis.

(See also Figs 16.2–16.4.)

HELPERR is a clinical tool providing a structured framework and an accepted approach to shoulder dystocia management (AAFP, 2004). Unfortunately when reciting the mnemonic, the assumption appears that all women give birth lying semi-recumbent or in lithotomy, and therefore it is important to stress the importance of individual clinical judgement as to which manoeuvre is employed first.

H   Help!
E   Evaluate for episiotomy
L   Legs hyperflexed (McRoberts manoeuvre)
P   Pressure suprapubic
E   Enter the vagina for internal manoeuvres
R   Remove the posterior arm
R   Roll on to all fours

Whilst AAFP (2004) suggests that there is no indication that one manoeuvre is superior to another, Baskett and Allen (1995) suggest that McRoberts is the most successful, whilst Kovavisarach (2006) suggests that the all fours position is extremely effective. However, the order of each manoeuvre is left to the attending clinicians' discretion with importance attributed to the effective application of each manoeuvre (AAFP, 2004) rather than to the order in which the manoeuvres are conducted. Thirty to sixty seconds is the recommended time span allocated to each manoeuvre (AAFP, 2004). All manoeuvres can be repeated if delivery is not achieved.

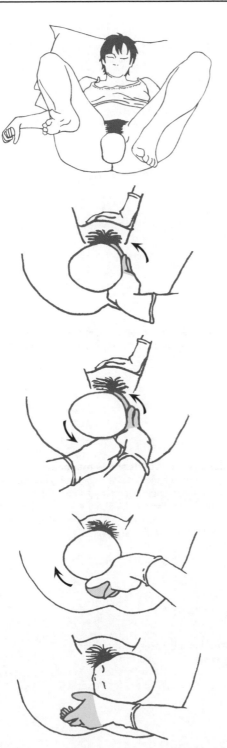

(a) **McRoberts manoeuvre** (end view)
The women is encouraged to abduct ber thighs towards her chest.

(b) **McRoberts and Rubins I** (suprapubic pressure)
- An assistant stands on the same side as the fetal back to apply downward, lateral pressure or rocking above the lateral shoulder.

Internal manoeuvres/Rubins II
- Approach the anterior shoulder from behind.
- Push it towards the fetal chest to reduce the shoulder girdle or move into the oblique diameter.

(c) **McRoberts, Rubins II and the Woods screw manoeuvre**
- Use both hands, place two fingers behind the anterior shoulder and two in front of the posterior shoulder.
- Attempt to rotate the shoulders as indicated, into the oblique diameter.

(d) **Reverse Woods screw manoeuvre**
- Place the fingers behind the posterior shoulder.
- Attempt rotation as shown.

(e) **Removal of posterior shoulder**
- Insert a well-lubricated hand.
- Locate the fetal arm and flex at the elbow; sweep arm out across the fetal chest.

Fig. 16.3 Manoeuvres for shoulder dystocia with the woman in a semi-recumbent position and the fetal position left occipitoanterior (LOA).

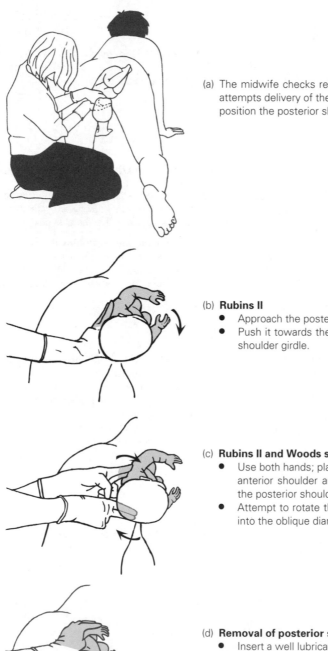

(a) The midwife checks restitution has occurred and attempts delivery of the posterior shoulder. In this position the posterior shoulder is uppermost.

(b) **Rubins II**
- Approach the posterior shoulder from behind.
- Push it towards the fetal chest to reduce the shoulder girdle.

(c) **Rubins II and Woods screw manoeuvre**
- Use both hands; place two fingers behind the anterior shoulder and two fingers in front of the posterior shoulder.
- Attempt to rotate the shoulders as indicated, into the oblique diameter.

(d) **Removal of posterior shoulder**
- Insert a well lubricated hand
- Locate the arm and flex at the albow, sweep arm out across the fetal chest.

Fig. 16.4   Manoeuvres for shoulder dystocia with the woman in an all fours position and the fetal position left occipitoanterior (LOA).

Help summoned immediately. Activate emergency bell, call emergency team via switchboard or dial 999 if at homebirth/birthing centre.

Evaluate for episiotomy. Episiotomy can improve access to conduct manoeuvres, but it will not in itself release the bony impaction of the shoulder (Nocon, 2000; AAFP, 2004). Episiotomy causes perineal trauma, and is almost impossible to perform once the head has delivered; some midwives therefore question its necessity (Gaskin, 1990). The Management of Obstetric Emergencies and Trauma group (MOET, 2003) recommends using an individual clinical judgement approach.

Legs hyperflexed (McRoberts manoeuvre). The woman lies in a flat supine position and abducts her thighs, pulling her knees to her chest, thus raising her coccyx off the bed and flattening her sacral promontory (see Figs 16.2 and 16.3a). The McRoberts manoeuvre facilitates delivery in over 40% of cases, and over 50% when used in conjunction with external pressure (AAFP, 2004).

Pressure applied externally suprapubically (also known as Rubins I manoeuvre). The clinician stands on the same side as the baby's back and directs pressure towards the maternal midline (Coates, 1995; AAFP, 2004) in a downward, lateral pressure, or rocking with the palm of the hands over the baby's anterior shoulder in order to reduce the bisacromial diameter and shift the impacted shoulder. If the direction of pressure is incorrectly applied towards the symphysis bone it will only impact the baby's shoulder further on the pelvic bone. Suprapubic pressure and McRoberts manoeuvre employed together can improve success rates (Gherman *et al.*, 1997).

Enter. Internal manoeuvres can be attempted whatever the mother's position and include Woods screw and Rubins II (Figs 16.3 and 16.4). These manoeuvres are painful for the woman and difficult and uncomfortable for the midwife.

- **Rubins II** (see Figs 16.3b and 16.4b). Insert the lubricated fingers of one hand (always posteriorly as there is more space) and apply pressure on the impacted anterior shoulder from behind, thus pushing the anterior shoulder towards the fetal chest and reducing the bisacromial diameter. Apply Rubins I external pressure simultaneously unless the woman is on all fours.
- **Woods screw** manoeuvre can be combined with Rubins II (AAFP, 2004). Insert the fingers of the second hand so that they are in front of the posterior shoulder (see Figs 16.3c and 16.4c). You can internally push/rotate the baby towards the symphysis pubis, thus rotating the baby into the oblique which frees the anterior shoulder from the pubic bone.
- **Reverse Woods screw.** Place fingers from behind on to the posterior aspect of the posterior shoulder and attempt to rotate the baby towards the symphysis pubis (see Figs 16.3d and 16.4d).

Remove the posterior arm. To deliver the posterior shoulder, insert the whole lubricated hand into the vagina to locate the baby's posterior arm and elbow. Flex the arm at the elbow and sweep across the fetal chest and out. Avoid excessive traction on the arm if possible, as the shoulder should have now disimpacted and delivery should normally follow (AAFP, 2004).

Roll onto all fours. Depending on the woman's mobility, midwives may consider this position change before the more interventionist manoeuvres as it is so successful (RCOG, 2005).

Turning onto all fours, sometimes referred to as the Gaskin manoeuvre, may dislodge the impacted shoulder (AAFP, 2004) by allowing unrestricted movement of the pelvis including the coccyx. The baby's weight on the symphysis helps widen the anterior-posterior pelvic diameter. The posterior shoulder (now nearest the ceiling) usually delivers first in this scenario. Anecdotally, in all fours delivery position, midwives report that there is sometimes enough room to insert the hand, along the curve of the sacrum and to splint, then free, the posterior shoulder. The all fours position may be impossible/impractical for women with a dense epidural block.

Last resort procedures

Whilst being unpleasant to undertake these procedures are preferable to fatality.

- **Clavicle fracture (cleidotomy).** Press upwards on the centre of the clavicle (AAFP, 2004); try using two fingers placed on the clavicle and pushing with the thumb between them. The bone should snap easily (Davis, 1997; RCOG, 2005), allowing release of the shoulder.
- **Cephalic replacement/Zavanelli manoeuvre** (RCOG, 2005). Turn the baby's head back to occipitoanterior or occipitoposterior (depending on the baby's original position for delivery). Flex the baby's head, push it back into the vagina and proceed to immediate CS. This manoeuvre has delivered varying success.

Aftercare

Post-birth counselling. The couple may benefit from debriefing at a time that is appropriate (Mapp, 2005). They may prefer to discuss this with the person(s) present at the delivery, and may wish to see a consultant obstetrician to discuss any long-term effects and the prospects for future pregnancies.

Documentation. Solicitors can frequently find fault in the documented management of shoulder dystocia, questioning whether the care followed recognised manoeuvres. Good practice and documentation help prevent litigation.

The AAFP (2004) recommends that documentation should include the following:

- Team members present
- Manoeuvres performed and duration of event
- Venous and arterial cord PH recordings
- On which of the baby's arms manoeuvres were performed

The RCOG (2005) also recommends recording
- Time of delivery of the head
- The direction the head is facing after restitution
- Time of delivery of the body
- Condition of the baby (Apgar score)
- What time attending staff arrived

Inverted uterus

This is the inversion of the uterus into the vagina during the third stage of labour. It is a rare but life-threatening complication due to the risk of significant haemorrhage and shock (AAFP, 2004).

Incidence and facts

- 1:2000 to 1:50 000 births (Kroll & Lyne, 2002).
- Kroll and Lyne (2002) suggest that the variation in statistics is dependent on third-stage management and the level of reporting.

Associated risk factors

- Mismanagement of the third stage of labour (Peña-Martin, 2007), e.g. fundal pressure and overzealous cord traction.
- Uterine atony, fundal implantation of the placenta or congenital weakness of the uterus has been identified as risk factors (AAFP, 2004), also placenta accreta or a short umbilical cord (Kroll & Lyne, 2002).

Signs and symptoms

See Box 16.2.

Box 16.2   Signs and symptoms of uterine inversion.

Uterus
  Inability to palpate uterus abdominally (WHO, 2003).
  The uterus may be visible as a shiny, bluish-grey mass protruding at the vagina (AAFP, 2004).

Haemorrhage
  The most common sign is haemorrhage, but the woman's rapid collapse appears to be out of proportion to the amount of blood lost (AAFP, 2004).

Profound shock
  Rapid shock may be partially attributed to a vasovagal, neurogenic response due to traction of the ovaries and fallopian tubes (AAFP, 2004) (see Box 16.4).

Pain
  Intense lower abdominal pain caused by traction on the ovaries and peritoneum and may be accompanied by a bearing-down sensation (Kroll & Lyne, 2002).

Practice recommendations

Treatment for uterine inversion consists of two main components: replacement of the uterus and treatment of shock (Beringer & Patteril, 2004).

- **Call for help** and/or transfer to hospital.
- **Replace the uterus promptly** (see Box 16.3). If not, or if attempts fail, a cervical restriction ring and/or an oedematous womb may result, preventing replacement (Kroll & Lyne, 2002). Betamimetics (uterine muscle relaxants) or general anaesthesia may then be required (AAFP, 2004).
- **Do not attempt to remove the placenta if it is adherent** to the uterus, as this may cause haemorrhage (WHO, 2003).
- **Treat for shock** (see Box 16.4).

- If immediate replacement of uterus is unsuccessful:
  - ○ **Prepare for theatre.**
  - ○ **Place the uterus in the vagina** if possible or hold by hand close to the vagina to minimise pulling on internal structures.
  - ○ **Withhold oxytocics** until the uterus is replaced (WHO, 2003).
  - ○ **Administer strong analgesia,** e.g. morphine.

Box 16.3   Replacing an inverted uterus.

Prompt manual replacement
- Apply gentle pressure with three or four fingers at the centre of the uterine fundus and push up until the uterus reverts (AAFP, 2004).
- Ensure the entire uterus is completely fed up through the cervix and hold in place for at least 5 minutes or until a firm contraction occurs (Kroll & Lyne, 2002).
- The woman will find the inversion painful and replacement can be agonising (Kroll & Lyne, 2002).

Placenta
Only after the uterus is replaced can an oxytocic be administered and the placenta carefully delivered (Campbell & Lees, 2000; Magill-Cuerden, 2001).

Aftercare

- An indwelling catheter for 24 hours avoids distension of the bladder (Silverton, 1993).
- Refer for physiotherapy to discuss pelvic floor muscle care and lifting/straining strategies.
- The mother may remember little of events, but her partner will have seen her sudden collapse. Offer the couple the option of seeing an obstetrician to discuss what happened, and why and to discuss any long-term effects of her collapse and future pregnancies.

Maternal collapse/shock

Shock is characterised by circulatory failure to maintain adequate perfusion of the vital organs (WHO, 2003). Blood is directed to vital organs; the peripheral circulation shuts down and if not corrected rapid progressive deterioration occurs. Due to increased circulatory volume during pregnancy initial compensation occurs, but by the time the BP drops and tachycardia is evident the situation is serious.

The types of shock in pregnancy and after birth can be broadly divided into two categories:

Haemorrhagic

Ante/postpartum haemorrhage (commonest cause)
Uterine inversion or rupture

Non-haemorrhagic

Pulmonary or amniotic embolism

Endotoxic shock (septicaemia)
Hypotension (regional anaesthesia or anaphylaxis)

Possible signs and symptoms of shock

- Pallor, blueness, central cyanosis, feeling cold to touch
- Tachycardia ± hypotension
- Anxiety and agitation, possibly vomiting
- Gasping for air (if severe)
- Drowsiness or unconsciousness
- Cardiac arrest can rapidly follow

See Box 16.4 for management of shock.

Box 16.4   Basic care for shock.

---

(1) Summon help.
(2) Ascertain the possible cause of shock:
   - Commence appropriate treatment.
   - Deliver the baby.
   - If at home or birthing centre, arrange urgent paramedic ambulance to hospital.
(3) Physical care:
   - Site two large gauge cannulae (a priority).
   - Take emergency bloods for:
     ○ group and cross-matching
     ○ full blood count
     ○ clotting studies; fibrinogen levels, prothrombin time (international normalised ratio) (PT(INR))/activated partial thromboplastin time (APTT).
   - Commence IV fluids.
   - Administer facial oxygen.
   - Observations:
     ○ pulse
     ○ blood pressure (BP)
     ○ pulse oximetry
(4) Serious collapse (see 'Maternal resuscitation', Chapter 17).
   Stay calm, think ABC:
   A = Airway
   B = Breathing
   C = Circulation
(5) Documentation. In hospital it is usually possible to assign a person to perform documentation of:
   - Vital signs.
   - Fluids charted, in and out including estimated blood loss.
   - Drugs given, dosages and times.
(6) Transfer to high-dependency area/intensive care unit:
   - Urinary catheter with urometer.
   - Central venous pressure line.
(7) In complete cardiac arrest of a pregnant woman, deliver the baby within 5 minutes. Obstetricians do not need to prepare a sterile field and should go for the quickest incision possible (Bobrowski, 1994).
(8) Communicate with the family.

Summary

Cord prolapse

- Call for help.
- Vaginal examination to apply pressure to the presenting part until delivery.
- Woman to adopt the all fours/knee-chest position, exaggerated Sims or Trendelen-burg.
- If at home/birthing centre, transfer to a consultant unit.
- Explain to the woman calmly what is happening and why.
- Consider as a last resort filling the woman's bladder with 400–700 ml saline.
- Emergency delivery: probable CS in first stage, spontaneous vertex delivery or in-strumental birth in second stage.

Amniotic fluid embolism

- Main symptoms: breathlessness, shock, followed by cardiac arrest (Fahy, 2001).
- Treat for sudden shock/collapse.
- High maternal mortality: proceed to urgent delivery of the baby.

Uterine rupture

- Prepare for theatre.
- Emergency delivery of baby.
- Haemorrhage control.
- Uterine repair in theatre.

Shoulder dystocia
Consider HELPERR mnemonic as a guide:

- H = Call for help
- E = Evaluate for episiotomy
- L = Legs hyperflexed (McRoberts manoeuvre)
- P = Pressure applied externally suprapubically
- E − Enter for internal manoeuvres
- R = Roll onto all fours
- R = Remove posterior arm

Uterine inversion

- Call for help.
- Replace the uterus promptly (see Box 16.3).
- Treat for shock (see Box 16.4).
- Offer analgesia.
- Withhold oxytocics until delivery of placenta.
- If unable to replace uterus prepare for theatre.

References

American Academy of Family Physicians (AAFP) (2004) Advanced Life Support in Obstet-rics (ALSO). In *Course Syllabus Manual*, 4th edn. American Academy of Family Physicians, Leawood, Kansas.

Bakshi, S. & Meyer, B.A. (2000) Indications for and outcomes of emergency peripartum hysterectomy: a five-year review. *Journal of Reproductive Medicine* **45** (9), 733–7.

Baskett, T.F. & Allen, A.C. (1995) Perinatal implications of shoulder dystocia. *Obstetrics and Gynaecology* **86**, 14–17.

Beringer, R.M. & Patteril, M., (2004) Puerperal uterine inversion and shock. *British Journal of Anaesthesia* **92** (3), 439–41.

Bobrowski, R. (1994) In *High Risk Pregnancy: Management Options*, 2nd edn (James, D.K., Steer, P.J., Weiner, C.P. & Goink, B., eds), pp. 959–82. WB Saunders, London.

Brown. L. (2002) Shoulder dystocia: auditing the development of guidelines for shoulder dystocia. *British Journal of Midwifery* **10** (11), 671–5.

Campbell, S. & Lees, C. (2000) Obstetric emergencies. In *Obstetrics by Ten Teachers*, 17th edn (Campbell, S. & Lees, C., eds), pp. 303–17. Edward Arnold, London.

Coates, T. (1995) Shoulder dystocia. In *Aspects of Midwifery Practice* (Alexander, J., Levy, V. & Roch, S., eds). Macmillan, Basingstoke.

Confidential Enquiry into Maternal and Child Health (CEMACH) (2004) *Why Mothers Die 2000–2002. The Sixth Report of Confidential Enquiries into Maternal Deaths in the United Kingdom*. RCOG Press, London.

Confidential Enquiry into Stillbirths and Deaths in Infancy (CESDI) (1998) *Confidential Enquiry into Stillbirths and Deaths in Infancy, 5th Annual Report*. Maternal and Child Health Research Consortium, London.

Davis, E. (1997) *Hearts and Hands: A Midwife's Guide to Pregnancy and Birth*, 3rd edn. Celestial Arts, Berkeley, California.

Davis, S. (1999) Amniotic fluid embolism and isolated disseminated intravascular coagulation. *Canadian Journal of Anaesthesia* **46** (5), 456–9.

Deering, S., Poggi, S., Cedonia, C., Gherman, R. & Satin. A. (2004). Improving resident competency in the management of shoulder dystocia with simulation training. *Obstetrics and Gynaecology* **103** (6), 1224–8.

Department of Health (DoH) (2004) *The National Service Framework for Children, Young People and Maternity Services*. (Standard. 11). Department of Health, London.

Enkin, M. (2000) Labor and birth after a previous caesarean section. In *A Guide to Effective Care in Pregnancy and Childbirth*, 3rd edn (Enkin, M., Keirse, M.J.N.C., Neilson, J., Crowther, C., Duley L., Hodnett, E. & Hofmeyr, J., eds), pp. 359–71. Oxford University Press, Oxford.

Fahy, K.M. (2001) Amniotic fluid embolism: a review of the research literature. *Australian Journal of Midwifery* **14** (1), 9–13.

Gaskin, I. (1990) *Spiritual Midwifery*. The Book Publishing Co., Summertown, Tennessee.

Gherman, R.B. (2002) Shoulder dystocia: an evidence based evaluation of the obstetrical nightmare. *Clinical Obstetrics and Gynaecology* **45**, 345–61.

Gherman, R.B., Goodwin, T.M., Souter, I., Neumann, K., Ouzounian, J.G. and Paul, R. (1997) The McRoberts manoeuvre for the alleviation of shoulder dystocia: how successful is it? *American Journal of Obstetrics and Gynaecology* **176** (3), 656–61.

Johnson, A. (2005) Obstetric brachial plexus palsy: the medico-legal view. *The Obstetrician and Gynaecologist* **7**, 259–65.

Kovavisarach, E. (2006) The "all-fours" manoeuvre for the management of shoulder dystocia. *International Journal of Gynaecology and Obstetrics* **95** (2), 153–4.

Kroll, D. & Lyne, M. (2002) Uterine inversion and uterine rupture. In *Emergencies around Childbirth – A Handbook for Midwives* (Boyle, M., ed.), pp. 89–95. Radcliffe Medical Press, Oxford.

Magill-Cuerden, J. (2001) Clinical file: case study. *The Practising Midwife* **4** (1), 29.

Managing Obstetric Emergencies and Trauma (MOET) (2003) *Course Manual* (Cox, C., Johanson, R., Grady, K. & Howell, C., eds). RCOG Press, London.

Mapp, T. (2005) Feelings and Fears Post Obstetric Emergencies. *British Journal of Midwifery* **13** (1), 36–40.

McGeown, P. (2001) Practice recommendations for obstetric emergencies. *British Journal of Midwifery* **9** (2), 71–4.

Mortimore, V. & McNabb, M. (1998) A six year retrospective analysis of shoulder dystocia and delivery of the shoulders. *Midwifery* **14**, 162–73.

Murphy, D.J. & MacKenzie, I.Z. (1995) The mortality and morbidity associated with umbilical cord prolapse. *British Journal of Obstetrics and Gynaecology* **102** (10), 826–30.

National Health Service Litigation Authority (2003) Supplement on obstetric brachial plexus injury. *National Health Service Litigation Authority Journal* **2**, 105–7.

National Institute for Health and Clinical Excellence (NICE) (2004) *Caesarean Section. Clinical guideline 13.* NICE, London.

Nocon, J.J. (2000) Shoulder dystocia and macrosomia. In *Best Practice in Labour Ward Management* (Kean, L., ed.), pp. 167–86. WB Saunders, Edinburgh.

Pasternak, J.F. (1993) Hypoxic-ischaemic brain damage in the term infant. Lessons from the laboratory. *Pediatric Clinician North America* **40**, 1061–72.

Paxton, A., Maine, D., Freedman, L., Fry, D. & Lobis, S. (2005) The evidence for emergency obstetric care. *International Journal of Gynaecology and Obstetrics* **8** (2), 181–93.

Peña-Martin, G. & Comunián-Carrasco, G. (2007) Fundal pressure versus controlled cord traction as part of the active management of third stage of labour. *Cochrane Database of Systematic Reviews*, Issue 4, Art No. CD00546.

Poggi, S. (2004) In Athukorala, C. Middleton, P. Crowther, C.A. Intrapartum interventions for preventing shoulder dystocia. *Cochrane Database of Systematic Reviews*, 2006 Issue 4. Art No. CD005543.

Prabulos, A.M. & Philipson, E.H. (1998) Umbilical cord prolapse. Is time from diagnosis to delivery critical? *Journal of Reproductive Medicine* **43** (2), 129–32.

Royal College of Paediatrics and Child Health (RCOG) (2005) *Shoulder Dystocia. Green-Top Guideline No. 42.* RCOG, London.

Royal College of Paediatrics and Child Health (RCOG) (2007) *Birth After Previous Caesarean Green-Top Guideline No. 45.* RCOG, London.

Silverton, L. (1993) *The Art and Science of Midwifery.* Prentice Hall International, London.

Simpkin, P. & Ancheta, R. (2005) *The Labor Progress Handbook*, 2nd edn. Blackwells, Oxford.

Squire, C. (2002) Shoulder dystocia and umbilical cord prolapse. In *Emergencies Around Childbirth – A Handbook for Midwives* (Boyle, M., ed.). Radcliffe Medical Press, Abingdon.

Walsh, D. (2007) Managing shoulder dystocia: 'on your back' or 'all-fours'? *British Journal of Midwifery* **15** (5), 254.

Weston, R. (2001) When birth goes wrong. *The Practising Midwife* **4** (8), 10–12.

World Health Organisation (WHO) (2003) Integrated management of pregnancy & childbirth. *Managing Complications in Pregnancy & Childbirth: A Guide for Midwives & Doctors.* Geneva, 2003.

17 Neonatal and maternal resuscitation

Nick Castle

Introduction

Midwives must be able to resuscitate both the newborn baby and the mother, and therefore they should receive annual neonatal and maternal resuscitation training. This training should also cover standard adult resuscitation.

Incidence and facts

- In the developed world around 5–10% of newborn babies require some degree of intervention at birth; typically active stimulation. This number is higher in the developing world (Ergenekon *et al.*, 2000).
- 1% of babies >2.5 kg require assisted ventilation and 20% of these need intubation.
- Occasionally babies are born unexpectedly 'flat', but this can be managed effectively by basic resuscitation techniques (Palme-Kilander, 1992). Only 0.2% of 'low-risk birth' babies require assisted ventilation, and only 10% of these require intubation (Palme-Kilander, 1992).
- It has been estimated that up to 800 000 newborn babies who currently die could be saved by timely basic resuscitation techniques (Zideman *et al.*, 1998), primarily prompt aerating of the lungs (Biarent *et al.*, 2005; Resuscitation Council UK, 2005b).
- Anticipation is the most important aspect of resuscitation; equipment and personnel should be assembled as soon as possible for suspected problems.

Risk management: anticipation

Many situations may result in a newborn baby requiring active resuscitation (Box 17.1). Also, any unexpected birth in the community or the emergency department, although usually uneventful, may present problems.

Box 17.1   Resuscitation anticipation: Risk factors.

Antenatal risk factors
- Maternal diabetes
- Pre-eclampsia/essential hypertension
- Chronic maternal illness (e.g. cardiovascular, thyroid, pulmonary, renal and neurological)
- Previous stillbirth or neonatal death
- Antepartum haemorrhage
- Oligo/polyhydramnios
- Size versus dates discrepancy/reduced fetal movements
- Alcohol or drugs misuse
- Other drugs, e.g. lithium carbonate, magnesium and adrenergic-blocking drugs
- No antenatal care

Intrapartum risk factors
- Preterm birth
- Prolonged rupture of membranes/infection, e.g. chorioamnionitis
- Abnormal fetal heart rate, e.g. bradycardia, tachycardia and prolonged decelerations
- Meconium-stained liquor
- Breech or malpresentation
- Recent maternal opioid analgesia (<4 hours)
- Cord prolapse
- Placenta praevia/abruption
- Fetal abnormality
- Instrumental or operative delivery
- General anaesthetic
(RCPCH & RCOG, 1997; AHA *et al.*, 2000)

Once a 'high-risk' birth is identified, a clinician trained in newborn resuscitation (e.g. paediatrician or advanced neonatal practitioner) should be summoned before birth (Royal College of Paediatrics and Child Health & Royal College of Obstetricians and Gynaecologists (RCPCH & RCOG), 1997). Midwives caring for women at home or in a birthing centre should be aware of factors that can influence the baby's condition at birth and that may necessitate transfer. For a list of community midwife's resuscitation equipment, see Box 17.2.

Box 17.2   Resuscitation equipment for home birth.

Baby resuscitation equipment
- Suction device
- O_2 funnel
- Self-inflating 500 ml bag-mask-valve device
- The use of the 500 ml BVM device in association with a slow, steady and controlled breath will reduce the risk of under-ventilation and/or barotrauma. The traditional 240 ml BVM device is no longer recommended as it is difficult to provide a slow constant inflation pressure (Zideman *et al.*, 1998)
- Oxygen cylinder with variable flow meter

Maternal resuscitation equipment
- Suction device
- Oxygen mask (medium concentration)
- Pocket mask with one-way valve and various oral airways

Box 17.2 *(Continued)*

> - BVM device (optional – as the above pocket mask using oxygen is effective for basic life support)
> - Oxygen cylinder with variable flow meter
>
> **Miscellaneous:** towels, torch, watch/stop watch, stethoscope
>   **Access to phone** to call for assistance
>   For further details refer to Chapter 6, p. xx.

Basic neonatal resuscitation

All previous newborn resuscitation guidelines have been superseded by the consensus document on resuscitation (Biarent *et al.*, 2005). Successful neonatal resuscitation is based on anticipation, environmental control, assessment, stimulation, effective ventilation and, rarely, cardiac compressions with intubation and drug administration. Resuscitation involves a number of processes that occur simultaneously. Each step will be considered separately, although the initial assessment and stimulation should occur as one swift action (see Fig. 17.1).

Environment

It is essential that the newborn baby does not become cold, as acidosis is worsened by hypothermia (Tyson, 2000). Skin-to-skin contact immediately following birth is effective at maintaining/increasing the baby's body temperature. In a hospital or birthing centre, an overhead heater, typically incorporated into a resuscitaire, should be available. Such equipment is not available in the community, so the attending midwife should minimise draughts, ensure that the area is warm and that warmed towels are available. Although this is common sense, it is typically simple procedures that are forgotten during the initial phase of any resuscitation attempt.

Assessment

A rapid assessment of tone, colour, respiratory rate, heart rate, and gut instinct that things are not right, will indicate the need to instigate resuscitation procedures. A stepwise approach is recommended in the assessment of the newborn that may require resuscitation, and this includes active stimulation and opening the airway.

ABC of neonatal resuscitation

(A) Airway. Place the newborn on a firm surface with the head in a neutral position. The newborn has a large head and a small neck, which can lead to airway obstruction. A gentle chin lift/jaw thrust may help.

(B) Breathing. Assess rate, rhythm and depth of ventilation – if the baby is apnoeic administer 'inflation breaths'. Administer supplementary oxygen if the baby is breathing but remains centrally cyanosed; otherwise it is not required.

(C) Circulation. Observe the baby's colour (if floppy and pale, circulation is inadequate) and record the baby's heart rate ideally using a stethoscope or by palpating the umbilical cord. Palpation is unreliable particularly if the heart rate is <100 bpm (Owen & Wyllie, 2004). Commence compression if heart rate is <60 bpm.

Dry the baby, remove any wet cloth and cover

▼

Initial assessment Start the clock or note the time Assess: COLOUR, TONE, BREATHING, HEART RATE (and reassess every 30 seconds)

▼

If not breathing…. **Control the airway** Head in the neutral position Consider chin lift /jaw thrust

▼

Support the breathing If not breathing, or heart rate <100bpm give FIVE INFLATION BREATHS (each 2–3 seconds long) Confirm a response: increase in HEART RATE or visible CHEST MOVEMENT

▼

If there is no response, ask yourself: Is the baby's head in the neutral position? Do I need chin lift /jaw thrust? Do I need longer inflation time? Do I need a second person's help with the airway? Is there an obstruction in the oropharynx – do I need suction? What about an oropharyngeal (Guedal) airway?

▼

When the chest is moving Continue the ventilation breaths if no spontaneous breathing

▼

Check the heart rate If undetectable or <60 bpm and NOT increasing, then

▼

Start chest compressions *Do this only when good ventilation has been established* 3 chest compressions to 1 breath

▼

Reassess after 30 seconds If heart rate improved, stop chest compressions but continue ventilation if not breathing If bradycardic continue ventilation and chest compressions Consider venous access and drugs at this stage

▼

AT ALL STAGES ASK…. Do I need help? Would tracheal intubation be more effective? Is the baby looking cyanosed – do I need supplementary oxygen?

Fig. 17.1   Neonatal life support algorithm (adapted from the Resuscitation Council, UK).

Stimulation

Drying and warming the baby provides adequate stimulation whilst preventing heat loss, but if this fails to generate a response then instigate resuscitation procedures (Biarent *et al.*, 2005). Avoid more aggressive forms of stimulus: they are not a substitute for effective resuscitation.

Suction

There is no role for routine suctioning as it can delay ventilation, causes airway trauma and may lead to vagal-induced bradycardia (Resuscitation Council UK, 2005b). Consider it only if ventilation is unsuccessful.

The initial five breaths

These 'inflation breaths' are designed to inflate and expand the lungs and remove amniotic fluid (Biarent *et al.*, 2005). If delivered effectively, these vital initial breaths can restore spontaneous breathing. They are delivered slowly with constant pressure (maximum pressure <30 cm of water (Biarent *et al.*, 2005)) held for 2–3 s. Do not deliver short, sharp, fast ventilations: this is ineffective and a common reason for failed initial resuscitation (see Table 17.1 for means of ventilation).

Table 17.1 Means of ventilation.

Device	Advantages	Disadvantages	Comments
Mouth-to-mouth	• Easy to learn • Provides a good seal	• Socially unpleasant • Difficult to provide additional oxygen	• This is a priority skill to learn but in a hospital basic airway devices should be available
Pocket mask	• Easy to learn • Provides a good seal • Can be used by one person • Some types have O_2 ports	• Requires training to use effectively • Maximum O_2 is 50% (at 10–15 l/min)	• This is the ideal first response device as it is easy and effective • Ideal for community midwifery use
Bag-valve-mask device	• Can provide high flow O_2 • Less tiring for rescuer	• Difficult to use: often results in under-ventilation • Usually unavailable at the bedside	• This is a device for anaesthetic staff or a two-person midwife technique, i.e. one securing mask to face, the other slowly squeezing the bag

National Institute for Health and Clinical Excellence (NICE) (2007) recommends that the initial breaths should be administered using air. However, if the baby fails to respond despite effective inflation breaths, then supplementary oxygen should be provided. A centrally cyanosed baby with a heart rate >100 bpm who continues to 'gasp' will respond rapidly with stimulation and oxygen therapy (Zideman *et al.*, 1998). Oxygen can be administered via a funnel, a facemask or a cupped hand over the baby's face. It is important not to waft oxygen over the baby as this will actively cool it, and a bag-valve-mask (BVM) device should not be used to deliver oxygen to a spontaneously breathing baby as it increases respiratory workload (American Heart Association *et al.*, 2000).

Following the initial breaths, reassess the baby. At this point the baby will either (a) have improved and be spontaneously breathing/crying, (b) remain apnoeic but with a heart rate >60 bpm or (c) be apnoeic with a heart rate <60 bpm.

Ventilation should continue at a faster rate of 30 breaths/min (allow 1 second for inspiration and 1 second for expiration). Commence cardiac compressions in all babies with a heart rate <60 bpm and reassess the baby every 30 seconds.

Table 17.2 Reasons for no response to assisted ventilation.

Problem	Possible cause	Action
Poor technique	• Ventilating too fast	• Slow down: administer the first breaths over 2–3 s, then subsequent breaths at 30 breaths/min.
Chest not rising	• Poor seal • Wrong size bag-valve-mask device • Airway obstructed	• Readjust mask position • Use a 500 ml BVM • Reposition head: consider chin lift/jaw thrust • Consider suction if thick meconium – although there is no proof of its efficacy (Resuscitation Council UK, 2005b) • Consider using an oral airway
Pressure release valve activated (this valve reduces the risk of pulmonary barotrauma)	• Airway obstructed • Ventilating too fast	• As above: reposition head, consider suction and/or oral airway • Slow down (see 'poor technique' above)

N.B. Occasionally you may need to override the pressure relief valve by pressing on the valve (some BVMs have a clip for this purpose). However this is rarely required, especially with a 500 ml BVM.

Refer also to Fig. 17.1 for neonatal life support resuscitation algorithm and Table 17.2 for trouble-shooting technique when a baby does not respond to ventilation.

Ongoing neonatal resuscitation/complications

Compressions

International guidelines indicate that cardiac compressions should be commenced once effective ventilation has been instigated but the heart rate remains <60 bpm. The ratio of breaths to compression is set at 3:1 emphasising the importance of ventilation. It is difficult for the single-handed resuscitator to maintain an effective respiratory rate whilst also performing compression (Whyte *et al.*, 1999; Biarent *et al.*, 2005), so this process is improved by the presence of a second trained person. Although rarely required, endotracheal intubation facilitates asynchronised compression/ventilations, which improves coronary artery perfusion, but it should only be considered if a skilled intubator is available.

Cardiac compression technique

- **Two-finger method.** Place the tips of two overlaid fingers just below the nipple line in the centre of the baby's chest. This is the preferred method for the lay public and the single-handed midwife.
- **Two-thumb method.** Encircle the baby's chest with your hands, placing two overlaid thumbs just below the baby's nipples in the centre of the chest. The two-thumb technique is the preferred method for resuscitating all babies <1 year old (Biarent *et al.*, 2005).

All midwives should be able to perform both resuscitation techniques, as the two-thumb method is not suitable for single-person resuscitation.

The umbilical cord

It is routine practice to cut the umbilical cord immediately at delivery although Prendiville and Elbourne (2000) have demonstrated that delaying this process by at least 30 seconds can increase the transmission of maternal blood volume by up to 50%. Whilst NICE (2007) recommends immediate cord clamping as they cannot exclude a risk of hyperbilirubinaemia, it is worth speculating that an anaemic baby could potentially benefit from the extra blood. The umbilicus should be cut long >10 cm to facilitate cannulation.

Meconium aspiration

Suctioning the baby prior to delivery of the baby's chest is ineffective and no longer recommended (Vain *et al.*, 2004). Suctioning should only be considered in the apnoeic 'flat baby' where there is thick meconium obstructing the baby's airway, although there is no evidence that even this prevents meconium aspiration (Resuscitation Council UK, 2005a).

Intubation

Intubation is rarely required (Palme-Kilander, 1992). It is a complex skill to learn and difficult to maintain. Therefore the emphasis is on effective BVM ventilation and not intubation. There are still a number of situations where intubation remains useful:

- Prolonged ventilation/difficult BVM ventilation.
- Surfactant administration.
- Special circumstances, e.g. diaphragmatic hernia.
  The rarity of neonatal intubation reduces the opportunity for staff to maintain clinical skills. In circumstances where BVM ventilation is proving ineffective/impossible, a laryngeal mask airway has been successfully used (Esmail *et al.*, 2002). Currently there is insufficient data to support the routine use of laryngeal mask airways during neonatal resuscitation (Biarent *et al.*, 2005), but it is an interesting area for consideration for improving resuscitation/ventilation in units without access to experienced intubators.

Drugs

Drugs have a very limited role in neonatal resuscitation (see Table 17.3).

- **Adrenaline** is the main resuscitation drug for the neonate who, despite effective ventilation and cardiac compressions, has a heart rate <60 bpm (Biarent *et al.*, 2005). Adrenaline should be administered intravenously (umbilical vein or cannula), although it can be administered via the intraosseous route. Administration via the endotracheal tube (ETT) is no longer recommended, but if this route is used higher doses are required (100 µg/kg) (Biarent *et al.*, 2005).

Table 17.3   Neonatal resuscitation drugs.

Drug	Dose/concentration	Route	Typical dose
Adrenaline	10–30 µg/kg 0.1–0.3 ml/kg of 1:10 000 (1 mg in 10 ml)	Intravenous (IV)	0.3–0.9 ml of 1:10 000
Sodium bicarbonate	1–2 ml/kg of 4.2% solution	IV only	3–6 ml of 4.2% solution
Naloxone	10 µg/kg (IV) 60 µg/kg (IM)	IV dose can be repeated A single one dose of 200 µg IM can be given	30 µg IV bolus Or A single 200 µg IM dose
10% dextrose	2.5 ml/kg	IV only	5–7.5 ml

- **Sodium bicarbonate** is reserved for a baby who has not responded to effective ventilation and cardiac compressions despite adrenaline (Biarent *et al.*, 2005). There is little evidence to support its routine use.
- **Normal saline** is the preferred fluid for use in the resuscitation of the newborn (Biarent *et al.*, 2005). A fluid challenge should be administered over at least 5 minutes if hypovolaemia is suspected or where initial attempts at resuscitation have failed.
- **Dextrose** should be administered to 'flat babies' who have a capillary blood sugar <2 mmol and have not responded to the initial 'five breaths'.
- **Naloxone** is rarely required and should only be considered once the baby has been effectively ventilated, has a good cardiac output but remains apnoeic where the mother has received opioids in labour. However, do not give it if there is a history of maternal opioid abuse (AHA *et al.*, 2000).

Extremely preterm babies

This is an emotive issue as neonatal intensive care has improved the outcome for even the smallest newborn (Van Reempts & Van Acker, 2001) (see Chapter 12). Refer to local policy on very low birth weight babies and babies born around the 24th week. If in doubt implement resuscitation as estimated gestational dates can be inaccurate.

Termination of neonatal resuscitation

The likelihood of successful neurological outcome following 10 minutes of advanced neonatal life support is extremely low (Haddad *et al.*, 2000), and therefore termination of resuscitation efforts in the lifeless baby is typically considered at this point (Biarent *et al.*, 2005).

Maternal resuscitation

Incidence and facts

- Cardiac arrest in pregnancy has been estimated at 1:30 000 pregnancies.
- In the UK, the peri-mortem/post-mortem caesarean section (CS) rate is 1:170 000 deliveries: road traffic accident is the most common reason (Whitten & Montgomery, 2000).

Basic life support

The emphasis of basic life support (BLS) during pregnancy is on airway management, assisted ventilations and cardiac compressions. The anatomical and physiological changes associated with pregnancy make resuscitation more difficult (see Box 17.3), and therefore require changes to established resuscitation procedures (Soar *et al.*, 2005). The main difficulties during pregnancy include an increased risk of aspiration/regurgitation, higher than normal oxygen demand and the woman needing to be in the tilted left lateral position.

Box 17.3   Pregnancy factors affecting maternal resuscitation.

Difficult intubation
- Full dentition
- Large breasts
- Raised thoracic cage or flared rib cage
- Neck obesity/oedema
- Supraglottic oedema

Difficult chest compression
- Left lateral tilt positions (to avoid inferior vena caval occlusion)
- Flared rib cage
- Raised diaphragm

Respiratory
- Increased tidal volume requirements and O_2 demand
- Reduced chest compliance
- Reduced functional residual capacity

Cardiovascular
- Incompetent gastro-oesophageal sphincter
- Increased intragastric pressure
- Increased risk of regurgitation

The ABC of maternal resuscitation

(Refer to Fig. 17.2.)

(A) Airway. Check for foreign bodies and then open the airway with a 'head tilt-jaw lift' manoeuvre. The jaw thrust manoeuvre can be used in conjunction with an airway adjunct (e.g. oropharyngeal airway) to facilitate effective ventilation.

(B) Breathing. All breaths should be given slowly to reduce the risk of gastric distension (Soar *et al.*, 2005) regardless of device used.

(C) Circulation. The compression/ventilation ratio is 30:2 prior to intubation. Following intubation, ventilation and cardiac compression are performed asynchronously with 10 breaths and 100 compressions per minute (Soar *et al.*, 2005).

The left lateral tilt position

To minimise the effects of aortocaval compression, all visibly pregnant critically ill women must be placed in a left lateral tilt position. This can be achieved using a wedge,

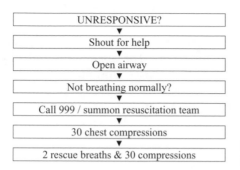

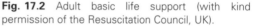

Fig. 17.2 Adult basic life support (with kind permission of the Resuscitation Council, UK).

using upturned chairs (if patient is on the floor) or by using the human wedge approach. The technique requires minimal training and patient movement to use. The general principles are to ensure the patient achieves a 30° left lateral tilt and that the wedge is non-compressible during chest compressions.

Advanced life support

The technique is the same regardless of the woman being pregnant (see Fig. 17.3), with one significant change: emergency peri-/post-mortem CS. The choice of drugs remains the same regardless of pregnancy. Drugs for maternal resuscitation are given in Table 17.4.

Advanced airway management

Maternal airway protection during cardiac arrest is vital to reduce the risk of pulmonary aspiration. The difficulties associated with intubating a pregnant woman require that an experienced/skilled intubator and equipment for failed intubation should be available.

Defibrillation

Immediate defibrillation to reverse ventricular fibrillation (VF) or pulseless, ventricular tachycardia (VT) remains vital, as no other intervention will be successful in restoring a normal cardiac rhythm. The risk to the unborn baby is extremely low and is greatly outweighed by the maternal benefits.

Emergency caesarean section

Emergency CS is directly linked to the successful resuscitation of the mother as well as the newborn and is an integral part of maternal resuscitation (Whitten & Montgomery, 2000). It is vital that there is no delay in performing this emergency procedure. Do not move the mother in cardiac arrest to an operating theatre, as this will waste time, adversely affect BLS: bring the equipment to the woman. Equally, full theatre-style sterility will not be possible and will also waste time. It has been suggested that delivery of the baby within 4 min of cardiac arrest may save the life of the baby (Boyle, 2002), although the mother's condition is always the priority.

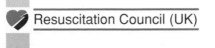 Resuscitation Council (UK)

Adult Advanced Life Support Algorithm

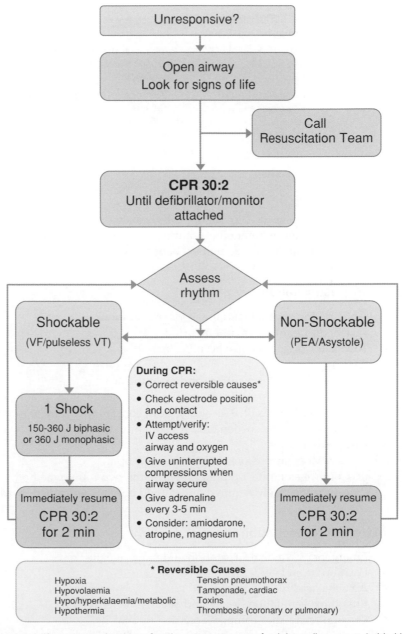

Fig. 17.3 Advanced life support algorithm for the management of adult cardiac arrest (with kind permission of Resuscitation Council, UK).

Table 17.4 Adult resuscitation drugs.

Drug	Dose/route	Rationale	Frequency
Adrenaline	1 mg 1:10 000 IV or double ETT dose via	To improve cerebral and coronary artery perfusion	1 mg every 3 min
Atropine	3 mg IV or double dose via ETT	To increase heart rate by blocking parasympathetic nervous system	Once only
Amiodarone	300 mg IV bolus, then further 150 mg if required	To increase reversal of VF or VT following defibrillation	One or two doses if resistant VF/VT
Calcium chloride	10 ml/10% solution IV only	To protect the heart from hyperkalaemia or magnesium overdose	Until QRS complexes narrow
Sodium bicarbonate	1 mmol/kg (1 ml/kg of 8.4%) typically 50 ml bolus IV of 8.4%	Treatment of acidosis in intubated patients during prolonged cardiac arrest, treatment of hyper-kalaemia and treatment of tricyclic antidepressant overdose	Depending on clinical situation

Summary

For a midwife to be able to safely perform resuscitation of both the mother and the newborn baby, a combination of training, clinical assessment skills and the ability to identify and treat the at-risk mother/baby are vital.

Infant resuscitation

- Anticipation of problems allows for preparation.
- Warm, draught-free environment.
- Towels for drying the newborn.
- **Airway**
  - Place baby on firm surface and open the airway.
- **Breathing**
  - First five breaths (2–3 seconds): slow, constant pressure to inflate lungs.
  - Consider gentle suction only if ventilation unsuccessful.
- **Circulation**
  - Cardiac compressions if heart rate <60 bpm.
  - Compression rate 3:1; preferably use the two-thumb method.
  - Intubation rarely required and should only be performed by trained staff.

Maternal resuscitation

- Emergency CS aids resuscitation and may save the baby.
- Position in left lateral tilt.
- Airway: head tilt and jaw lift.
- Breathing: ventilation slowly and effectively delivered.
- Circulation: cardiac compressions at a ratio of 30:2.

References

American Heart Association, Resuscitation Council (UK), European Resuscitation Council *et al.* (2000) International guidelines 2000 for cardiopulmonary resuscitation and emergency cardiovascular care – an international consensus on science. *Resuscitation* **46** (special issue) xix–xx, 293–301, 401–16.

Biarent, D., Bingham, R., Richmond, S., Maconochie, I., Wyllie, J., Simpson, S., Nunez, A. & Zideman, D. (2005) European guidelines council guidelines for resuscitation Section 6. Paediatric life support. *Resuscitation* **67** (Suppl. 1), S97–134.

Boyle, M. (2002) *Emergencies Around Childbirth: A Handbook for Midwives.* Abingdon, Radcliffe.

Ergenekon, E., Koc, E., Atalay, Y. & Soysal, S. (2000) Neonatal resuscitation course experience in Turkey. *Resuscitation* **45** (3), 225–7.

Esmail, N., Saleh, M. & Ali, A. (2002) Laryngeal mask airway versus endotracheal intubation for Apgar score improvement in neonatal resuscitation. *Egypt Journal of Anesthesiology* **18**, 115–21.

Haddad, B., Mercer, B., Livingstone, J. & Sibai, B. (2000) Outcomes after successful resuscitation of babies born with Apgar scores of at 1 and 5 min. *American Journal of Obstetrics and Gynaecology* **182**, 1210–14.

National Institute for Health and Clinical Excellence (NICE) (2007) *Clinical Guideline 55: Intrapartum Care.* National Institute for Health and Clinical Excellence, London.

Owen, C. & Wyllie, J. (2004) Determination of heart rate in the baby at birth. *Resuscitation* **60**, 213–7.

Palme-Kilander, C. (1992) Methods of resuscitation in low Apgar score newborn infants – a national survey. *Acta Paediatrica* **81**, 739–44.

Prendiville, W. & Elbourne, D. (2000) The third stage of labour. In *A Guide to Effective Care in Pregnancy and Childbirth*, 3rd edn (Enkin, M., Keirse, M.J.N.C., Neilson, J., Crowther, C., Duley, L., Hodnett, E. & Hofmeyr, J., eds), pp. 300–309. Oxford University Press, Oxford.

Resuscitation Council UK (2005a) *Adult Life Support.* Available at: www.resus.org.uk/pages/als.pdf (accessed March 2008).

Resuscitation Council UK (2005b) *Neonatal Life Support.* Available at: www.resus.org.uk/pages/nls.pdf (accessed March 2008).

Royal College of Paediatrics and Child Health & Royal College of Obstetricians and Gynaecologists (RCPCH & RCOG) (1997) *Resuscitation of Babies at Birth.* BMJ Publishing, London.

Soar, J., Deakin, C D., Nolan, J.P., Abbas, G., Alfonzo, A.J., Handley, A.J, Lockey, D., Perkins, G.D. & Thies, K. (2005) Section 7. Cardiac arrest in special circumstances. *Resuscitation* **67** (1), S135–71.

Tyson, J. (2000) Immediate care of the newborn infant. In *A Guide to Effective Care in Pregnancy and Childbirth*, 3rd edn (Enkin, M., Keirse, M.J.N.C., Neilson, J., Crowther, C., Duley L., Hodnett, E. & Hofmeyr, J. eds), pp. 417–28. Oxford University Press, Oxford.

Vain, N., Szyld, E., Prudent, L., Wiswell, T., Aguilar, A. & Vivas, N. (2004) Oropharyngeal and nasopharyngeal suctioning of meconium-stained neonates before delivery of their shoulders: multicentre, randomised controlled trial. *Lancet* **364**, 597–602.

Van Reempts, P. & Van Acker, K. (2001) Ethical aspects of cardiopulmonary resuscitation in premature neonates: where do we stand? *Resuscitation* **51** (3), 225–32.

Whitten, W. & Montgomery, L. (2000) Postmortem and perimortem caesarean sections: what are the indications? *Journal of the Royal Society of Medicine* **93**, 6–9.

Whyte, S., Sinha, A. & Wyllie, J. (1999) Neonatal resuscitation – a practical assessment. *Resuscitation* **40** (1), 21–5.

Zideman, D., Bingham, R., Beattie, T., Bland, J., Bruinsstanssen, M. & Frei, F. (1998) Recommendations on resuscitation of babies at birth. *Resuscitation* **37** (2), 103–10.

18   Induction of labour

Mary-Lou Elliott

Introduction

Induction of labour (IOL), although a common procedure, can present challenges for both mothers and clinicians (National Institute for Health and Clinical Excellence (NICE), 2001).

Once women have passed their due date, frustration, anxiety and boredom leave them vulnerable to the suggestion of IOL. Midwives can be of great support during this time, encouraging positive thinking and suggesting natural methods for stimulating labour. Being overdue can be viewed positively as getting some extra personal time before the baby's arrival (Robertson, 1997).

The recommendation of IOL can begin an anxious time for many women who have planned for a normal labour and birth. Feelings of disappointment and loss of control can also occur if their intended place of birth changes from home or birthing centre to an unfamiliar consultant unit. The midwife has an important role to play in educating women about IOL and providing the information needed to make informed choices about whether/when to consent to procedures, the types of interventions possible and the support available during labour and birth.

Definition

IOL can be viewed as any procedure or intervention that starts off labour rather than allowing it to commence spontaneously. Although natural and alternative methods of induction can be used, the term *IOL* in this chapter generally refers to surgical and/or pharmacological methods.

253

Incidence and facts

- Approximately 20% of women in the UK have labour induced (NICE, 2001).
- 33% of women induced stated they would have valued more information about the reasons for and process of IOL (Nuutulia *et al.*, 1999).
- Despite an increased risk of operative delivery and sometimes a more painful labour, women undergoing IOL for premature rupture of membranes (PROM) tend to have fewer negative comments than those undergoing expectant management, and feel more satisfaction and less worry with the experience (Hodnett *et al.*, 1997). This could stem from a decrease in anxiety and the relief obtained from a proactive approach to finally getting their baby born.
- NICE (2001) recommend IOL for all women with pregnancies 41/40.
- IOL for post-41/40 nulliparous pregnancies may reduce perinatal mortality without increasing caesarean section (CS) rates (NICE, 2001), but the evidence base is controversial.

IOL is usually recommended when it is agreed that the risk of continuing the pregnancy outweighs the risk of intervention to induce birth. An exception, however, may be IOL for maternal request, where the mother's desire for delivery may be at odds with clinical opinion. IOL should only be considered when vaginal birth is felt to be the appropriate mode of delivery.

Possible indications

- Prolonged pregnancy
- Pre-labour rupture of membranes >24 hours (NICE, 2007)
- Pre-eclampsia
- Cholestasis
- Diabetes
- Stabilised unstable lie
- Suspected intrauterine growth restriction
- Intrauterine death or severe fetal abnormality (termination of pregnancy)
- Rhesus isoimmunisation
- Congenital fetal abnormality requiring early treatment
- Severe maternal condition, e.g. advanced cancer
- Genital herpes (while inactive)
- Previous stillbirth
- Previous large baby (>4 kg)
- Maternal request

IOL should only be offered with caution to women with the following:

- Previous CS or uterine scar
- High parity
- Polyhydramnios
- Uncertain due date

Contraindications:

- Placenta praevia or vasa praevia

- Malpresentation
- Fetal compromise
- History of hypertonic labour following prostaglandin
- No consent for IOL

Insufficient evidence exists for recommending IOL for multiple pregnancy, macrosomia or history of precipitate labour.

Risks and side effects

The concept of IOL as 'routine' is a dangerous one; it should always be approached with caution. In women with particular risk factors, induction should not take place on an antenatal ward but on labour ward where the woman and baby can be more closely monitored. This is advisable for women with relevant risk factors including suspected fetal growth compromise, previous CS and high parity (NICE, 2001).

One of the less easily measurable risks of IOL may be the effect on a woman's sense of control. Once she has initially consented to IOL, she may be offered little subsequent choice in continuing on to the next 'inevitable' procedure, leading to a cascade of interventions (Royal College of Midwives (RCM), 2005). Anxiety and loss of control may lead to increased stress levels which can have physiological consequences for labour (see Chapter 1). It must of course be remembered that prolonged pregnancy can also be stressful, so for some women induction actually gives them a sense of relief.

Other risks include the following:

- Membrane sweeping can cause minor bleeding but does not result in an increased incidence of membrane rupture or infection (NICE, 2001).
- Repeated vaginal examinations (VEs) can be painful, so perform them only when essential. Hibitane obstetric cream is not recommended for VEs as its chlorhexidine component can cause soreness.
- Whilst there is no conclusive evidence that prostaglandin-induced labour is more painful than spontaneous onset (NICE, 2001), some anecdotal accounts suggest otherwise. Prostin sometimes causes vaginal soreness (NICE, 2001). Intravenous (IV) oxytocin infusion appears to causes more painful contractions, perhaps due to their more intense onset, and as a result many women in this situation will opt for epidural anaesthesia.
- Hypertonic uterine contractions caused by oxytocics and/or prostaglandins can lead to fetal oxygen deprivation, uterine rupture and maternal and/or perinatal death (Smith *et al.*, 2004). Close fetal and maternal surveillance is therefore essential. Induction and labour for women with high parity or previous CS carries a small but significant risk of uterine rupture even in the absence of hypertonic contractions (see Chapter 11).
- Response to prostaglandins and oxytocics is unpredictable, and midwives should observe women for tachycardia, nausea, vomiting, diarrhoea, water intoxication and headache (Hawkins, 2000).

- The CS risk evidence is controversial. Some studies suggest that IOL for uncomplicated post-term pregnancies increases the risk of CS delivery, length of hospital stay, use of epidural and non-epidural anaesthesia, neonatal resuscitation, neonatal intensive care unit admission and phototherapy (Seyb *et al.*, 1999; Maslow & Sweeny, 2000; Boulvain *et al.*, 2001). Cochrane meta-analysis (Gulmezoglu *et al.*, 2006) and NICE (2001) however state that a policy of routine IOL for post-term pregnancies >41/40 is associated with no difference in CS delivery compared with conservative management. The Royal College of Obstetricians and Gynaecologists (RCOG) (2001) suggests that the CS rate is in fact lower with IOL, and all agree there is no difference in use of epidural anaesthesia, instrumental delivery or fetal heart rate abnormalities.

Information giving and informed consent

Midwives are in a unique position to fully explain what IOL entails and answer any questions the woman and her partner may have. MIDIRS provides an informed choice leaflet entitled 'Prolonged Pregnancy' (www.infochoice.org) and most trusts provide information leaflets containing contact numbers, should women have further questions following the initial discussion.

An obstetrician's recommendation of IOL can be very difficult to refuse, but women should be made aware that they have the right to decline. Midwives can be in a difficult position, since they may be supporting a woman's right to refuse intervention whilst there may sometimes be very good reasons for recommending IOL (e.g. high-risk medical problems like pre-eclampsia).

If a woman chooses to decline post-dates IOL, conservative management should be offered, i.e. maternal vigilance of fetal movements, and twice weekly liquor volume scans and cardiotocographs (CTGs) (NICE, 2001).

Determining expected date of delivery

Midwives will be familiar with the various methods of determining expected date of delivery (EDD). Consideration to the length of the menstrual cycle will enhance accuracy, and this is important in avoiding unintentional preterm IOL. Research shows that using ultrasound scan to calculate EDD results in fewer pregnancies considered post-term if the biparietal measurement is performed between 13/40 and 22/40 (Gardosi *et al.*, 1997), but women may feel undermined if scan dates do not correspond to dates of which they are certain.

IOL for social reasons

Some women may wish to be induced even though there are no medical or post-dates indications. Midwives should discuss the risks of early/unnecessary IOL, but where resources allow, maternal request for IOL at term may be considered when there are compelling psychological or social reasons and the woman has a favourable cervix. Social induction is unlikely to be supported if there are contraindications to IOL or staffing/resource issues.

Induction for post-term pregnancy

NICE (2001) recommends offering induction beyond 41/40 for women with uncomplicated pregnancies, but compliance with this recommendation varies among trusts. Without IOL:

- by 40/40   58% will give birth
- by 41/40   74% will give birth
- by 42/40   82% will give birth

18% will remain undelivered after 42/40 without IOL.

The incidence of stillbirth increases with gestation (NICE, 2001):

- at 37/40   1:3000
- at 42/40   3:3000
- at 43/40   6:3000

There is no current evidence to suggest that IOL before 41/40 improves fetal or maternal outcomes, but IOL after this time has been found to decrease rates of stillbirth and neonatal death in otherwise uncomplicated pregnancies (Hartman & King, 2001). Cochrane review by Gulmezoglu *et al.* (2006) concludes that there is only a very slightly increased perinatal mortality beyond 41/40 and states 'the absolute risk is extremely small' and that women should be counselled on both relative and absolute risks.

IOL versus expectant management for PROM at term

Premature rupture of membranes at term:

- Occurs in 6–19% of term pregnancies (NICE, 2001).
- 86% of women with PROM will go into spontaneous labour within 24 hours; the rate of spontaneous labour will then increase by 5% per day (NICE, 2001).
- NICE (2007) recommends IOL by 24 hours post-PROM.

Women induced after 24 hours were less likely than those managed expectantly to develop chorioamnionitis and endometritis, with no difference in instrumental or CS rates or adverse neonatal outcome (NICE, 2007). Neonatal infection rates were marginally reduced by early IOL in one study quoted by NICE. Women should be given information to make an informed choice on this issue; neonatal outcomes are not very different with either method (Dare *et al.*, 2006).

Assessing the cervix

The Bishop score is a subjective assessment of cervical ripeness for IOL that describes cervical effacement, consistency, position, dilatation and descent of the fetal presenting part. The score is determined by VE: a score of 6 or above viewed as favourable for IOL. Despite dilatation alone having been found to be a better determinate of successful IOL and vaginal delivery than the combined components of the Bishop score (Williams *et al.*, 1997), it is still routinely used. Ultrasound scan has been shown to be of value in the prediction of successful IOL but is not widely used. (Rane *et al.*, 2004).

Methods of induction

Natural methods

Women seem open to natural methods of inducing labour once their due date has arrived. Most natural methods have had little research into their effectiveness, but anecdotal reports show varying levels of success. Natural methods include the following:

- Breast/nipple stimulation: Kavanagh *et al.* (2005) state that this appears effective in inducing labour and reducing postpartum haemorrhage but recommends caution in high-risk groups as the results can be dramatic.
- Sexual intercourse: this is a difficult and delicate area to study and research is so far inconclusive.
- Exercise, e.g. brisk walking.
- Eating spicy foods, e.g. curry.
- Eating fresh pineapple.
- Membrane sweeping.

NICE (2001) recommends membrane sweeping/stripping from term, a safe and effective method of reducing post-term pregnancy in low-risk women. The procedure is usually performed by a midwife who gently inserts a finger into the cervix and rotates it 360°, separating the membranes from the lower uterine segment. This aims to increase production of prostaglandins in the hope that amniotomy or oxytocic drugs can be avoided. Serial sweeping every 48 hours until labour commences results in consistent reduction in post-term pregnancy regardless of Bishop score (Boulvain *et al.*, 2005). Women's satisfaction is generally high despite the procedure's discomfort, with most happy to accept it again in the future (de Miranda *et al.*, 2006).

Complementary/alternative methods

Unless specifically trained in alternative methods, midwives would be wise to direct women to qualified practitioners, advising them to be cautious before using any of the methods discussed.

- Acupuncture/acupressure/moxibustion (this is also used for turning breeches)
- Reflexology
- Visualisation and meditation
- Hypnosis
- Herbal remedies
- Homeopathic remedies
- Castor oil

There are few studies into the above methods of IOL, but numerous websites and texts exist which explore their use.

Surgical/pharmacological methods

- Amniotomy or artificial rupture of membranes (ARM)
- Prostaglandin
- IV oxytocin

ARM

- ARM involves risk and constitutes a definite commitment to delivery. See Chapter 2 for risks, benefits and contraindications.
- There is insufficient evidence to recommend ARM alone as a method of IOL (Bricker and Luckas, 2007), so even if the cervix is sufficiently dilated to allow ARM, it is usually good practice to give at least one dose of prostaglandin first to ripen the cervix. However, many midwives believe that multigravid women with a high Bishop score may respond favourably to ARM alone, and this may prevent further intervention, so a decision should be made on an individual basis after discussion with the woman.
- CTG monitoring is not indicated, and water birth is not contraindicated following ARM induction once labour has been established if all else appears normal.
- ARM plus IV oxytocin within 1 hour results in a shorter latent phase of labour (Moldin and Sundell, 1996) although the optimal time interval between ARM and syntocinon is not clear.
- ARM is not automatically indicated following prostin if the woman is contracting and VE confirms progress.

Prostaglandins

- Prostaglandin (PGE2) vaginal tablets or gel soften or 'ripen' the cervix. Tablets are significantly cheaper and just as effective as gel (NICE, 2001).
- Oral prostaglandins have gastrointestinal side effects and lack evaluation casting doubts over their safety, so are rarely used (Hawkins, 2000).
- Prostaglandins given prior to ARM increase its effectiveness (NICE, 2001).
- Prostaglandin IOL alone results in a decreased incidence of operative delivery and an increased chance of delivery within 24 hours compared with oxytocin IOL alone (Enkin *et al.*, 2000). The woman's ability to remain mobile and upright in labour may play a part in this.
- Although misoprostol has been reported to be a safe and effective IOL drug (Surbek *et al.*, 1997), it is not currently licensed for obstetric use. NICE (2001) and Gaskin (2001) suggest that certain risks have not yet been fully evaluated.

Oxytocin

- IV oxytocin (Syntocinon) is used to stimulate contractions if prostin and ARM have not achieved good labour progress.
- It should be administered via a controlled infusion pump/syringe driver with a non-return valve.
- Women who have had prostaglandins may respond dramatically to oxytocin and experience severe contractions (NICE, 2001). Continuous electronic fetal monitoring (EFM) is recommended during oxytocin induction to observe for uterine hypertonus, hypercontractility and/or fetal distress (NICE, 2001).

Care of a woman during IOL

Although IOL is a significant intervention in the normal process of labour, the midwife can do much to support the woman in her wish for a normal birth. Once the reason for IOL is understood and all agree that it is desirable, it is important to ascertain the woman's understanding of the process. Discuss how much she would actually like to know about the procedure (does she really want to see an amnihook?), and to provide further explanation and written information if necessary. The midwife should be aware that the woman may be in a high state of anxiety, especially if IOL is indicated for a fetal concern.

Midwives can give reassurance and explanations about the length of time it may take to get labour established, which may sometimes mean several days. If IOL has to be postponed after starting due to a busy labour ward, further explanation and support will be needed for both women and their birth partner/s. Midwives familiar with distressed women in antenatal beds who are well over their due dates and desperate to give birth recognise the need for sensitivity should this situation arise.

Partners and birth supporters should be included whenever possible so that all members of the 'birthing team' can work together to achieve a satisfying experience for the woman. Familiarisation with the birth setting, advice regarding suitable clothing, refreshment, meals and rest periods will enhance the experience. Where possible, the woman should not be separated from her support, and her midwife should give extra support if she is alone at any time.

Although usually done on delivery suite, IOL can be initiated on the antenatal ward alongside other women undergoing the procedure if there are no complications in the pregnancy (NICE, 2001).

General labour care applies as with spontaneous labour. Consent issues are just as important, and just because a woman has agreed to IOL, her consent for subsequent VEs and interventions is no less important. The midwife's documentation should show evidence of a clear plan of care, progress of the labour and drugs used in the IOL process.

Midwifery care for starting IOL

- Review notes/history to ascertain EDD and rule out contraindications.
- Discuss the procedure with the woman and her partner(s) and gain consent. Make time to answer any questions and advise on coping mechanisms for 'prostin pains'/early labour, such as warmed wheatgerm bag, a warm bath or going for a distracting walk.
- Ensure the IOL has been authorised and prostaglandin written up. Prostaglandins must be prescribed by a doctor. The midwife is responsible for ensuring the correct dose is administered safely.
- Ask woman to empty her bladder.
- Ensure the woman's privacy.
- Commence CTG pre-procedure to ascertain fetal well-being.
- Assess cervix and explain Bishop score.
- Administer appropriate dose of prostaglandin or ARM depending on Bishop score. The gel/tablet is inserted into the posterior vaginal fornix at regular intervals; NICE recommends 6-hourly but the optimal time is unknown. Maximum recommended tablet dosage is 6 mg for all women. Maximum gel dosage is 4 mg for a nulliparous and 3 mg for other woman (NICE, 2001).

- Continue CTG until unequivocally satisfactory (typically 30–60 min), but once labour is established intermittent monitoring is recommended following prostaglandin IOL in the absence of other risk factors (NICE, 2001).
- Ensure maternal and fetal surveillance is implemented, should continuation of IOL be delayed.
- Women should be warned of side effects and advised to inform the midwife of symptoms such as very strong, frequent and painful contractions, sudden nausea and vomiting or if anything is worrying them.
- Intermittent FH monitoring is perfectly acceptable after initial CTG (NICE, 2001), and therefore labour in water is an option. It is sensible to ensure that labour is truly established first as early immersion can slow labour (see Chapter 7).
- Inform obstetrician if lack of progress or any problems.

Continuing IOL: care with IV oxytocin

If the woman has not established in labour, she will naturally feel disappointed: remember she may have had up to five doses of prostaglandin over several days and be tired and despondent. The next option to discuss is oxytocin, informing her she still has the option to decline. Women have occasionally been known to go home and return several days later in spontaneous labour or for further IOL.

- ARM is recommended prior to IV oxytocin if possible as it makes IOL much more effective (NICE, 2001).
- Ensure that oxytocin has been authorised and prescribed. It should not be started <6 hours after prostaglandin due to the combined uterotonic effects (NICE, 2001).
- Discuss analgesia prior to commencing IV oxytocin as it is likely to be more painful: the woman may be happy to wait and see how she copes.
- Oxytocin regimes may vary among trusts but all must be monitored closely.
  - Site IV cannula and commence oxytocin infusion.
  - Infusion rate is 1–2 mU/min, increasing at 30-min intervals (NICE, 2001).
  - The minimum dose possible should be used, aiming for 3–4 contractions every 10 min. If overcontracting reduce the infusion (NICE, 2001).
  - Continuous EFM is recommended (NICE, 2007).
  - If severe hypercontractility and/or fetal compromise is suspected, discontinue the infusion immediately and suggest the woman adopts a lateral position and summon an obstetrician. If the situation does not resolve tocolysis may be considered and/or the delivery expedited. Although not licensed for use in obstetrics, the beta-sympathomimetic drugs, salbutamol via inhaler and terbutaline 0.25 mg subcutaneously, can be administered and are effective in reversing the effects of oxytocics (Hawkins, 2000).
- The women's wishes and consent should be elicited at every stage of the induction process. Clear explanations and support are vital.

Summary

- 20% women experience IOL which many find stressful.
- Many women are open to trying natural/complementary IOL methods.

- Pharmacological/surgical IOL involves risk: it is never 'routine'.
- IOL can take several days and can be wearing for all involved.
- Informed choice throughout the IOL process is vital.
- Pharmacological IOL is usually more painful than spontaneous onset of labour.
- The main risks of prostaglandin and oxytocin are hypercontractility and fetal distress.
- Continuous EFM during oxytocin IOL is recommended.
- Discontinue oxytocin infusion if hypercontracting or suspected fetal compromise.

Recommended reading

Clement, S. (1998) *Psychological Perspectives in Pregnancy and Childbirth.* Churchill Livingstone, London. Have suggested to M-Lou she cuts this.

Tiran, D. & Mack, S. (2000) *Complementary Therapies for Pregnancy and Childbirth*, 2nd edn. Bailliere Tindall, London.

References

Boulvain, M., Marcoux, S., Bureau, M., Fortier, M. & Fraser, W. (2001) Risks of induction of labour in uncomplicated term pregnancies. *Paediatric and Perinatal Epidemiology*, **15** (2), 131–8.

Boulvain, M., Stan, C. & Orion, O. (2005) Membrane sweeping for labour. *Cochrane Database of Systematic Reviews*, Issue 1.

Bricker, L. & Luckas, M. (2007) Amniotomy alone for induction of labour. *Cochrane Database of Systematic Reviews*, Issue 4.

Dare, M., Middleton, P., Crowther, C, Flenady, V. & Varatharaju, B. (2006) Planned early birth versus expectant management (waiting) for prelabour rupture of membranes at term (37 weeks or more). *Cochrane Database of Systemic Reviews*, Issue 1.

de Miranda, E., Van Der Bom, JG., Bonsel, G.J., Bleker, O.P. & Rosendaal, F.R. (2006) Membrane sweeping and prevention of post-term pregnancy in low-risk pregnancies: a randomised controlled trial. *BJOG: An International Journal of Obstetrics and Gynaecology*, **113** (4), 402–408.

Enkin, M., Keirse, M., Neilson, J., Crowther, C., Duley, L., Hodnett, E. & Hofmeyr, J. (2000) *A Guide to Effective Care in Pregnancy and Childbirth*, 3rd edn. Oxford University Press, Oxford.

Gardosi, J., Vanner, T. & Francis, A. (1997) Gestational age and induction of labour for prolonged pregnancy. *British Journal of Obstetrics and Gynaecology* **104** (7), 792–7.

Gaskin, I.M. (2001) The dark side of US obstetrics' love affair with misoprostol. *MIDIRS Midwifery Digest* **11** (2), 205–209.

Gulmezoglu, A., Crowther, C. & Middleton, P. (2006) Induction of labour for improving birth outcomes for women at or beyond term. *Cochrane Database of Systematic Reviews*, Issue 4.

Hartman, K. & King, V. (2001) Commentary – elective induction of labour: complicating the uncomplicated? *Paediatric and Perinatal Epidemiology* **15** (2), 138–9.

Hawkins, D.F. (2000) *Prescribing Drugs in Pregnancy. A Guide to Preconception Counselling and Use of Medicines in Pregnancy, Labour and the Puerperium*, Euromed Communications.

Hodnett, E.D., Hannah, M.E., Weston, J.A., Ohlsson, A., Myhr, T.L., Wang, E.E., Hewson, S.A., Willan, A.R. & Farine D. (1997) Women's evaluations of induction of labor versus expectant management for prelabor rupture of the membranes at term. *Birth* **24** (4), 214–20.

Kavanagh, J., Kelly, A. & Thomas, J. (2005) Breast stimulation for cervical ripening and induction of labour. *Cochrane Database of Systematic Reviews*, Issue 3.

Maslow, A.S. & Sweeny, A.L. (2000) Elective induction of labor as a risk factor for caesarean delivery among low-risk women at term. *Obstetrics and Gynecology* **95** (6), 917–22.

Moldin, P.G. & Sundell, G. (1996) Induction of labour: a randomised clinical trial of amniotomy versus amniotomy with oxytocin infusion. *British Journal of Obstetrics and Gynaecology* **103** (4), 306–12.

National Institute for Health and Clinical Excellence (NICE) (2001) *Clinical Guideline D – Induction of Labour*. National Institute for Health and Clinical Excellence, London.

National Institute for Clinical Excellence (NICE) (2007) *Clinical Guideline 55: Intrapartum Care*. National Institute for Clinical Excellence, London.

Nuutulia, M., Halmesmaki, E., Hiilesmaav, E. & Ylikorkala, O. (1999) Women's anticipation of and experiences with induction of labour. *Acta Obstetricia et Gynecologica Scandinavica* **78** (8), 704–709.

Rane, S.M., Guirgis, R.R., Higgins. B. & Nicolaides, K.H. (2004) The value of ultrasound in the prediction of successful induction of labour. *Ultrasound in Obstetrics and Gynecology* **24** (5), 538–49.

Robertson, A. (1997) *The Midwife Companion*. ACE Graphics, Camperdown, Australia.

Royal College of Midwives (RCM) (2005) *Campaign for Normal Birth*. Royal College of Midwives. Available at: http://www.rcmnormalbirth.org.uk (accessed November 2007).

Royal College of Obstetricians and Gynaecologists (RCOG) (2001) *Induction of Labour: Clinical Guideline 9*. RCOG, London.

Seyb, S.T., Berka, R.J., Socol, M.L. & Dooley, S.L. (1999) Risk of caesarean delivery with elective induction of labor at term in nulliparous women. *Obstetrics and Gynecology* **94** (4), 600–607.

Smith, G., Pell, J., Pasupathy, D. & Dobbie, R. (2004) Factors predisposing to perinatal death related to uterine rupture during attempted vaginal birth after caesarean section. *BMJ* **329**, 375–7.

Surbek, D.V., Boesiger, H., Hoesli, I., Pavic, N. & Holzgreve, W. (1997) A double-blind comparison of the safety and efficacy of intravaginal misoprostol and prostaglandin E2 to induce labor. *American Journal of Obstetrics and Gyanecology* **177** (5), 1018–23.

Williams, M.C., Krammer, J. & O'Brien, W.F. (1997) The value of the cervical score in predicting successful outcome of labor induction. *Obstetrics and Gynecology* **90** (5), 784–9.

19 Pre-eclampsia

Annette Briley

Introduction

Pre-eclampsia is a condition peculiar to pregnancy, characterised by raised blood pressure (BP) and proteinuria. It can be associated with seizures (eclampsia) and multi-organ failure in the mother, while fetal complications include intrauterine growth restriction (IUGR) and placental abruption (Shennan & Chappell, 2001).

Pre-eclampsia leads to increased maternal and fetal mortality and morbidity. In the developed world it is a leading cause of maternal death, and in the UK most deaths have been consistently associated with suboptimal care, particularly by intrapartum care providers (Department of Health (DoH), 1996; CEMACH, 2004).

Underlying pathophysiology of pre-eclampsia

Pre-eclampsia is associated with abnormal implantation of the placenta and concomitant shallow trophoblastic invasion (Pijnenborg, 1994) leading to reduced placental perfusion. The maternal spinal arteries (also known as the uterine arteries) fail to undergo their normal physiological vasodilatation; blood flow may be further impeded by atherotic changes causing obstruction within the vessels.

This pathology causes increased resistance in the uteroplacental circulation with impaired intervillus blood flow resulting in ischaemia and hypoxia, manifested in the second half of pregnancy (Graham *et al.*, 2000).

A similar picture of inadequate trophoblastic invasion exists in pregnancies complicated by IUGR in women with no pre-eclampsia. This suggests that the maternal syndrome of pre-eclampsia must be associated with other features.

Incidence

The incidence of pre-eclampsia varies according to population characteristics and the definitions used to describe it (Davey & MacGillivray, 1988; Chappell *et al.*, 1999; Briley *et al.*, 2006).

UK definition. BP 140/90 or more on two occasions (at least 4 hours apart and within 1 week) with ++ protein or 3.0 g/24 hours or more (International Society for the Study of Hypertension in Pregnancy).

Australasian definition. Hypertension of 140/90 or more with either proteinuria 300 mg/24 hours, protein creatinine ratio ≥30 mg/mmol, dipstick ++ or any other multi-system complication.

Some authors feel that the Australasian definition is more appropriate for the clinical management of a pre-eclamptic woman, since, for example, a hypertensive women with low platelets would meet their definition of pre-eclampsia.

- The true incidence is unknown, but is estimated at <5% in most populations. It may be 6–8% in some nations (Lain & Roberts, 2002; Rumbold *et al.*, 2006). Some studies indicate an incidence as low as 2.2%, even in a primigravid population, which is known to have a higher prevalence (Higgins *et al.*, 1997).
- Up to 20% of all pregnant women will be hypertensive during pregnancy. Of these fewer than 10% will suffer serious disease.
- Pregnancy-induced hypertension (elevated BP with no proteinuria and no pregnancy-related pathology) is approximately three times more common than pre-eclampsia (Shennan & Chappell, 2001)
- In the UK fewer than 10 maternal deaths occur each year, but in the developing countries 50 000 maternal deaths are attributed to eclampsia and a similar number to pre-eclampsia (Duley, 1992).

Facts

- All midwives will see women with pre-eclampsia throughout their professional lives.
- All pregnant women with a headache, severe enough to seek advice, or with new epigastric pain, should have their BP and urine checked as a minimum (Confidential Enquiry into Maternal and Child Health (CEMACH), 2004).
- The International Society for the Study of Hypertension in Pregnancy has adopted the term 'gestational hypertension' to describe all hypertensive women, with or without proteinuria, who were normotensive with no proteinuria before pregnancy.
- Antenatal women with pre-eclampsia require close monitoring. Placental insufficiency is a common problem with early-onset pre-eclampsia, and this can lead to IUGR in 30% pre-eclamptic pregnancies (Royal College of Obstetricians and Gynaecologists (RCOG), 2006) and sometimes placental abruption and fetal demise.
- Late-onset hypertension (>37 weeks gestation) rarely results in serious morbidity for mother or baby. However, hypertension that presents early results developing pre-eclampsia in most women (Shennan & Chappell, 2001).

- In severe pre-eclampsia the main causes of maternal death are cerebral haemorrhage and adult or acute respiratory distress syndrome (DoH, 2001). Therefore, management during the intrapartum period concentrates on BP control and fluid balance. Around 50% of UK deaths due to eclampsia involve substandard care, i.e. insufficient involvement of a consultant obstetrician and inadequate treatment leading to intercranial haemorrhage (CEMACH, 2004).

Associated risk factors

- There is a well-established genetic link; a family history of a mother or sister with pre-eclampsia increases risk four- to eightfold (Lie *et al.*, 1998).
- Paternal influence was first reported in 1983 (Need *et al.*, 1983) with women reported to be at twice the risk of developing pre-eclampsia if their partner has previously fathered a pre-eclamptic pregnancy. Subsequent studies have reported similar associations (Dekker, 2002).
- A new partner returns a woman's risk to that of a primigravida (McCowan *et al.*, 1996).
- Assisted conception particularly with donor gametes increases risk (Wang *et al.*, 2002).
- Strickland *et al.* (1986) reported women being ten times more likely to develop pre-eclampsia in their first pregnancy, with miscarriages and terminations of pregnancy offering some protection. Other authors have also referred to pre-eclampsia as a 'disease of primiparity' (Government Office for Science (GOS), 2007).
- Multiple pregnancies more than double the risk (Duley *et al.*, 2001).
- Maternal age >35 years adds risk. Historically women under 20 have been reported to be at increased risk, although a recent study of women under 19 when they delivered showed a very low pre-eclampsia rate, even though most participants were primigravidae (the ATE study: data publication pending 2008). Obesity (body mass index ≥30) increases the risk fourfold (Shennan *et al.*, 1996; Poston *et al.*, 2006). The UK has the highest levels of obesity in Europe, with recent government reports suggesting that current figures will be increased further by 2050 (GOS, 2007).
- Underlying maternal medical conditions increase risk, e.g. chronic hypertension and renal disease (Poston *et al.*, 2006) insulin resistance and glucose intolerance including gestational diabetes (Duley *et al.*, 2001; Ramsay *et al.*, 2006).
- The impact of multiple risk factors needs further research; however, a retrospective cohort study in Scotland reported a rate of pre-eclampsia in obese primiparous women as 3.9% compared with 1.6% in multiparous obese women (Smith *et al.*, 2007), suggesting that these two risk factors together increase risk. In the Vitamins in Pre-eclampsia trial (Poston *et al.*, 2006) women with multiple risk factors had a risk ratio of 1.18 (confidence interval 95%, 0.87–1.60) again suggesting a cumulative impact of more than one risk factor.

Ongoing research:

- A large multicentre study looking at the genetic components of women with the disease failed to identify a specific gene in women with pre-eclampsia (the GOPEC Consortium, 2005). With technological advances it may be possible to further identify those at risk in the future.

- An international screening study is currently underway, looking for biomarkers to predict those at risk of developing pre-eclampsia early in pregnancy to provide a window of opportunity for potential prophylactic measures and stratify antenatal care (www.maps-study.com).

Signs and symptoms

Clinicians cannot rely on BP and proteinuria alone to diagnose pre-eclampsia, as these are only signs of clinical end-organ damage. Just under 50% of all women presenting with pre-eclampsia will have had no previous hypertension or proteinuria (Douglas & Redman, 1994; Milne *at al.*, 2005). The diagnosis must be considered in women with fetal involvement or other signs, such as:

- Epigastric pain
- Headache/visual disturbances
- Intrauterine growth restriction
- Note: Oedema is no longer considered a reliable sign of pre-eclampsia, except for rapid-onset facial oedema.

Severe pre-eclampsia is considered in the presence of the following:

- Severe hypertension (>160/110 mm Hg) or
- Hypertension with additional symptoms, such as:
  - Headache
  - Visual disturbance
  - Epigastric pain
  - Brisk reflexes or clonus
  - Platelet count below 100 ($\times 10^9$/l)
  - Aspartate transaminase (AST) or alanine transaminase (ALT) >50 IU/l (there is significantly increased maternal morbidity above 150 IU/l) (RCOG, 2006).

All women presenting in the antenatal period with hypertension and proteinuria will have some or all of the following:

- **BP** and protein **urinalysis**.
- **Blood tests** (see also 'Pre-eclampsia' under the heading 'Blood tests for specific conditions and blood pictures' on p. 317, Chapter 23).
  - **Full blood count.**
  - **Platelet count.** Endothelial dysfunction results in platelet dysfunction. If the platelet count is >50×10^9/l, haemostasis is likely to be normal, but delivery is often considered if the platelet count falls below 100.
  - **Clotting studies** if the platelets are <100×10^9/l (RCOG, 2006). Necessary because pre-eclampsia can cause disseminated intravascular coagulation.
  - **Uric acid** or **urate levels**. These are used to assess the severity of the disease and its progression. However, severe disease can occur in the presence of low, normal and high uric acid concentrations (Lie *et al.*, 1998).
  - **Plasma urea** and **creatinine** concentrations. Raised levels of these are generally associated with late renal involvement and serious disease. They are not a useful

early indicator of disease severity, but should be obtained longitudinally to assess the progression of renal involvement.
  ○ **Liver function tests.** Pre-eclampsia can cause liver problems, e.g. subcapsular haematoma, rupture and hepatic infarction.
- **Symphysial fundal height** (accurately measured) and/or **ultrasound** assessment of fetal growth.
- **Cardiotocograph (CTG).** This may give some information about fetal well-being but has no predictive value (RCOG, 2006).
- **Liquor volume assessment** (amniotic fluid index or AFI).
- **Umbilical artery Doppler** analysis.
- In some units a **uterine artery Doppler** waveform assessment may also be carried out, although its value has yet to be clarified (RCOG, 2006). These tests have ±20% positive prediction value (but a 99% negative predictive value), which according to NICE guidelines make it an ineffective test for widespread implementation (National Institute for Health and Clinical Excellence (NICE), 2006). However, in some units it is regularly used either prior to or after the onset of hypertension.

A plan of care will be devised depending on findings. If conservative management is agreed, the woman must be advised to quickly report any pre-eclamptic symptoms. Some women may wish to monitor their own BP at home; any device used should be checked for accuracy.

Many women find it difficult to believe in the potential seriousness of pre-eclampsia, as they often feel quite well unless they are at a significant stage of compromise. It can be difficult to get a balance between clarifying the risks and frightening the woman. Written material may back up explanations, and/or referral to the APEC website, which uses clear language to explain this complex condition.

Box 19.1 summarises BP and urine testing.

Box 19.1   Diagnostic BP and urine criteria for severe pre-eclampsia.

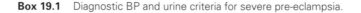

Diastolic/systolic BP (see also 'Signs and symptoms').
- Diastolic BP ≥90 mm Hg on two or more occasions at least 4 hours (and less than 7 days) apart
- Diastolic BP ≥110 mm Hg on one occasion
- Systolic >160 mm Hg or diastolic ≥110 mm Hg or a MAP >125 mm Hg (DoH, 2001)
- BP ≥140/90 mm Hg with proteinuria (≥0.3 g/day or ≥2+)

Mean arterial pressure
- MAP between 125 and 140 mm Hg for >45 min requires medical referral and treatment
- MAP ≥140 mm Hg for >15 min, urgent medical aid and treatment is required
- MAP >150 mm Hg represents serious risk of cerebral autoregulatory dysfunction and subsequent risk of cerebral haemorrhage.

Proteinuria
- One 24 hours collection with total protein excretion ≥300 mg[a]/24 hours, or
- Two 'clean-catch midstream' or catheter specimens of urine collected ≥4 hours apart, measuring 2 or more ++ on reagent strip

[a] Some units only diagnose pre-eclampsia when proteinuria exceeds 500 mg/24 hours.

BP measurement

Care with BP measurement is essential. There is abundant evidence in the literature to suggest that this is often poorly performed, commonly impacting on practice. Factors to consider include the following:

- **Equipment.** Mercury sphygmomanometry remains the 'gold standard' for measuring BP. However due to safety concerns regarding the use of mercury, most units no longer have these machines available in clinical areas. Use a mercury sphygmomanometer for the first reading if possible, and if any uncertainty (CEMACH, 2004; RCOG, 2006). If one is not available cross-check with another validated automated device for increased accuracy (RCOG, 2006). Aneroid machines are commonly used and are reliable when maintained. They require regular calibration to ensure accuracy. There are numerous automated devices available although very few have been validated for use in pregnancy, and even fewer validated as accurate in pre-eclampsia. Most automated devices under-record BP in pre-eclampsia.
- **Cuff size.** Always use the appropriate size cuff. The standard bladder (23 cm × 12 cm) is too small for at least 25% pregnant women. Undercuffing may overestimate BP by >10 mm Hg leading to hypertension overdiagnosis. Overcuffing has the opposite (although smaller) effect by underestimating BP by <5 mm Hg (Shennan & Shennan, 1996).
- **Maternal positioning.** Ensure the woman is sitting comfortably and positioned correctly with the mercury scale at heart level. If using an automated device, ensure that she is positioned as per manufacturer's instructions. Do not talk to the woman and discourage her from speaking during the BP measurement.
- **Digit preference/digit avoidance.** Rounding the final digit of the BP to 0 occurs in >80% BP measurements in antenatal care. Operators also tend to avoid the digits that require action, e.g. they record a diastolic of 88 rather than 90.
- **Korotkoff sounds.** During measurement deflate the cuff at 2–3 mm/second. This prevents overdiagnosis of diastolic hypertension. Korotkoff 4 (the fading or changing of sound) is *no longer recommended* due to problems with reproducibility. RCOG (2006) now recommends using Korotkoff 5 (the disappearance of sound).
- **Multiple readings.** This may be necessary as there are natural variations in BP (RCOG, 2006).

Urine testing

During urine testing discrepancies can arise with the interpretation of proteinuria. False negatives are common when using dipstick urinalysis. Some of these are being reduced by the use of automated dipstick readers in some units. This is a relatively inexpensive method of limiting operator bias. But in general:

- 24 hours urine collections should be used to confirm diagnosis if significant proteinuria unless imminent delivery is indicated by other symptoms (RCOG, 2006).
- Women with proteinuria >300 mg in 24 hours should be considered at risk.

- New innovations in bedside automated devices relating proteinuria to creatinine have not yet been fully evaluated, but may aid clinical practice in the near future (RCOG, 2006).

Care during labour

Most units have a protocol for the management of the severely pre-eclamptic women in labour. All midwives should know where it is. It should be updated as new evidence becomes available.

The decision to deliver will depend on maternal and fetal condition and gestational age. These factors will influence the place and mode of delivery, which ideally will take place in a consultant unit with neonatal facilities (DoH, 1996). Multidisciplinary communication and documentation regarding the management of labour, test results and decisions are essential to ensure a high standard of care. It is important that the midwife caring for the woman should have experience in providing high-risk care and if not should be supported and supervised by a more experienced colleague.

Preterm birth

Pre-eclampsia is a major cause of (usually iatrogenic) prematurity, accounting for 15% of all preterm births, and 25% of all babies born at very low birth weights (<1.5 kg) (Macintosh, 2003). Therefore, many babies born to pre-eclamptic mothers will be admitted to a neonatal unit. If <34 weeks gestation, maternal corticosteroids should be administered to reduce neonatal respiratory problems (Guinn *et al.*, 2001).

If time allows, liaise with the woman and her family and the neonatal unit; this may include a visit or meeting the staff. Some women may require transfer to a specialist neonatal unit: this is likely to be very frightening for the woman and her family. If delivery is imminent and neonatal facilities not available, the baby may require urgent transfer soon after delivery. Take time to explain what is happening and why: this may offer some reassurance.

Psychological support

Due to the intense surveillance and increased intervention during labour and birth, the midwife may easily focus on the woman's physical condition and forget about her emotional needs.

A relaxed environment may have a physiological as well as psychological effect, as stress will not help the woman's condition. Providing appropriate lighting and minimising noise can promote an atmosphere of calmness. There may still be choices that women can make if they are well enough.

Women with pre-eclampsia can become seriously ill very quickly, and this can be very frightening for them and those around them. They will need reassurance and a clear calm explanation of what is happening and what interventions are being offered. Whilst informed choice is not always possible, in emergency situations emotional support is essential.

Monitoring the maternal and fetal condition in moderate/severe pre-eclampsia

Blood pressure

- BP every 15 min (see Box 19.1).
- Be aware that the devices used, cuff size, positioning and technique are subject to inaccuracies (see 'BP measurement' on p. 269).
- Many labour wards (and high dependency units) use mean arterial pressure (MAP) to guide management.

Fluid balance

- Women who are severely ill are unlikely to want to eat in labour, but most will require oral fluids.
- All women with moderate to severe pre-eclampsia should have an intravenous cannula sited for administration of fluids and medication.
- Maintain a strict fluid balance chart. Fluid management is critical: local protocols may advise restricting fluids in labour to a predefined volume.

Antacids are usually recommended in labour in women with pre-eclampsia due to the increased risk of caesarean section.

Monitoring the fetal heart. Continuous CTG is recommended (NICE, 2007) for monitoring the fetal heart rate and any abnormalities in the trace reported and action taken including fetal blood sampling, where appropriate (see Chapters 3 and 23).

Analgesia. General comfort measures include verbal reassurance, touch, massage and comfortable positions (within the restrictions of monitoring equipment). These simple non-invasive measures may promote a feeling of being supported and cared for which should help the woman cope with a medicalised labour and delivery. Epidural may be recommended because it causes vasodilatation which can lead to a reduction in BP and attenuate surges. An established effective epidural is also advantageous should an operative delivery be indicated. The ultimate choice is the woman, and if she makes an informed decision to decline epidural/spinal anaesthesia the midwife must support her in that decision. Policies vary between units, but if the woman's platelet count is considered low ($\leq$80), an epidural may be inadvisable.

Intubation (general anaesthetic) should be avoided because it causes hypertension and laryngeal oedema.

Second stage

- Management will be determined by maternal and fetal condition. If both allow, a spontaneous vaginal delivery is the mode of choice. In moderate to severe pre-eclampsia there is a low threshold for intervention leading to instrumental delivery.
- Ensure that appropriate medical aid is available and that there are two midwives caring for this woman throughout the delivery.
- Monitor the BP closely: it may be unrealistic to check after each contraction, but in severe pre-eclampsia every 5–10 minutes is sensible.
- Involuntary pushing, whilst not discouraged, is not actively encouraged until the presenting part is visible on the perineum.

- Active pushing is contraindicated as it involves directed, prolonged breath holding and bearing down which alters heart rate and increase stroke volume.
- Avoid the supine position: it compresses the distal aorta and reduces blood flow to the uterus and lower extremities (Sleep *et al.*, 2000). It also prolongs the second stage, causes a reduction in circulating oxytocin, reducing the frequency and strength of contractions and can lead to fetal heart rate abnormalities (Gupta *et al.*, 2004). Left lateral and other alternative positions are preferable.

Drugs used in the treatment of severe hypertension

If the woman has not delivered, colloids are usually infused before treatment is started to maintain uteroplacental circulation preventing hypotension and fetal distress.

Antihypertensive treatment should be started in women with a systolic blood pressure over 160 mm Hg or a diastolic blood pressure over 110 mm Hg, but may be introduced at lower BP measurements in women with other symptoms of the disease. Drugs used in the acute management of severe hypertension include oral or intravenous (IV) labetalol, oral nifedipine or IV hydralazine.

In moderate hypertension, effective treatment may enable the continuation of the pregnancy – reducing some of the neonatal complications of prematurity.

Note: Atenolol, angiotensin-converting enzyme (ACE) inhibitors and angiotensin receptor-blocking (ARB) drugs *should be avoided* because they have adverse fetal side effects. Similarly, diuretics are contraindicated in hypertension and should only be used in cases of pulmonary oedema.

Nifedipine

Local guidelines may vary, but recommended dosage is 10–20 mg orally (*not* sublingually as this can cause precipitous hypotension) repeated every 30 minutes to a maximum dose of 50 mg (Sibai, 2003).

Hydralazine

Hydralazine is widely used in the acute management of women with hypertension and is titrated against BP. A recent review for the RCOG (2006) guidelines suggests that other drugs may be preferable to hydralazine, but the currently available evidence is not strong enough to preclude its use. It is given:

- 5 mg IV in fluid
- Repeated every 20 min (at 5 mg IV)
- Maximum cumulative dose of 20 mg (four doses of 5 mg IV over 80 min) (DoH, 2001)

Labetalol

Labetalol has the advantage that it can be given initially by mouth in severe hypertension and then, if needed, intravenously. Dosage is as follows:

- 100 mg BD orally
- 20 mg IV at 10 min intervals

- Increasing to 40, 80 and 80 mg
- Maximum cumulative dose of 300 mg (four doses of 20, 40, 80, 80 mg over 40 min) (DoH, 2001)
- Avoid in asthmatic women (RCOG, 2006)

Magnesium sulphate

Magnesium sulphate should be considered if it is felt that there is a real risk of fitting (eclampsia); often when a decision to deliver has been made, or in the immediate postnatal period (RCOG, 2006). It has been demonstrated to reduce the risk of seizures in pre-eclampsia (Duley *et al.*, 2002). It is also advisable after any seizure (see later on p. 274)

Care of a woman receiving drug treatment for severe hypertension

- Monitor closely ensuring BP falls gradually. Rapid reduction will adversely affect the uteroplacental circulation and lead to fetal distress.
- Monitor the fetal heart for signs of fetal compromise.
- Low threshold for central venous pressure (CVP) line.

Fluid balance management

Women with pre-eclampsia have leaky capillary membranes and a predisposition to low albumin levels; therefore if fluid administration is excessive or unmonitored they are prone to developing pulmonary oedema. General guidelines include the following:

- Maintenance of strict fluid balance charts.
- These women are strongly advised to have a urinary catheter inserted.
- A urometer should be used to accurately record output per hour. 100 ml urine excreted over 4 hours is commonly said to be sufficient to maintain renal function, although RCOG (2006) states that there is no evidence that maintaining a specific urine output prevents renal failure: oliguria is common in pre-eclampsia and should resolve as the condition improves (RCOG, 2006).
- Most protocols limit colloid fluid intake to 85 ml/hour unless the woman haemorrhages in which case fluid restriction is inappropriate (RCOG, 2006).

Management of eclampsia

When pregnant women fit due to pre-eclampsia it is known as eclampsia. This suggests that it is different from other sorts of convulsions, such as those due to epilepsy, but this is not the case. In the event of a fit it is important to stabilise the mother before delivering the baby. Remember that eclampsia is an absolute indication for an urgent delivery once the maternal condition is stabilised. It is extremely important that the midwife explains everything that is happening to the woman and her partner/relatives.

Note: If a pregnant woman presents as semi-conscious or drowsy, non-eclamptic convulsions should be considered: conditions such as epilepsy are more likely to be the cause than eclampsia. However if there is no history of previous convulsions always assume a fit in pregnancy is due to eclampsia.

Incidence

- Fewer than 1% of women with pre-eclampsia will have an eclamptic fit (Shennan & Chappell, 2001).
- 1.6% of women who have an eclamptic fit will die, and 35% will have a major complication (RCOG, 2006).

Facts

- Prophylactic use of anticonvulsants (other than magnesium sulphate therapy for severe pre-eclampsia where a fit is predicted (RCOG, 2006)) is controversial and local policies vary (Duley *et al.*, 2002; Poston *et al.*, 2006).
- The Collaborative Eclampsia Study (Duley *et al.*, 1995) showed that magnesium sulphate administration following a convulsion, when compared with diazepam and phenytoin, resulted in significantly less maternal ventilation, pneumonia and fewer ITU admissions.

Signs and symptoms preceding an eclamptic fit

Sometimes eclampsia is preceded by the woman feeling:

- Unwell
- Headache
- Epigastric pain
- Blurred vision
- Nauseated, she may vomit
- Confusion, irritability and disorientation

However, often there is no warning.
   Further medical examination or blood tests may also reveal the following:

- Signs of clonus (jerkiness) (but brisk tendon reflexes are not predictive of fitting (RCOG, 2006))
- A tender liver
- Abnormal liver enzymes (ALT or AST rising to above 70 IU/l)
- Platelet count falling to below 100×10^9/l
- HELLP syndrome

Care during/following an eclamptic fit

Immediate action:

- Keep calm.
- Summon help, including medical aid; do not leave the woman alone.
- Pull the emergency bell if in hospital, dial 999 if at home.
- Think ABC: airway, breathing, circulation.
- Ensure the woman is in a safe environment.
    ○ Remove obvious dangers
    ○ Do not try to restrain the woman or put anything in her mouth

- Ensure that, once the fit has finished, the woman is in the left lateral position and administer oxygen via a face mask: these measures may maximise uteroplacental blood flow.
- Note the time and duration of the fit. Most fits are self-limiting but occasionally they are much harder to control, or recurrent.

Subsequent action:

- Maternal observations
  - Assess airway and breathing
  - Check pulse
  - BP
  - Pulse oximetry (if available)
  - Assess proteinuria (catheter sample)
- **Gain IV access** (some unit protocols suggest two IV cannulae) to enable IV drug administration and blood to be taken.
- **Monitor the fetus.** Perform a CTG.
- **Catheterise** so urinary output can be accurately monitored.
- **Reassure**
  - Talk calmly and quietly to the woman through the fit and afterwards to reassure her, even though she may appear semi-conscious.
  - Reassure the woman's partner and other relatives where possible; they will be very frightened.
- **Plan for delivery.** Once stabilised, unless there is a fetal bradycardia, there is no immediate urgency to deliver (RCOG, 2006), and a delay of several hours may occur to ensure the best care is available. The woman's condition must always take priority over the fetal condition.
- **Documentation.** Record accurately all events, including the details of the time and duration of the fit.

Drug treatment for eclampsia: magnesium sulphate anticonvulsant therapy

Magnesium sulphate is the therapy of choice to control seizures; diazepam and phenytoin should *no longer* be used as first-line drugs (Collaborative Eclampsia Trial, 1995). The intravenous route is associated with fewer adverse effects.

- A loading dose of 4 g should be given by infusion pump over 5–10 min
- Followed by a further infusion of 1 g/hour maintained for 24 hours after the last seizure or 24 hours after delivery

Subsequent seizures should be treated (according to local protocol) with either:

- a further bolus of 2 g magnesium sulphate, or
- an increase in the infusion rate to 1.5 g or 2.0 g/hour.

Subsequent seizures can also be treated with alternative agents such as diazepam or thiopentone, but only as single doses; the prolonged use of diazepam is associated with an increase in maternal death (Collaborative Eclampsia Trial, 1995).

If convulsions persist, intubation may be necessary to protect the airway and maintain oxygenation; in these cases the woman needs transfer to intensive care facilities where intermittent positive pressure ventilation is available (RCOG, 2006).

Care of the woman receiving magnesium sulphate infusion

Monitor for magnesium sulphate toxicity:

Fluid balance. Urinary output should be monitored hourly. Magnesium sulphate is mostly excreted in the urine. Urine output should be closely observed, and if less than 20 ml/hour the magnesium infusion should be stopped.

Reflexes. Magnesium sulphate toxicity can be assessed clinically as it causes a loss of deep tendon reflexes. If patella reflexes are absent stop the infusion.

Observe the woman for other signs of magnesium sulphate toxicity, i.e. nausea, hot flushes, confusion, weakness, blurred vision and slurred speech.

Respiration. Monitor respiration rate hourly. If <14 breaths/min and/or pulse oximetry is <95% oxygen saturation, the magnesium sulphate therapy should be stopped. If respiratory depression occurs, calcium gluconate 1 g (10 ml) over 10 min can be given.

Blood levels. Blood should be taken for magnesium levels 1 hour after commencing the maintenance dose and repeated 6-hourly. The therapeutic range is 2–4 mmol/l.

- If serum urea >10 mmol/l, or magnesium levels >4 mmol/l, then the dose needs to be *reduced*.
- If magnesium levels are <1.7 mmol/l, the dose needs to be *increased*.

Postnatal BP management for women with pre-eclampsia or eclampsia

Monitoring of BP and antihypertensive medication should be continued after delivery. Some women may require treatment for up to 3 months postpartum.

Women with persisting hypertension and proteinuria at 6 weeks postnatal check may have underlying renal disease and may require further investigation.

Women with severe pre-eclampsia or eclampsia need to be closely observed postnatally. Up to 44% of eclampsia occurs postpartum, especially at term (Milne *et al.*, 2005) and it has been reported up to 4 weeks postnatally, although the incidence falls dramatically after the 4th postnatal day (RCOG, 2006). The timing of transfer home needs to take account of the risk of late seizures. Most women with severe pre-eclampsia or eclampsia will need inpatient care for at least 4 days following delivery. Usually following delivery the BP falls; however, it generally rises again around 24 hours postpartum. Any woman with pre-eclamptic symptoms in the postnatal period, even without any history of pre-eclampsia, must be carefully monitored and referred for investigation.

Currently, there is insufficient evidence to recommend any particular antihypertensive postnatally. Drugs prescribed for breastfeeding women may include labetalol, atenalol and nifedipine, either singularly or in combination. Methyldopa is best avoided postnatally due to its link with depression.

Follow-up

- An assessment of BP and proteinuria by the GP at the 6-week postnatal check is recommended. If hypertension or proteinuria persists, then further investigation is recommended.
- Women experiencing severe pre-eclampsia or eclampsia should be offered a formal postnatal review to discuss the events of the pregnancy.
- Preconception counselling should be offered prior to any subsequent pregnancy, to discuss the events that occurred, risk factors and any preventative therapies.

HELLP syndrome

HELLP syndrome (H = haemolysis, EL = elevated liver enzymes, LP = low platelets) is a severe complication of pre-eclampsia. The severity of HELLP syndrome is not dependant on the severity of hypertension. HELLP syndrome has also been reported in normotensive women.

Incidence

- HELLP occurs in 0.2% of all pregnancies.
- It is more common in women with proteinuric hypertension (4–12% of women with pre-eclampsia or eclampsia).

Underlying pathophysiology

Impaired liver function is an element of HELLP syndrome (see Chapter 23).

Haemolysis. This is the breakdown of red blood cells causing the release of haemoglobin into the blood plasma. It is a normal process, as the life span of each red blood cell (RBC) is about 120 days. Normally the process is slow enough for the RBCs to be removed by the liver, spleen and bone marrow. However, when the process occurs more rapidly and RBC production is unable to keep up, the resultant reduction in the number of circulating RBCs causes microangiopathic haemolytic anaemia.

Elevated liver enzymes. HELLP syndrome impairs liver function. Women commonly complain of epigastric pain caused by obstruction of blood flow in the hepatic sinusoids by intravascular fibrin deposition.

Low platelets. Platelets are the first line of defence against bleeding. They work by:

- Plugging holes in capillaries (primary haemostasis).
- Initiating coagulation.
- As the blood escapes through bigger holes, eventually platelets become an integral part of most clots.

Thrombocytopenia is due to the increased consumption of platelets.

Signs and symptoms of HELLP

- HELLP syndrome is commonly diagnosed when the results of pre-eclampsia blood tests are reviewed.

- Women may complain of epigastric pain.
- Women may bleed excessively (for example, from cannula site) and the blood fails to clot.

Care of women with HELLP syndrome

Once HELLP syndrome is evident *urgent delivery* is required. However this is problematic due to:

- Problems with low platelets, therefore regional blocks are contraindicated.
- The woman is a poor candidate for general anaesthesia as intubation increases BP.
- The woman will bleed excessively at caesarean section.
- The woman already has a coagulopathy, with reduced intravascular volume; therefore, a postpartum haemorrhage is particularly problematic.

Consequently management includes the following:

- Low threshold for CVP line.
- It is imperative to accurately record fluid balance.

Corticosteroids have been used in HELLP syndrome. There is evidence to suggest that they lead to a more rapid resolution of the biochemical and haematological abnormalities; however, there is no evidence that they reduce morbidity (Clenney *et al.*, 2004).

Summary

- Signs and symptoms of pre-eclampsia may include any of the following:
  - BP $\geq 160/110$ mm Hg or MAP ≥ 125 mm Hg
  - BP $\geq 140/90$ mm Hg with proteinuria (≥ 0.3 g/day or $\geq 2+$)
  - Headache, nausea, confusion, blurred vision, epigastric pain, brisk reflexes and clonus
  - Platelets $<100 \times 10^9/l$ and/or ALT/AST >50 IU/l
- Drug treatment may include nifedipine, labetalol, hydralazine and magnesium sulphate.

First-stage labour care for severe pre-eclampsia

- BP check every 15–20 min in first stage, more frequently in second stage.
- Consider MAP instead of systolic/diastolic.
- Strict fluid balance chart:
  - Hourly urine output (100 ml/4 hours)
  - Limit fluid intake (approx 85 ml/hour)
- IV access, possibly CVP line.
- 4-hourly antacids.
- CTG is recommended.
- Epidural/spinal may help lower BP.
- Psychological support for woman and birth partner(s).

Second-stage labour care for severe pre-eclampsia

- BP check every 5–10 min.
- Avoid active (sustained breath holding) pushing and supine position.
- Low threshold for instrumental delivery.
- Avoid general anaesthetic.

Eclamptic fit

- Eclampsia is an indication for urgent delivery.
- Action: get help, think ABC, give O_2, remove dangers and allow the fit to pass.
- Post-fit: maternal observations, IV access, CTG and catheterise.
- Plan for delivery – soon, but not as emergency unless fetal compromise suspected.
- The woman always has priority over the baby.

Useful contact

Action on Pre-eclampsia (APEC)   Website: www.apec.org.uk

References

Bower, S., Bewley, S. & Campbell, S. (1993) Improved prediction of pre-eclampsia by two stage Doppler screening of uterine arteries using the early diastolic notch color Doppler imaging. *Obstetrics and Gynecology* **82**, 78–83.

Briley, A.L., Poston, L. & Shennan, A.H. (2006) Vitamin C and E and the prevention of pre-eclampsia. *The New England Journal of Medicine* **355** (10), 1065.

Chappell, L.C., Seed, P.T., Briley, A.L. Kelly, A.J., Lee, R., Hunt, B.J., Parmar, K., Bewley, S.J., Shennan A.H., Steer, P.J. & Poston, L. (1999) Prevention of pre-eclampsia by antioxidants: a randomised trial of vitamin C and vitamin E in women at increased risk of pre-eclampsia. *Lancet* **347**, 810–16

Clenney, T.L. & Viera, A.J. (2004) Corticosteroids for HELLP (haemolysis, elevated liver enzymes low platelets) syndrome. *British Medical Journal* **329**, 270–72.

Collaborative Eclampsia Trial (1995) Which anticonvulsant for women with eclampsia? Evidence from the collaborative eclampsia trial. *Lancet* **345** (8963), 1455–63; erratum in *Lancet* 1995, **346**, 258.

Confidential Enquiry into Maternal and Child Health (CEMACH) (2004) *Why Mothers Die (CEMACH). The Sixth Report on Confidential Enquiries into Maternal Deaths in the United Kingdom, 2000–2002.* HMSO, London.

Davey, D.H. & MacGillivray, I. (1988) The classification and definition of the hypertensive disorders of pregnancy. *American Journal of Obstetrics and Gynecology* **158**, 892–8.

Dekker, G. (2002) The partner's role in the etiology of pre-eclampsia. *Journal of Reproductive Immunology* **57** (1–2), 203–15.

Department of Health (DoH) (1996) Why Mothers Die, 1991–1993. *Report on Confidential Enquiries into Maternal Deaths in the United Kingdom.* Department of Health, HMSO, London

Department of Health (DoH) (2001) Why Mothers Die, 1997–1999. *The Fifth Annual Report of the Confidential Enquiry into Maternal Deaths in the United Kingdom.* HMSO, London.

Douglas, K.A. & Redman, C.W.G. (1994) Eclampsia in the United Kingdom. *British Medical Journal* **309**, 1395–400.

Duley, L. (1992) Maternal mortality associated with hypertensive disorders of pregnancy in Africa, Asia, Latin America and the Caribbean. *British Medical Journal* **99**, 547–53.

Duley, L., Carroli, G., Belizan, J. & Villar, J. (1995) Which anticonvulsant for women with pre-eclampsia- evidence from the collaborative eclampsia trial. *Lancet* **345**, 1455–63.

Duley, L., Henderson-Smart, D., Knoght, M. & King, J. (2001) Antiplatelet drugs for prevention of pre-eclampsia and its consequences: systematic review. *British Medical Journal* **322**, 329–33.

Duley, L. & The MAGPIE Collaborative Group (2002) Do women with pre-eclampsia and their babies benefit from magnesium sulphate? The Magpie Trial: a randomised placebo controlled trial. *Lancet* **359**, 1877–90.

GOPEC Consortium (2005) Disentangling fetal and maternal susceptibility for pre-eclampsia: a British multicenter candidate-gene study. *American Journal of Human Genetics* **77**, 127–31.

Government Office for Science (GOS) (2007) *Foresight: Tackling Obesities: Future Choices Project*. Department of Innovation, Universities and Skills, London.

Graham, C.H., Postovit, L.M., Park, H., Canning, M.T. & Fitzpatrick, T.E. (2000) Adriana and Luisa Castellucci Award Lecture 1999: The role of oxygen in the regulation of trophoblast gene expression and invasion. *Placenta* **21**, 443–50.

Guinn, D.A., Atkinson, W., Sullivan, L. Lee, M., MacGregor, S., Parilla, B., Davies, J., Hanlon-Lundgerg, K., Simpson, L., Stone, J., Ogasawara, K. & Maraskas, J. (2001) Single vs weekly courses of antenatal steroids for women at risk of preterm delivery. *Journal of the American Medical Association* **286**, 1581–7.

Gupta, J.K. & Hofmeyr, G.J. (2004) Position for women during second stage of labour. *The Cochrane Database of Systematic Reviews*, Issue 1.

Higgins, J.R., Walshe, J.J., Halligan, A., O'Brien, E., Conroy, R. & Darling, M.R. (1997) Can 24 hour ambulatory monitoring blood pressure measurement predict the development of hypertension in primigravidae? *British Journal of Obstetrics and Gynaecology* **104**, 356–62.

Lain, K. & Roberts, J. (2002) Contemporary concepts of the pathenogenesis and management of pre-eclampsia. *Journal of the American Medical Association* **287**, 3183–5.

Lie, R.T., Rasmussen S., Brunborg, H., *et al.* (1998) Fetal and maternal contributions to risk of pre-eclampsia: population based study. *British Medical Journal* **316**, 1343–7.

Macintosh, M. (2003) *Project 27/28: An Enquiry into Quality of Care and Its Effect on the Survival of Babies Born at 27–28 Weeks*. TSO, London.

McCowan, L., Buist, R.G., North, R.A. & Gamble, G. (1996) Perinatal morbidity in chronic hypertension. *British Journal of Obstetrics and Gynaecology* **103**, 123–9.

Milne, F., Redman, R., James Walker, J., Baker, P., Bradley, J., Cooper, C., de Swiet, M., Fletcher, G., Jokinen, M., Murphy, D., Nelson-Piercy, C., Osgood, V., Robson, S., Shennan, A., Tuffnell, A., Twaddle, S. & Waugh, J. (2005) The pre-eclampsia community guideline (PRECOG). How to screen for and detect onset of pre-eclampsia in the community. *British Medical Journal* **330**, 576–80.

National Institute for Clinical Excellence (NICE) (2007) *Clinical Guideline 55: Intrapartum Care*. National Institute for Clinical Excellence, London.

National Institue of Clinical Health and Excellence (NICE) (2006) *Antenatal Guidelines*. DoH, London.

Need, J.A., Bell, B., Meffin, E. & Jones, W.R. (1983) Pre-eclampsia in pregnancies with donor insemination. *Journal of Reproductive Immunology* **5**, 329–38.

Pijnenborg, R. (1994) Trophoblastic invasion. *Reproductive Medicine Review* **3**, 53–73.

Poston, L., Briley, A.L., Seed, P.T. & Shennan, A.H. (2006) Vitamin C and E in women at risk of pre-eclampsia (VIP trial): randomised placebo-controlled trial. *Lancet* **367** (9267), 1534.

Ramsay, J., Greer, I. & Sattar, N. (2006) ABC of obesity. Obesity and reproduction. *British Medical Journal* **333**, 1159–62.

Royal College of Obstetricians and Gynaecologists (RCOG) (2006) *The Management of Severe Pre-eclampsia/eclampsia Guideline 10A.* RCOG Press, London.

Rumbold, A.R., Crowther, C.A., Haslam, R.R., Dekker, G.A. & Robinson, J.A., for the ACTS Study Group (2006) Vitamins C and E and the risks of pre-eclampsia and perinatal complications. *New England Journal of Medicine* **354**, 1796–1806.

Shennan, A.H. & Chappell, L.C. (2001) Pre-eclampsia. *Contemporary Clinical Gynaecology and Obstetrics* **1**, 353–64.

Shennan, A.H., Gupta, M., Halligan, A., Taylor, D.A. & de Swiet, M. (1996) Lack of reproducibility of korotkoff phase IV by mercury sphygmomanometry. *Lancet* **347**, 139–42.

Shennan, C. & Shennan, A. (1996) Blood pressure in pregnancy: the need for accurate measurement *British Journal of Midwifery* **4** (2), 102–8.

Sibai, B. (2003) Diagnosis and management of gestational hypertension and severe pre-eclampsia. *Obstetrics and Gynaecology* **102**, 181–92.

Sleep, J., Roberts, J. & Chalmers, L. (2000) The second stage of labour. In *A Guide to Effective Care in Pregnancy and Childbirth*, 3rd edn (Enkin, M., Keirse, M.J.N.C., Neilson, J., Crowther, C., Duley L., Hodnett, E. & Hofmeyr, J., eds), pp 289–99. Oxford University Press, Oxford.

Smith, G.C.S., Shah, I., Pell, J.P., Crossley, A. & Dobbie, R. (2007) Maternal obesity in early pregnancy and risk of spontaneous and elective preterm deliveries: a retrospective cohort study. *American Journal of Public Health* **97** (1), 157–62.

Strickland, D.M., Guzick, D.S., Cox, K., Grant, N.F. & Rosenfeld, C.R. (1986) The relationship between abortion in the first pregnancy and development of pregnancy-induced hypertension in the subsequent pregnancy. *American Journal of Obstetrics and Gynecology* **154**, 146–8.

Wang, J., Knottnerus, A., Schuit, G., Norman, R., Chan, A. & Dekker, G. (2002) Surgically obtained sperm, and risk of gestational hypertension and pre-eclampsia. *Lancet* **359** (9307), 673–4.

20   Stillbirth and neonatal death

Cathy Charles and Barbara Kavanagh

Introduction

Perinatal loss has been described as a life crisis for both parents and professionals alike (Gardner, 1999). The death of a baby is not uncommon at one every 200 births, but most staff feel uncomfortable dealing with it. It is difficult to develop expertise in something which occurs so sporadically (Cartwright & Read, 2004), and certain midwives who volunteer more readily than others may get called on each time, risking burnout.

Death is not the expected outcome of pregnancy, and parents can be left stunned. The loss of their baby may be some parents' first experience of death (Rajan, 1992). They have to face not only the loss of the person whom they have helped to create, but also the loss of future ambitions, hopes and dreams. These parents undergo intense grief reactions. These feelings are very similar to any other form of bereavement (Golding, 1991), and although every experience of grief is personal and intense, this is a normal healthy response to loss. Typical symptoms may include shock, numbness, disbelief, emptiness, a sense of failure, anger and guilt. There may also be a recurrence of feelings related to any previous loss.

The midwife provides support in the very early stages of the grieving process, when denial, guilt and anger may be most in evidence (Butler, 2000). Kohner (1995) stresses that this is a difficult and demanding time for professionals. What they say and do may be critically important. Their words and actions are frequently remembered by parents for years to come, and may influence their memories and their grieving.

Definition

A stillbirth is defined as a baby delivered without life after 24 weeks of pregnancy. The stillbirth rate is the number of stillbirths per 1000 live births and stillbirths (Confidential Enquiry into Maternal and Child Health (CEMACH), 2007).

The Royal College of Obstetricians and Gynaecologists (RCOG, 2005) has decided recently that a baby known to have *died before* 24 weeks but *born after* 24 weeks (e.g. early death of a twin who is then born with its live sibling near term) should no longer be registered as a stillbirth.

The perinatal mortality rate is defined as the number of stillbirths and early neonatal deaths (those occurring in the first week of life) per 1000 live births and stillbirths (CEMACH, 2007).

Incidence and facts

- The stillbirth rate in England, Wales and Northern Ireland was 5.5 per 1000 births in 2005. Perinatal mortality was 8.2 per 1000 (CEMACH, 2007).
- CEMACH (formerly Confidential Enquiry into Stillbirths and Deaths in Infancy (CESDI) from 1992 to 2002) is committed to improving outcomes in maternal and infant health. There has been a significant downward trend in intrapartum-related deaths (CEMACH, 2007).
- Although the last 50 years have seen dramatic improvements in social welfare and maternity care, almost 1% of women entering the second half of pregnancy will lose their baby (Fox *et al.*, 1997).
- The immediate care a woman receives during a stillbirth can affect her emotional status at least 3 years after delivery (Radestad *et al.*, 1998).

Predisposing factors for stillbirth

The main causes of stillbirth are broadly classified by CEMACH (2007) as severe/lethal congenital anomalies (16%), antepartum haemorrhage (8%) and intrapartum cause (7%). Over 50% are unexplained.

Predisposing factors (see Box 20.1) are a complex area. It is often impossible to separate maternal and fetal factors. Some are social and very hard to address. Others are disease specific and more controllable. Generally, however, predisposing factors have poor predictive value.

There is no helpful mortality rate for home births. Most home stillbirths and neonatal deaths are unplanned home births, usually preterm: presumably due to rapid labour and the mother is unable to get to hospital in time. Twenty-five per cent of these home births are unbooked pregnancies (CEMACH, 2007).

Diagnosing fetal death and decision making

The beginning of the grieving process

When a fetus or baby dies, parents should be told at once (Kohner, 1995). Delay will inevitably cause greater stress. Confirmation should ideally take place with both parents

Box 20.1   Predisposing factors for stillbirth and neonatal death.

Antenatal
- Maternal age <20 or >40 (CEMACH, 2007).
- Body mass index >30 (CEMACH, 2007).
- Social deprivation doubles the risk (CEMACH, 2007).
- Ethnicity: women of black and Asian origin have approximately double the risk (CEMACH, 2007). Women with refugee status may be three times more at risk (Lanchandani *et al.*, 2001).
- Placental problems: e.g. praevia, abruption and intrauterine growth retardation.
- Maternal disorder: e.g. pre-eclampsia, infection, diabetes and cholestasis.
- Prolonged pregnancy >41/40.
- Multiple pregnancy.
- Isoimmunisation.

Intrapartum
- Cord compression/accident.
- Uterine rupture.
- Placental abruption.

Newborn conditions
- Prematurity: by far the largest category.
- Low birth weight.
- Birth trauma.
- Infection.
- Congenital malformation.
- Accident.
- Sudden infant death syndrome.

N.B. A large number of stillbirths and neonatal deaths are *unexplained* and occur with *no* predisposing factors.

---

present. The attitudes and empathy of midwives and doctors at the outset of this traumatic experience will influence from the beginning the grieving process, and the memories they take away with them. Two doctors should be present for confirmation of intrauterine death and real-time ultrasound should be performed (National Institute for Health and Clinical Excellence (NICE), 2007a) by a practitioner skilled in real-time imaging and able to discuss the findings openly with the mother (Fox *et al.*, 1997).

Good communication and honesty are essential. Full explanations should be given by midwives and doctors. Lovell (1983), cited in Moulder (1999), noted that some women were critical of the way staff handled the diagnosis of an intrauterine death or an abnormality; a succession of different staff were involved; staff were ill prepared and some unable to conceal their own distress at the diagnosis. When a mother first understands that death has occurred, there is a sense of shock and numbness temporarily preventing her from being overwhelmed by the full impact of the event (Jones, 1997). Some health professionals may find it difficult to know what to say at this point. If a partner is present, it may be appropriate to give them a few moments alone before they are faced with painful decisions. A trained interpreter should be made available to women who do not have fluent English.

The distress of the father is sometimes comparatively disregarded (Stillbirth and Neonatal Death Society (SANDS), 2007). He may feel distraught with grief, angry, helpless, even guilty (Bennett *et al.*, 2005) and deeply disturbed by his partner's distress. He may suppress this, feeling he must not show the depth of his grief to staff or even sometimes his partner through fear of upsetting her further. Make it clear that he is not just there as a supporter: ask him how he is and include him in all information giving, acknowledging that he too is a bereaved parent.

Planned termination for fetal abnormality may make it easier for staff to reconcile the death (Walpole, 2002) but it may not be easier for any parents. They are likely to grieve like any other parents, and guilt at having chosen to end their baby's life may compound their suffering.

Decision making and choices

Parents will be looking for guidance from staff. Supporting grieving parents to make important decisions at a time of unbearable sorrow and anguish is one of the most challenging roles undertaken by a midwife (Thomas, 1999). The midwife should have a caring, sensitive and non-judgemental attitude, acknowledging the importance of the loss. Basic counselling/listening skills are very helpful. It can be stressful to give control and choice to parents if their decisions differ from those that professionals would make on their behalf (Kohner, 1995).

Decision making can be very hard for the mother at this time. Due to the impact of overwhelming shock and disbelief, midwives and doctors may have to repeat themselves and reiterate questions, as information is not always retained if given only once. This is made worse if the woman is in pain.

Mode of delivery

It may be possible to discuss in advance the options and support available for labour and birth. A woman whose baby has died in utero may be shocked to learn that she is advised to have a vaginal birth. It is a frightening thought to give birth to a dead baby. Her first reaction may be that she requests to have a caesarean section. Take time to listen to her reasons for this and discuss her worries about vaginal birth. Gently point out that caesarean delivery is thought to affect a woman's physical and mental recovery, in particular her ability to identify and accept the loss of her baby.

Induction or expectant management

Unless the cause of the fetal death threatens the mother's life, late fetal death seldom possesses a threat to maternal physical welfare (Howarth & Alfirevic, 2001). There is a small risk of disseminated intravascular coagulation and postpartum haemorrhage if the mother carries a dead baby for several weeks, but generally awaiting spontaneous labour is safe.

However, Radestad *et al.* (1996) noted increased anxiety in women who were induced more than 24 hours after diagnosis of death in utero, and suggest that birth should occur as soon as feasible after the diagnosis. Delaying birth on the other hand may give some parents time to come to terms with the situation. The decision of whether or not to induce rests with the parents themselves and that choice must be respected and supported.

Induction of labour following late intrauterine death differs from other inductions: fetal well-being is no longer an issue, so side effects and complications need only be considered from the maternal perspective. Also most planned inductions with a live baby occur near term, while inductions for fetal death present over a wide range of gestational ages (Howarth & Alfirevic, 2001).

Place of birth

Whilst most women give birth in a consultant unit following intrauterine death, the parents may choose otherwise. Thomas (1999) suggests that in the presence of an experienced midwife this sad event, occurring in the security of the home away from all the noise and intrusion of the hospital, can give parents positive memories and a sense of controlling events rather than events controlling them.

Midwives in a community unit/birthing centre or at home may be less experienced in caring for a stillbirth, but in one sense the birth is like any other. Postnatally there is rarely any urgency, so blood samples and paperwork can usually be undertaken slowly. Consent for any post-mortem must be signed by a doctor, but this does not have to be done straightaway. A supervisor of midwives can be an invaluable resource, and consultant unit staff are often happy to give telephone advice.

A doctor will still need to certify death, and some general practitioners (GPs) may be unwilling to be involved, since they are uncertain what to enter on the certificate as 'cause of death'. Cases have been known where a GP feels obliged to report this technically 'unexplained death' to the police, and this can involve a lot of unnecessary bureaucracy and distress which a hospital birth will avoid (Charles, personal communication). A doctor is usually involved in taking skin biopsies from the baby (if requested), which may be awkward at home.

These are just practical considerations, and should not discourage midwives from supporting women who choose to give birth at home.

Midwifery care in labour

Compassion and individualised care

The woman needs sensitive care from a midwife who is not afraid of her or her baby, and who shows respect and regards the baby as a precious, delicate little person. A study of late pregnancy loss by Moulder (1999) found that trust between the woman and her midwife was of key importance.

The diversity of women's needs must be understood. Touch, for example, may help some women during stillbirth, but not others (Butler, 2000). Cultural differences may affect reaction to loss; it is important not to make assumptions (Schott & Henley, 1996; Nallon, 2007). The mother may be unwilling to see or hold her baby due to a specific religious or cultural prohibition against seeing a dead body. Equally, be aware that whilst she may technically belong to a religious group, she may hold uncertain or ambivalent views and not wish to follow any rigid practice.

Ideally, the birth should take place away from the main busy delivery suite area, in a quiet, calm atmosphere.

Observations

Prior to induction (if necessary) for intrauterine death, check blood pressure, pulse and temperature and test urine for proteinuria to exclude pre-eclampsia.

If the fetus may have been dead for some time, then take maternal blood for a platelet count and clotting studies as disseminated intravascular coagulation could be a problem. One-third of women with abruption and fetal demise develop some degree of coagulopathy (American Academy of Family Physicians (AAFP), 2004).

Once labour has commenced observations are as per normal labour (see Chapter 1).

Fetal heart monitoring is obviously not required. The absence of the baby's heartbeat serves as a painful and constant reminder to the mother and midwife that there is to be a tragic outcome to this labour.

Analgesia

Distress is worsened by the fact that the woman must undergo labour, which is both psychologically and physically painful (Smith, 1999). Radestad *et al.* (1998) report that women undergoing stillbirth use more analgesia than women delivering a live baby and describe the labour and birth as unbearably physically hard. The woman must be reassured that support and adequate pain relief will be available to her at any time. Any maternal pyrexia/infection will be a contraindication to epidural anaesthesia (Swanson & Madej, 1997). This information must be shared with the mother, otherwise if refused a promised epidural she may feel let down by the midwife.

The birth of the baby

Giving comfort and support to the bereaved parents at this time of enormous sadness will help create a positive birth experience.

A slow and gentle birth will minimise damage: the skin is often very fragile. A baby who has been dead for some time may be macerated: parents should be gently prepared for this possibility.

Small premature babies presenting by the breech can have a slow head delivery. Babies who have died often deliver slowly due to absent tone. This can be distressing and parents will need extra support at this time.

Clarify, well in advance if possible, whether the mother wishes to have her baby given straight to her. If not the baby could be wrapped in a small towel (not paper as it will be difficult to remove from the baby's skin later) and then offered to the parents to hold.

Third stage of labour

If the dead baby has been retained in utero for several weeks or in cases of suspected placental abruption (or other risk factors – see page 208 in haemorrhage chapter), the mother is at increased risk of postpartum haemorrhage. Particular risk factors may have been identified at confirmation of fetal death and by blood tests for infection and clotting studies. In such cases active management of the third stage is advised.

Following birth, the placenta should be transported according to local pathology guidelines. This varies between hospitals; some pathologists request the placenta is sent dry, others request it is transported in formaldehyde.

Immediate care following birth: precious moments with the baby

The meeting with and parting from the baby is a unique time.

Attitudes to pregnancy loss have undergone a revolution in recent years. Many feel that it is good to offer the parents involvement with their dead baby (Matthews *et al.*, 2002; Hughes & Riches, 2003; SANDS, 2007). They should be aware that they can have as much time on their own with their baby as they wish. However, they should not be *forced* to view, hold, caress, or kiss the baby (SANDS, 2007). Such actions do not appear to reduce the risk for anxiety or depression (Radestad *et al.*, 1996). Hughes *et al.* (2002) found that holding a dead baby had a negative impact on many mothers and their next-born child, and suggested that parents should not be pressurised into holding their dead baby or be told that mourning would be more difficult if they did not have this contact. SANDS (2007) also recommend that women should not be forced to view, hold, caress or kiss the baby. Unfortunately NICE (2007b) have slightly misinterpreted Hughes *et al*'s study since NICE state that "it is now considered unhelpful for women to see and hold their babies (after stillbirth) unless they particularly wish to do so." This was not a conclusion of the study and Turton (2008), who was one of the researchers, states that some – although far from all – parents did value contact with their baby. The only conclusion from all this is that the midwife should treat women/couples as individuals and try to anticipate and respond to their particular needs and wishes as far as they can be gauged.

If the parents wish to hold the baby (and most will), fears may be minimised by advising them beforehand how the baby will look and feel: e.g. it will feel floppy and may have some movement of the skull bones (Dyer, 1992).

Creating memories and mementos

Memories help to facilitate mourning. The added difficulty when grieving for a stillborn baby is that parents have not had the time to get to know their baby. There is no known person to talk about. To assist parents to grieve normally, the most should be made of what is available to create special memories for them (Greaves, 1994).

Many maternity units have recognised this need and provide memory booklets (often supplied by SANDS the Stillbirth and Neonatal Death Society), to contain mementos. Footprints and handprints can be taken, put on to card and placed in the booklet. Include locks of hair, name bands, the tape measure and the baby's personal details such as weight and measurements.

Most parents have a camera with them for the birth. If not, some units offer a camera for use by the parents; they can be given the film to develop in their own time. Hospital policy may recommend a polaroid photograph is placed in the mother's notes. Parents should be told that polaroid photos will eventually fade, especially if exposed to light.

If they wish, parents can bathe and dress their baby in clothes they have chosen; this process may take a long time and should not be hurried. If the parents wish another family member, or member of staff could do this.

The sensation of smell can be an emotional trigger. Dusting clothes, shawls and soft toys with baby powder and placing keepsakes in a plastic bag will preserve the smell for many years, providing powerful memories.

Offering an entry in the hospital's book of remembrance can give the parents comfort: they may wish to visit subsequently to view this in the hospital chapel.

Some parents may not wish to have any mementos of their baby for personal, cultural or religious reasons. Whilst these views would seem to be contrary to facilitating the grief process, they should not be viewed as abnormal or wrong (Schott & Henley, 1996). Unless there is an obvious cultural reason, it may be helpful to suggest that mementos are taken and filed away in the medical records, so that the parents could ask for them at a later stage if they wished. Some parents may take time to assimilate the experience and subsequently regret the absence of mementos.

Other members of the family, such as siblings and grandparents, may wish to see the baby so they can create their own memories and say their own goodbyes. Parents need to be prepared for the honesty that children can show. This may be a confusing time for them. They have often been looking forward to the birth of their baby brother or sister. They sometimes ask unexpected questions; guiding the parents to be honest is the best course of action. Children are very accepting of death as long as they are able to participate and share the experience with their family (Dyer, 1992).

Ongoing care in the postnatal period

Checklists, tests and paperwork

There are various maternal tests that can be undertaken to try to identify the cause of fetal death. Obstetricians and hospitals vary in the blood tests they offer. (Refer to Chapter 23, p. 19) Maternal and paternal genetic tests may also be offered, and possibly follow-up genetic counselling.

Checklists are used to avoid important tasks being overlooked and to prevent the parents being asked the same questions repeatedly. A checklist example is given in the Appendix. Schott and Henley (1996) argue that a checklist can sometimes be used inflexibly and can become an end in itself, rather than a way of ensuring that the needs of the parents are met. Focusing on a checklist may be a way of depersonalising the situation and minimising the time spent with parents.

Post-mortem (autopsy)

Many parents want to know the cause of their baby's death, though they may find the idea of a post-mortem distressing. Staff may fear to approach the subject, although the urge to protect parents is often misplaced:

> 'The worst thing possible had happened – my baby had died. You couldn't tell me anything that was more upsetting than that' (Henderson, 2006).

Since Alder Hey (Redfern, 2001) some parents are reluctant to allow a post-mortem on their baby, and the perinatal pathology service is experiencing recruitment and retention difficulties (Rose *et al.*, 2006). This unsatisfactory situation may lead staff to discourage parents from having an autopsy. Post-mortems have declined from 58% all deaths in 1993 to 39% in 2005 (CEMACH, 2007).

A coroner may order a post-mortem, particularly if the death is unexpected or resulted from an accident. Parents often hope that a post-mortem will give them the reason for their baby's death, but they should be aware that this is very often not the case: only around 20% yield a cause of death (CEMACH, 2007).

Post-mortem must be discussed very gently, giving clear unbiased information. Explanation of the procedure may help. The Department of Health (DoH) (2003a) has an information leaflet for parents. The NHS consent form (DoH, 2003b), revised following Alder Hey (DoH, 2003c) in trying to cover all eventualities, is very long and detailed; there is no perfect answer to the problem of giving full information and gaining full consent without overloading and distressing parents.

Post-mortem may be full or limited. Less invasive tests, e.g. X-rays, CT scans and tissue samples, may also be offered although they yield less information than a full post-mortem. If parents wish to have a post-mortem or have any major tissue samples (e.g. brain biopsy) returned for burial with the baby, they should be warned that this may delay the funeral, possibly by some weeks.

It is also helpful if the midwife notes anything unusual noted after the birth and records this in the notes and on the pathology request form, e.g. a true knot in the cord, a broken cord blood vessel and a pale baby's body with a very contused face (which might indicate the cord was very tight around the neck). Many such 'abnormalities' may be incidental, but observations at the time may be helpful. Do not assume that the pathologist will observe everything: they will appreciate comments made by clinicians at the time. Later on, by the time a placenta has been handled by pathology technicians, and perhaps a piece of placenta has been cut off for microscopic examination, a key diagnostic finding such as a small nick in a blood vessel may have been masked. Avoid however being drawn into speculation on the cause of the baby's death.

Registering the baby's death

Box 20.2 describes the various certification steps required for registering a baby's death prior to burial or cremation.

Spiritual beliefs and funeral arrangements

Formal burial or cremation is a legal requirement for all babies who are stillborn or die after birth. A funeral can provide a focus for grieving families to mourn. Attendance at the funeral by staff involved with the baby's birth is often valued by both families and the staff themselves.

Many parents may have had little or no contact with death and have never had to think about making funeral arrangements. Rajan (1992) reports women being deeply hurt when asked how they would like the baby 'disposed of'. This is such a sensitive issue and it should be handled with great respect.

The spiritual and religious outlook of individuals often takes on more importance during bereavement (Jones, 1997). Asking the bereaved couple if they wish to see a hospital chaplain, or other religious person if appropriate, may help them to reach any

Box 20.2 Registering a baby's death.

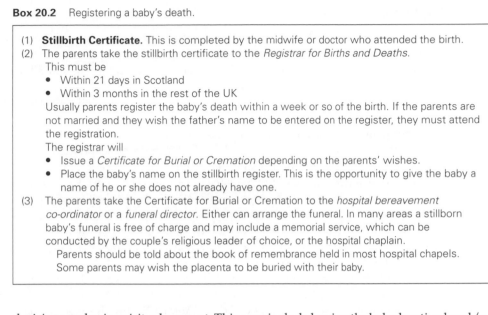

(1) **Stillbirth Certificate.** This is completed by the midwife or doctor who attended the birth.
(2) The parents take the stillbirth certificate to the *Registrar for Births and Deaths*.
This must be
   - Within 21 days in Scotland
   - Within 3 months in the rest of the UK
Usually parents register the baby's death within a week or so of the birth. If the parents are not married and they wish the father's name to be entered on the register, they must attend the registration.
The registrar will
   - Issue a *Certificate for Burial or Cremation* depending on the parents' wishes.
   - Place the baby's name on the stillbirth register. This is the opportunity to give the baby a name of he or she does not already have one.
(3) The parents take the Certificate for Burial or Cremation to the *hospital bereavement co-ordinator* or a *funeral director*. Either can arrange the funeral. In many areas a stillborn baby's funeral is free of charge and may include a memorial service, which can be conducted by the couple's religious leader of choice, or the hospital chaplain.
   Parents should be told about the book of remembrance held in most hospital chapels.
   Some parents may wish the placenta to be buried with their baby.

decisions and gain spiritual support. This may include having the baby baptised and/or named although this may not be suitable for every faith and culture. Hospital chaplains are usually a wonderful source of information and support. Most are extremely sensitive and will not dwell on religious matters if the parents do not wish it. However, even the most atheist parents may wish to speak some words over their baby to say goodbye. A few formal words spoken by a chaplain, such as: 'We cry for James today, for the life he will not have and the hopes we had for him. We are so sad to say goodbye to this beautiful boy' may help parents to have some sense of a 'rite of passage', and encourage tears to fall.

Staying in hospital

Naturally many women find it painful to see newborn babies and mothers or pregnant women. Many may wish to leave hospital within a few hours of birth. Radestad *et al.* (1998) suggest that differences in the length of stay after fetal death may depend on the mother's opinion of the maternity hospital environment.

If a mother wishes to stay, or is too unwell to leave, if possible let her choose the kind of postnatal room she would like. Most will want a single room. Many large hospitals have a designated room with an en-suite bathroom and a double bed so that the father can stay. Parents should be able to spend as much time as they want with their baby on the postnatal ward.

The option of taking the baby home

It is important to offer choice. Parents may not realise that they can take their baby home before the funeral, allowing them to spend precious time together as a family before saying goodbye. Midwives may be uncomfortable with this idea and find it difficult to discuss this option with the parents. Nevertheless, the issue should not be avoided.

Going home

On discharge from hospital, appropriate information should be given to the parents. They must be reassured that they can return to see their baby whenever they wish before the funeral. Give them a contact number. Often the hospital chaplain is the ideal contact.

Inform the GP, the health visitor and the community midwife. Tell the parents you have done this, and that the community midwife will be contacting them the next day.

Information should also be given to the parents about support groups, up-to-date contact numbers and any other relevant advice including contraception.

Inform mothers that they will probably have the normal sensation of full breasts a few days after the birth. This sensation will peak at 35 days and may take some weeks to resolve completely. It can be distressing to realise that the breasts will produce milk, yet there is no baby to feed. Drugs like bromocriptine are hardly ever used these days as they have unpleasant side effects and there is little evidence to support their effectiveness. Suggest simple analgesia and minimal stimulation to alleviate breast engorgement. Simple remedies like cabbage leaves may help.

A consultant obstetrician appointment will be arranged for about 6 weeks' time. The parents need to know that this is a discussion about the baby's death and does not normally include a physical examination of the mother. Ensure this is not a maternity clinic appointment so the mother does not have to wait with pregnant/postnatal mothers; usually the gynaecology clinic is a better setting. A longer (often at least a double length) appointment is usually made.

Planning for a future pregnancy

Mothers may ask midwives about the timing of a future pregnancy, the risks involved and the chances of a live healthy baby. Gently inform her that difficulties can arise if the mother becomes pregnant while she is still mourning or during a time when she has not been able to mourn for her stillborn baby. The new pregnancy can hinder the completion of the mourning process, as it deprives the mother of time and space to mourn (Greaves, 1994). These circumstances can be made worse if the baby is born near the anniversary of the lost baby. However, some parents will be very keen to try for another baby as soon as possible. It must be remembered that this is a very personal decision, and the timing of another baby will be up to the couple.

Midwives should be aware of the special needs of parents undergoing a subsequent pregnancy. O'Leary (2005) suggests that:

- Women with uncomplicated pregnancies are often classified 'high-risk' because of their previous loss.
- Parents may be more anxious in labour and receive more intervention.
- Parents may experience joy on hearing a newborn cry, but also may feel numbness, denial and a sense of loss.
- A new baby can intensify, not diminish, grieving for the previous baby. This can be especially hard if the babies are the same sex.
- Staff should acknowledge the previous baby and ask if this new baby looks similar, just as they would with a previous live child.
- Grief for a lost baby does not go away, and the baby can never be 'replaced'.

'A new layer of grief surfaces when parents become pregnant and then again when they see their baby' (O'Leary, 2004).

Supporting staff

Cowan and Wainwright (2001) feel midwives are often emotionally unsupported, just as grieving mothers were ignored 20 years ago. There have been some recent studies into midwives' views:

- Midwives would value more training in perinatal bereavement (Cartwright & Read, 2004).
- Midwives often feel guilty when a baby dies, even if it is not their fault (Cowan & Wainwright, 2001).
- Staff may feel their ability to give good care is hampered by lack of time (Kaunonen, 2000).
- A midwife's personal circumstances may affect how she will cope (Cowan & Wainwright, 2001).
- Midwives report conflict in moving from a perinatal death to the next client expecting a happy birth (Moulder, 1999; Mander, 2000). They value 'time out' to recover before rushing into the next birth.
- Students usually want to be involved in perinatal death (Mitchell & Catron, 2002) although often trained staff think they should be protected (Nallon, 2007).
- Staff value the support of their colleagues, but also should be able to access professional support/counselling (Cartwright & Read, 2004) including debriefing (Nallon, 2007).

Summary

- What professionals do and say following perinatal death can affect the grieving process.
- Midwives should have a sensitive non-judgemental approach, with good listening skills.
- Give parents clear information and be prepared to repeat it.
- Parents may wish to touch or hold their baby, but they should not be forced to do this.
- Personal, cultural and religious beliefs must be respected.
- Memories and mementos will help parents mourn.
- A new birth can open up old scars.
- Caregivers themselves need emotional support and time for debriefing.

Useful contacts

Antenatal Results and Choices (ARC) Telephone: 020 7631 0285. Website: www.arc-uk.org

Child Bereavement Charity Telephone: 01494 446648. Website: www.childbereavement.org.uk

Stillbirth and Neonatal Death Society (SANDS) Telephone: 020 7436 5881. Website: www.uk-sands.org

The Miscarriage Association   Telephone: 01924 200799. Website: www.miscarriageas-sociation.org.uk

References

American Academy of Family Physicians (AAFP) (2004) *Advanced Life Support in Obstetrics (ALSO) Course Syllabus Manual*, Revised 4th edn. American Academy of Family Physicians, Leawood, Kansas.

Bennett, S., Litz, B., Lee, B. & Maguen, S. (2005) The scope and impact of perinatal loss: current status and future directions. *Professional Psychology: Research and Practice* **36** (2), 180–87.

Butler, M. (2000) Facilitating the grief process: the role of the midwife. *The Practising Midwife* **3** (36), 37.

Cartwright, P. & Read, S. (2004) Perinatal loss: working with bereaved families. *Primary Health Care* **14** (2), 38–41.

Confidential Enquiry into Maternal and Child Health (CEMACH) (2007) *Perinatal Mortality 2005 England Wales and Northern Ireland*. RCOG Press, London. Available at: www.cemach.org.uk (accessed March 2008).

Cowan, L. & Wainwright, M. (2001) The death of a baby in our care: the impact on the midwife. *MIDIRS Midwifery Digest* **11** (3), 313–6.

Department of Health (DoH) (2003a) *A Guide to the Postmortem Examination Procedure Involving a Baby or Child*. DOH, London. Available at: www.doh.gov.uk/tissue (accessed March 2008).

Department of Health (DoH) (2003b) *Consent to a Hospital Postmortem Examination on a Baby or Child*. DoH, London. Available at: www.doh.gov.uk/tissue (accessed March 2008).

Department of Health (DoH) (2003c) *Families and Post Mortems: A Code of Practice*. DoH, London. Available at: www.doh.gov.uk/tissue (accessed March 2008).

Dyer, M. (1992) Stillborn – still precious. *MIDIRS Midwifery Digest* **2** (2), 341–4.

Fox, R., Pillai, M., Porter, H. & Gill, G. (1997) The management of late fetal death: a guide to comprehensive care. *British Journal of Obstetrics and Gynaecology* **104**, 4–10.

Gardner, J. (1999) Perinatal death: uncovering the needs of midwives and nurses and exploring helpful interventions in the United States, England, and Japan. *Journal of Transcultural Nursing* **10** (2), 120–30.

Golding, C. (1991) *Bereavement*. Redwood Press, Melksham, Wiltshire.

Greaves, J. (1994) Normal and abnormal grief reactions: midwifery care after stillbirth. *British Journal of Midwifery* **2** (2), 61–5.

Henderson, N. (2006) Communicating with families about post-mortems: practical guidance. *Paediatric Nursing* **18** (1), 38–40.

Howarth, G.R. & Alfirevic, Z. (2001) Induction of labour following late fetal death (age 24 weeks) (protocol for a Cochrane Review). *The Cochrane Library*, Issue 4. Update Software, Oxford.

Hughes, P. & Riches, S. (2003) Psychological aspects of perinatal loss. *Current Opinion in Obstetrics and Gynaecology* **15** (2), 107–11.

Hughes, P., Turton, P., Hopper, E. & Evans, C. (2002) Assessment of guidelines for good practice in psychosocial care of mothers after stillbirth: a cohort study. *Lancet* **360** (9327), 114–8.

Jones, M. (1997) Mothers who need to grieve: the reality of mourning the loss of a baby. *British Journal of Midwifery* **5** (8), 478–81.

Kaunonen, M., Tarrka, M.T., Hautamaki, K. & Paunonen, M. (2000) The staff's experience of the death of a child and of supporting the family. *International Nursing Review* **47** (1), 46–52.

Kohner, N. (1995) *Pregnancy Loss and the Death of a Baby: Guidelines for Professionals.* Stillbirth and Neonatal Death Society (SANDS), London.

Lanchandani, S., Shiel, O. & MacQuillan, K. (2001) Obstetric profiles and pregnancy outcomes of immigrant women with refugee status. *Irish Medical Journal* **94** (3), 79–80.

Lovell, A. (1983) Some question of identity. *Social Science and Medicine* **17** (11), 755–61.

Mander, R. (2000) Personal grief: understanding the bereaved and their carers. In *Midwifery Practice: Core Topics 3* (Alexander, J., Roch, C. & Levy, V., eds), pp. 29–50. Macmillan Press, London.

Matthews, M., Kohner, K., Kersting, A., Fish, S., Baez, E., McCabe, A., Ambuehl, E., Brooks, D., Hughes, P., Turton, P., Hopper, E. & Evans, C. (2002) Psychological care of mothers after stillbirth. *Lancet* **360** (9345), 1600–602.

Mitchell, M. & Catron, G. (2002) Teaching grief and bereavement: involving support groups in educating student midwives. *Practising Midwife* **5** (8), 26–7.

Moulder, C. (1999) Late pregnancy loss: issues in hospital care. *British Journal of Midwifery* **1**, 244–7.

Nallon, K. (2007) Midwives' needs in relation to the provision of bereavement support to parents affected by perinatal death. Part two. *MIDIRS* **17** (1), 109–12.

National Institute for Health and Clinical Excellence (NICE) (2007a) *Clinical Guideline 55: Intrapartum Care.* National Institute for Health and Clinical Excellence, London.

National Institute for Health and Clinical Excellence (NICE) (2007b) *CG45 Antenatal and Postnatal Mental Health: Understanding NICE guidance.* National Institute for Health and Clinical Excellence, London.

O'Leary, J. (2004) Grief and its impact on prenatal attachment in the subsequent pregnancy. *Archives of Women's Mental Health* **7** (1), 7–8.

O'Leary, J. (2005) The baby who follows the loss of a sibling: special considerations in the postpartum period. *International Journal of Childbirth Education* **20** (4), 28–30.

Radestad, I., Nordin, C., Steineck, G. & Sjogren, B. (1998) A comparison of women's memories of care during pregnancy, labour and delivery after stillbirth or live birth. *Midwifery* **14**, 111–7.

Radestad, I., Steineck, G., Nordin, C. & Sjogren, B. (1996) Psychological complications after stillbirth – influence of memories and immediate management: population based study. *British Medical Journal* **312**, 1505–508.

Rajan, L. (1992) 'Not just me dreaming': parents mourning pregnancy loss. *Health Visitor* **65**, 354–7.

Redfern, M. (2001) *The Royal Liverpool Children's Enquiry report.* The Stationary Office, London.

Rose, C., Evans, M. & Tooley, J. (2006) Falling rates of perinatal post-mortem examination: are we to blame? *Archive of Diseases in Childhood – Fetal Neonatal Edition* **91** (6), F465.

Royal College of Obstetricians and Gynaecologists (RCOG) (2005) *Registration of Stillbirths and Certification of Pregnancy Losses before 24 Weeks of Gestation.* Good practice no 4. RCOG, London.

Schott, J. & Henley, A. (1996) Childbearing losses. *British Journal of Midwifery* **4** (10), 52.

Smith, S. (1999) The lost children. *Contemporary Nurse* **8** (1), 245–51.

Stillbirth and Neonatal Death Society (SANDS) (2007) *Pregnancy Loss and the Death of a Baby: Guidelines for Professionals.* SANDS, London.

Swanson, L. & Madej, T.H. (1997) The febrile obstetric patient. In *Clinical Problems in Obstetric Anaesthesia* (Russell, I.F. & Lyons, G., eds), pp. 123–31. Chapman and Hall, London.

Thomas, J. (1999) A baby's death – helping parents make difficult choices. *The Practising Midwife* **2** (7), 16–19.

Turton, P. (2008) To see or not to see: should parents hold their stillborn? *Midwives* April/May, 16.

Walpole, L. (2002) Perinatal loss: qualitative and quantitative explorations of midwives' experiences. In *Proceedings of the International Confederation of Midwives Conference 2002.* The Hague ICM, Vienna.

Appendix: Checklist following a pregnancy loss after 24 weeks

This is an example of a checklist that can be used following delivery of a stillbirth or neonatal death. Many maternity units will have devised their own form, which can be ticked, signed and dated as appropriate.

Mother's Name . . . .   Partner's Name . . . .
Unit No. . . . .   Telephone No. . . . .

	Please tick, sign and date where appropriate
1. Both parents informed of stillbirth death by:	Name: . . . .
2. Consultant Obstetrician and Supervisor of Midwives informed:	. . . . Consultant . . . . Supervisor
3. Parents given opportunity to see/hold the baby	
4. Momentoes offered to parents (please tick): Photographs: Other: Taken ☐ Lock of hair ☐ Accepted by parents ☐ Cot card ☐ Kept in notes ☐ Name band ☐ Foot/hand print ☐	
5. Religious advisor notified (if desired by parents). Baptism or other religious ceremony offered	
6. Consent for post-mortem requested? Consent given: Yes ☐ Declined ☐	
7. Inform mortician as soon as possible that consent for post-mortem has been obtained	
8. Date and time of post-mortem given?	
9. Post-mortem form completed by **medical staff**?	
10. GP informed: By telephone ☐ By letter ☐	
11. Notice of death form completed?	
12. Community midwife informed on day of discharge: By telephone ☐ By discharge letter ☐	
13. Health visitor informed?	
14. Apply 'teardrop' sticker to mother's notes?	
15. Anti-D given? Yes ☐ No ☐	
16. Rubella vaccination given? Yes ☐ No ☐	

Contd.

17. Bloods taken for investigation? Yes ☐ No ☐ (Note: not listed as may vary between hospitals)	
18. Mother given information regarding lactation?	
19. Contact groups discussed (if appropriate)? – SANDS – ARC – Miscarriage Association	
20. Parentcraft/Relaxation classes cancelled?	
20. At discharge, have TTO drugs been given? Yes ☐ No ☐ (TTO – to take out)	
22. Inform Consultant's Secretary of need for appointment as soon as possible and attach 'proforma' to notes Yes ☐ No ☐ Date of appointment	
23. Genetic counselling appointment made (if appropriate) Yes ☐ No ☐	
24. Death or Stillbirth certificate completed, explained and given to parents. Print name of Certifying Officer on counterfoil.	
25. Information on funeral arrangements given and discussed.	
26. Parents' decision on funeral arrangements: Hospital: Burial ☐ Cremation ☐ Informal service ☐ Private: Burial ☐ Cremation ☐	
27. Chapel service requested Yes ☐ No ☐	
28. Parents given information about The Book of Remembrance?	
29. Notify Bereavement Co-ordinator	
30. CEMACH form completed, signed and posted.	

When completed retain this checklist in mother's notes

21 Bullying and assertiveness

Hilary Field

Introduction

Interaction with others can be a cause of considerable stress in our lives. We may find that in some areas of life we succeed in communicating our needs and wishes confidently, effectively and honestly, yet find that in others we feel totally insignificant.

The Advisory Conciliation and Arbitration Service (Advisory, Conciliation and Arbitration Service (ACAS), 2006) characterise bullying as:

> 'Offensive, intimidating, malicious or insulting behaviour, an abuse or misuse of power through means intended to undermine, humiliate, denigrate or injure the recipient. Bullying or harassment may be by an individual, against an individual or involve groups of people. It may be obvious or it may be insidious. Whatever form it takes it is unwarranted and unwelcome to the individual.'

In an environment where the midwife gives care, in being supportive, empathic and acting as an advocate for women, she should be able to expect that support and empathy from colleagues. Midwives must reflect on their interactions with others and challenge beliefs so that they may continue to evolve professionally. This can be hard for victims of bullying to do, having lost their self-belief and confidence.

Incidence and facts

- 40% midwives admit to having been bullied and 68% report observing bullying (Tehrani, 2004).
- Bullying is a major reason for midwives leaving the profession (Ball *et al.*, 2002).
- Bullying can cause anxiety-related illness: increased sickness, depression, post-traumatic stress disorder (Tehrani, 2004) or even suicide (Hastie, 2006).
- Midwives who feel bullied may resist challenging the 'norm' in their working area and may be less willing to support women in their choices.

- Workplace bullying is prevalent within the hierarchy of the NHS (UNISOM, 2003) and can become an 'entrenched role' for some individuals (Hadikin, 2006)

What is a bully?

- Bullies are driven by a need to control. Despite a confident facade they often have low self-esteem.
- They may have been bullied themselves in the past, not necessarily in the work environment (Randle *et al.*, 2007).
- They may be experiencing bullying themselves from their managers or even their peers (Keeling *et al.*, 2006).
- They may not realise that they are behaving in a bullying way.
- Bullies may sometimes consider themselves a force to be reckoned with; someone to be revered (Keeling *et al.*, 2006) with good social skills which enable them to build a clique (Randle *et al.*, 2007).

Victims of bullying may experience

- Being unjustly scrutinised and criticised at work or becoming the subject of unfounded or malicious rumours.
- Being given impossible workloads compared to other people.
- Having work, ideas or initiatives credited to someone else, possibly even the bully.
- Being 'volunteered' without discussion and excluded from decision making, e.g. off duty changes, on calls.
- Verbal abuse, dismissive comments, threats, ridicule or being completely ignored (Hastie, 2006). It may be related to age, sex or race.
- Feeling that vital or necessary information is withheld from them (Georgiou, 2006).

Bullying can affect the care given to women

Midwives in authority (e.g. senior midwives and managers) have more power to influence conformity and obedience than junior midwives (Hollins Martin, 2006). Bullied midwives may be vulnerable to their influence, and adopt the habits and language of peers or seniors in order to avoid standing out and making themselves vulnerable. This may affect their care of women in labour.

If a woman's choices conflict with the norms of controlling staff, a midwife who lacks confidence is less likely to support her. While women may be offered the illusion of choice, disempowered midwives may not feel able to provide it.

A midwife may:

- Set up syntocinon on a woman with slightly slow progress against the woman's wishes because the senior midwife (who scares her) wants her to get the woman delivered quickly.
- Terminate the first breastfeed to weigh the baby and finish the case quickly as she has overheard colleagues say she is 'slow'.
- Do an admission cardiotocograph on a low-risk woman, although she knows it is poor practice, because everyone else does it and she is afraid to stand out.

- Find reasons for a woman not to use the birthing pool without having evidence to justify this because colleagues who are not happy with giving this care feel it is 'too risky' or alternative.
- Encourage a woman to lie semi-recumbent in labour or the second stage because that the norm on delivery suite.

Dealing with bullying

Workplaces have policies in place for reporting bullying. Victims need to know they can find help, feel supported and that the bullying behaviour will be appropriately understood and dealt with. However victims may be reluctant to report incidents, as they fear repercussions. This may particularly be the case when bullying has been very subtle in nature or when the midwife's manager is involved in bullying. In research funded by the Royal College of Midwives (Ball *et al.*, 2002), midwifery managers were considered to be part of the problem rather than supportive to victims (Keeling *et al.*, 2006).

Consider the following strategies:

- Seek information and support: search the internet, consult union representatives, staff counselling services or an independent body such as the Citizens Advice Bureau.
- Be prepared to report the bullying to a midwifery manager, supervisor of midwives or human resources department.
- Keep a diary of events and interactions: record dates and times of incidents and note any witnesses (RCN, 2005).
- Prepare others to support and defend you. You are probably not the only victim of the bully.
- Some forms of discriminatory bullying can be challenged via legislation, e.g. Sex Discrimination Act 1975, Race Relation Act 1976 and Disability Discrimination Act 1995.

It may be that attempts to challenge bullying through the organisation are of limited use; therefore, it is helpful for the individuals to make changes to their own attitudes and behaviour. In changing behaviour by becoming more assertive a victim can regain a sense of control, making a bully think twice before taking their usual stance. Being assertive can help reduce stress by allowing the victim to stand up for their rights, without being bullied or bullying others in return.

Victims can:

- Avoid being alone with the bully.
- Try to understand why the bully behaves as they do. Although this is difficult it may help to feel sympathy towards them.
- Have an honest talk with them in the presence of a colleague. Tell them about how their put-downs make you feel and how you need positive feedback as well as constructive criticism.
- Prepare in advance by practising how to respond to bullying behaviour; this will increase self-confidence.
- Be aware of the legislation that is in place within your workplace for reporting bullying.

- Ensure that you understand the bully's position, reasoning and needs and if not ask for clarification.
- Develop your assertiveness to help you regain confidence and self-belief.

Assertiveness

Assertiveness is simply effective communication, a skill that can be learnt like any other. By developing assertiveness victims cease to take on the role of 'passive' personality and can therefore moderate the influence of an aggressor. Individuals who are not naturally confident or assertive can still improve aspects of the way they communicate, giving the overall impression of greater confidence.

Individuals can work on developing their assertiveness through further reading, attending workshops, seminars, personal coaching or signing up for assertiveness training within their employing authority.

Assertiveness training will teach victims how to:

- Observe and correct their body language, maintain good eye contact, remain relaxed and breathe slowly.
- Use pre-rehearsed open responses such as: 'I can see that you are busy but could you tell me what is your evidence . . . (for what you have said or claimed)?' 'That is interesting/significant – I need a minute to think about what you have just said.'
- Challenge decisions that affect them which have been made without their contribution.

Summary

- Bullying can be endemic within large hierarchical institutions such as the NHS.
- Know your rights: workplaces have policies in place for reporting and dealing with bullies.
- Changing the bully is unlikely; changing yourself is the most effective way. Being more assertive allows you to be more confident in interpersonal situations.

Useful contacts

Andrea Adams Trust   (committed to preventing workplace bullying) Telephone: 01273 704 900. Website: www.andreaadmstrust.org
Bullying   Website: www.bullyonline.org

Further reading

Burnard, P. (2006) *Counselling Skills for Health Professionals*, 4th edn. Stanley Thornes, Cheltenham.
Randall, P. (1997) *Adult Bullying, Perpetrators and Victims*. Routledge, London.

References

Advisory, Conciliation and Arbitration Service (ACAS) (2006) *Bullying and Harassment at Work: Guidance for Employees*. Available at: http://www.acas.org.uk/index.aspx? articleid=797 (accessed March 2008).

Ball, L., Curtis, P. & Kirkham, M. (2002) *Why Do Midwives Leave?* The Royal College of Midwives, London. Available at: http://www.rcm.org.uk (accessed March 2008).

Georgiou, S. (2006) Stress at work. *RCM News and Appointments* (Mid-May), 4.

Hadikin, R. (2006) Mind the bully: using emotional intelligence. *The Practising Midwife* **9** (11), 32–3.

Hastie, C. (2006) Exploring horizontal violence. *MIDIRS Midwifery Digest* **16** (1), 25–30.

Hollins Martin, C.J. (2006) Are you as obedient as me? *Midwifery Matters* (Autumn), Issue110. Available at: http//www.radmid.demon.co.uk/obedience.htm (accessed March 2008).

Keeling, J., Quigley, J. & Roberts, T. (2006) Bullying in the workplace: what it is and how to deal with it. *British Journal of Midwifery* **14** (10), 616–21.

Randle, J., Stevenson, K. & Grayling, I. (2007) Reducing workplace bullying in healthcare organisations. *Nursing Standard* **21** (22), 49–56.

RCN (2005) *Bullying and Harassment at Work. A Good Practice Guide for RCN Negotiators.* RCN, London.

Tehrani, N. (2004) Bullying: a source of chronic post traumatic stress? Results from a study into the experience of workplace bullying. *British Journal of Guidance and Counselling* **32** (3), 357–66.

UNISON (2003) *Bullying at Work.* Available at: www.unison.org.uk/acrobat/13375.pdf (accessed March 2008).

22 Risk management, litigation and complaints

Cathy Charles

Introduction

The idea that something may go wrong with a birth and/or that a woman may choose to complain or litigate is anathema to those midwives who believe in the process of normal birth and who base their relationships with women on trust. Many midwives are uncomfortable with the concept of risk management, and there is a widespread belief that midwives are being pressured into practising defensively which is at odds with a caring attitude.

The mental distress caused to the injured individual and their family following an adverse event can be immense (Williams & Arulkumaran, 2004). It is easy however to forget the staff involved. A bad outcome can occur however well a midwife has practised. It is even more distressing if someone realises they have made a mistake.

This chapter is, however, intended to both inform and reassure. If midwives practise safely with a good knowledge base, communicate well with colleagues and women and keep good records, they will minimise their chances of an adverse outcome. An understanding of the principles of basic maternity clinical risk management will help all midwives to reflect on their care.

Incidence and facts

- 26% of English NHS litigation cases are maternity issues, but the costs account for 70% of the total NHS litigation sum paid out (Hepworth, 2003).
- A severely brain-damaged child may be awarded over £1 million costs (Williams & Arulkumaran, 2004).

- Despite scare stories there are very few obstetric litigation cases (40–50 between 2002 and 2005) (NHS Litigation Authority (NHSLA), 2007).
- In 2004 there were 2757 maternity complaints in England, Wales and Scotland (Symon, 2006).
- The most common cause of alleged negligence is cardiotocograph (CTG) misinterpretation (Williams & Arulkuraman, 2004).
- Most trusts now have clinical risk management teams to analyse and learn from adverse events.

Clinical risk management: learning from adverse events

Clinical risk management (CRM) is a way of identifying critical incidents and adverse outcomes, to establish if, why and where things went wrong. Root cause analysis can help distinguish individual mistakes by staff from 'latent failures' of the organisation. Lessons learned can help reduce the likelihood of recurrence.

Many midwives appear to believe that CRM exists solely to minimise the chances of litigation. While this may be the driver for health service managers to invest money in risk management services (Symon, 2001), it should not make midwives cynical about risk management in principle. Whatever the reason for its evolution, CRM encourages a willingness to learn from our mistakes in a logical and analytical way. This can help midwives to give better care to women, surely something that everyone can relate to.

Unfortunately, CRM in some trusts has been clumsily implemented by weak managers who are quick to leap to simplistic solutions and blame staff. It is vital to implement CRM in a supportive way, involving supervisors of midwives and not to simply make it part of a hierarchical way of controlling midwives. If not, risk management simply becomes another means of enforcing compliance with medicalised policies and protocols and eroding individual clinical judgement. Interpretation of national guidelines, such as those of National Institute for Clinical Excellence (NICE) or Royal College of Obstetricians and Gynaecologists (RCOG) can become very prescriptive, and midwives may feel they have 'transgressed' in failing to follow what are, after all, only guidelines, not mandatory practice. Although the midwifery voice is getting louder, the obstetric voice is very much the lead on most national guideline development.

The process of event analysis

Most adverse events occur for not just one but several reasons. The clinician giving the care may be just the last link in the chain of small events, which have led to the incident.

The midwife who links up an intravenous infusion to an epidural catheter may have done so for a complex number of reasons: it is helpful to look at the unit workload, common working practices in that area, training and updating opportunities, as well as the individual's competence (is this just a one-off aberration for that midwife?) and any obvious ill health issues. It would also be simple to make a practical change that would reduce the chances of a recurrence despite all these factors, e.g. making sure that the epidural tubing is a different colour from the intravenous tubing and labelled with 'epidural' stickers. Good incident investigators avoid coming to easy conclusions, but always remain vigilant for simple steps like this to reduce risk.

It is helpful to use a systematic approach to analyse adverse events. The National Patient Safety Agency (NPSA) (www.npsa.nhs.uk) has developed a Root Cause Analysis (RCA) toolkit, which can be supplied free to NHS staff, and a training programme to assist staff in analysis. Ideally all staff involved in an adverse event should meet to review what happened. Often if the case involves many different professionals, this is not practicable unless the outcome was particularly severe, e.g. maternal death.

A well-managed incident review can be a very positive experience. Staff may be able to dispel unfounded guilt, realise what went well or did not, express distress and benefit from the support of colleagues. Real insights into what, if anything, went wrong, and what might be learned to prevent a recurrence or mitigate its effects can improve care in future situations. Conversely, a poorly reviewed case can compound guilt, set staff against each other and fail to prevent a recurrence since nothing has been learned.

All staff can contribute to effective care review in many different ways. It is good to be involved in multidisciplinary case review, but informal methods are often underrated. Anecdotal discussion, including the ubiquitous 'coffee room chat', as staff offload their thoughts about recent cases, can be a rich source of insight, support and learning.

Most maternity units also have regular multidisciplinary open meetings to discuss interesting cases/near misses. These tend sometimes to be obstetric led, but midwives increasingly attend and present cases. Such meetings can provide good learning and enhance interprofessional understanding. They are, however, only a broad overview, not a systematic process. The danger is that the most assertive voice may dominate and inaccurate conclusions result. In serious incidents there is no substitute for calm methodical analysis of the notes, statements and verbal accounts.

Litigation

It is unfortunate that much maternity care is based on fear of litigation. Obstetric decision making in particular often tries to contain risk by taking the 'safest' line, i.e. intervene early before things go wrong, instead of giving the best care to a woman in labour. Midwives are affected by this fear too, but have overall as a profession somehow managed to resist, to an extent, this overwhelming pressure. This brings them into inevitable conflict with obstetricians at times. This generalisation does not of course take into account that there are many intelligent supportive obstetricians and risk-averse unsupportive midwives.

Women's rising dissatisfaction with their births (Lane, 2001) may be partly due to rising expectations, but it may also be due to genuine unhappiness at unjustified opposition to their wishes. Whereas some parents may be unhappy with insufficient action, litigation may also, potentially, arise from women denied the normal birth they expected due to unnecessary intervention (Royal College of Midwives (RCM), 2005). If this were to become commonplace, it might refocus the interventionist approach that currently erodes much maternity care.

CTGs are a real source of difficulty in litigation, as even experts disagree when interpreting traces. This is of course outside a midwife's control. Suffice to say, if midwives decide to perform CTGs, they must be very sure that they are able to interpret them: this is obvious in any case for good clinical care. Regular CTG training is now mandatory in most trusts and is a Clinical Negligence Scheme for Trusts (CNST) requirement. (Refer to Chapter 3 for CTG records and storage.)

It is commonly said that it is not so much *if* but *when* a midwife will have to stand up in court to explain his/her actions. This is nonsense. Fewer than 2% of medical negligence claims actually go to court (NHSLA, 2007) so most midwives will never have the experience of a court appearance. Whilst of course parents may need money to care for a disabled child, sometimes an injured party's initial impulse to sue may be part of a process of grieving and not always based on true negligence. Many want simply an explanation of what happened, an apology, and to prevent a recurrence (Vincent *et al.*, 1994). Other means, such as the complaints procedure, may serve these people better. Despite a widely held belief that people will litigate for the most minor issues, and that 'no win no fee' legal firms have fuelled this culture, in fact only a very tiny proportion of people sue. No solicitor wants to take on a case that has no chance of success. Consequently, most cases that get further than a preliminary letter have genuine issues to be addressed.

This chapter is not intended to document the process of litigation. There are many other resources which will do this: the NHSLA website has a brief guide for clinicians on clinical negligence litigation with a simple diagram showing the process of a claim.

Vicarious liability of employer

NHS employees are covered by vicarious liability, by which the law can hold one person or institution liable for the actions of another. So in theory a woman who chooses to sue for the negligent actions of a midwife will in fact sue the trust which employs the midwife, not the midwife herself. Concerns exist as to whether a trust board may try to recover part of the costs from the negligent employee, since this is possible in law, although extremely unlikely.

It is not possible, as is widely believed, for an employer to shirk vicarious liability when a midwife has worked later than his/her nominated shift. The midwife is still performing the work for which he/she has signed a contract with his/her employer, and staying on duty when responding to a particular need (e.g. a woman who gives birth just after the end of a shift period) is practising flexibly and sensitively (Jenkins, 1995). However voluntarily grossly exceeding sensible working hours is more of a grey area; this is unwise for all kinds of reasons, and a midwife who has worked excessive hours makes him/herself very vulnerable.

The liability position for independent midwives (IMs) is different, since they are self-employed and therefore personally responsible for obtaining professional indemnity insurance (PII). Controversially in 1994 the Royal College of Midwives withdrew its PII for independent midwives after a member's ballot (Anderson, 2007). The last commercial insurance provider for IMs withdrew in 2002. IMs therefore have no choice but to practise without insurance and have to inform their clients of this before they are engaged.

NHSLA and CNST

- The NHS Litigation Authority (NHSLA) has a litigation 'risk pooling' scheme, i.e. trusts pay into a central scheme which then meets the cost of any litigation. Without this scheme, one big litigation case could practically bankrupt a service.
- The NHSLA administers the Clinical Negligence Scheme for Trusts (CNST) who has produced Maternity Clinical Risk Management Standards to assess the way CRM

activities are organised. They focus on communication, clinical care and staffing levels.

- Trusts are assessed by CNST 1–3 yearly: those who demonstrate good practice get a discount on their CNST contributions. Such contributions can be over £1 million: a significant dent in the maternity budget.
- CNST standards are largely common sense and do not necessarily conflict with the desire of midwives to give flexible individualised care, although they are very policy/protocol driven. It is very important that midwives are involved in their trust's policy development groups to ensure that workable, sensible, flexible and evidence-based protocols are developed.

Records

The old maxims 'if you didn't write it down it didn't happen' or 'you are only as good as your written records' have some truth, as records are a key factor in demonstrating care. Records should be clear, accurate and readable when photocopied or scanned.

- Entries must be dated and signed (use the 24-hour clock) and signed, with the writer's name and position printed clearly alongside.
- Any error should be scored with a single line so it is still readable, and the correction dated, timed and signed.
- Records should be written as contemporaneously as possible. Any later entry should be clearly dated, timed and signed.
- Any consultations/referrals should be documented.
- Refer to Chapter 3 for CTG documentation.
- Try to avoid unnecessary detail: sometimes it can be almost impossible to extract relevant information from notes full of random wandering prose.
- Patients have a right to access their own records under the Data Protection Act 1998.
- Records must be retained for 25 years (United Kingdom Central Council (UKCC), 1998). Community and independent midwives will need to securely store their diaries and records for 25 years, or pass them on to their employer or local supervising authority (Nursing and Midwifery Council (NMC), 2004; Griffiths, 2007).

However, remember that records are only part of the picture. What will carry great weight in court is what the woman perceived, i.e. interactions with staff, verbal explanations given to her at the time and her *understanding* of what was happening during the incident. Remember: you may write 'Vaginal examination with consent' in the maternity notes, but if the woman has not given express consent, and explains this articulately in court, then the record may give scant protection. 'Poor practice and lack of communication are likely to be the underlying factors in litigation – and no amount of documentation will ever cover that up' (Morris, 2005).

Complaints

Many more midwives are likely to be involved in some way with a formal or informal complaint than litigation. Symon (2006) challenges however the assumption that complaints are rising and states:

'We should not conclude that complaints lurk around every corner. Given the number of women having babies in Britain the incidence of complaints is comparatively low.'

Sidgewick (2006) suggests that complaints tend to have four recurrent factors:

- Poor communication with client/family
- Poor communication between professionals
- Poor staffing
- Staff attitude

Complaints should be treated positively, as showing that people believe that the organisation should know about their concerns. The process can however be very upsetting: even the best midwives may at some point in their career have to read a distressing letter from someone they have cared for, cataloguing an unhappy experience. This can come as a real shock.

Most people tend to forgive well-intentioned mistakes when everyone is honest about what happened. A home visit from a manager and opportunity to retell the story may reassure many women that someone is listening, and that changes are being made to improve the experience for other mothers. However, the Parliamentary and Health Service Ombudsman for England (Health Service Ombudsman for England (HSOE), 2003) has noted that people may become more, not less, angry if a complaint is investigated clumsily, and this dissatisfaction may lead to litigation (Symon, 2006).

For the NHS complaints procedure, go to the Department of Health (DoH) website www.dh.gov.uk.

Writing a statement

It may feel intimidating to be asked to provide a statement to a supervisor, manager or a member of the risk management team. It is normal procedure now to collect statements from clinicians involved in an event with an adverse outcome, as a proactive way of gathering facts for case investigation. Most statements are only used for this purpose, although they are kept on file for any possible future litigation. In the unlikely case that litigation ensues, the trust's solicitor will sit down and prepare a formal statement with the clinician. Original statements written without such help may be a useful aide memoir for this process, but are rarely used in court.

The Royal College of Midwives (RCM, 1997) has produced guidance on statement writing.

Caring for the mother or father following an adverse event

This is a challenge for all involved. Any support will obviously depend on the nature of the adverse event: it is not possible to be prescriptive about this. If the baby has died, refer to Chapter 20 (perinatal loss) for how to support parents.

If you fear there may have been some error or omission which contributed to the outcome, you are in a difficult position. Honesty is of course normally the best policy with parents, but until you know the facts it is usually best to avoid speculation. Staff may feel guilty quite unjustifiably: a bad outcome does not necessarily mean that someone has done something wrong. It is natural that parents may feel they have to blame someone. It is possible to be supportive without lying: 'None of us at the moment know why this has happened' is often the honest truth.

Parents may feel angry towards staff following an adverse outcome, behaving in a distressed and hostile way. They may feel rejected or abandoned by staff: indeed this may not be paranoia, it may be actually happening. Midwives need to deal with their own feelings and resist the urge to avoid parents who may be expressing negative thoughts.

The midwife who feels he/she may be even partly responsible for any adverse event is in a particularly difficult position. Whilst it is natural and helpful to give parents the opportunity to ask questions about the birth, be aware that by 'explaining' what happened, midwives may, consciously or unconsciously, attempt to justify their own actions or those of others. Fear of the consequences of admitting blame may change the interaction too. There are no answers to these difficult dilemmas: midwives can only be aware of the problems and attempt to navigate their way through this difficult territory.

The Patient Advice and Liaison Service (PALS) can provide support and advice to parents who have experience an adverse event.

Midwives who need a confidential ear may wish to access staff support services for non-judgemental listening, e.g. RCM counselling service. See also 'Supporting staff' in Chapter 20.

Conclusion

Midwives face a challenge in offering competent, sensitive and responsive care to women without practicing defensively. Adverse events can shake our faith in midwifery. We can only do our best in trying to minimise them and learn from them. Despite everyone's best efforts, occasional bad outcomes will occur; the secret is to keep a sense of balance.

Summary

- There need be no conflict between woman-centred care and awareness of risk management issues.
- Adverse events distress everyone: staff can feel victims too.
- Almost everyone will have to write a statement at some point.
- Good analysis of adverse events can enable helpful learning.
- Very few staff will actually appear in court.
- NHS midwives are covered by their employer's vicarious liability. Independent midwives practise without insurance cover.
- Complaints may be a good sign of willingness to express dissatisfaction.
- Parents need sensitive support following an adverse event.

Useful contacts

Clinical Negligence Scheme for Trusts (CNST) on NHSLA Website
   Website: www.nhsla.com
Department of Health (DoH)   Website for complaints procedure. Website: www.dh.gov.uk
National Patient Safety Agency (NPSA)   Website: www.npsa.nhs.uk
NHS Litigation Authority (NHSLA)   Website: www.nhsla.com

Patient Advice and Liaison Service (PALS) Website: www.dh.gov.uk. For details of local services contact local hospital, clinic or general practitioner or phone NHS Direct 0845 46 47.

Root Cause Analysis (RCA) toolkit. Website: www.npsa.nhs.uk

Royal College of Midwives (RCM) 24-hour counselling service. Telephone: 0845 605 00 44.

References

Anderson, T. (2007) Is this the end of independent midwifery? *Practising Midwife* **10** (2), 4–5.

Griffiths, R. (2007) Record keeping: midwives and the law. *British Journal of Midwifery* **15** (5), 303–304.

Health Service Ombudsman for England (HSOE) (2003) *Annual Report 2002–3*. HMSO, London.

Hepworth, S. (2003) Clinical cases by speciality. *NHS Litigation Authority Journal* **2**, 4.

Jenkins, R. (1995) *The Law and the Midwife*. Blackwell Science, Oxford.

Lane, K. (2001) Fear of litigation: the tail that wags the dog. *Annual Conference of the Australian Sociological Association*. University of Sydney, Sydney.

Morris, S. (2005) Is fear at the heart of hard labour? *MIDIRS Midwifery Digest* **15** (4), 508–11.

NHS Confederation (2001) *Building a Safer NHS for Patients*. NHS Confederation Publications, London.

Nursing and Midwifery Council (NMC) (2004) *Midwives Rules and Standards*. Available at: www.nmc-uk.org (accessed March 2008).

Royal College of Midwives (RCM) (1997) *Statement Writing*. Available at: www.rcm.org.uk/info/docs/Statement%20 writing.doc (accessed March 2008).

Royal College of Midwives (RCM) (2005) RCM annual conference (guest speaker Janine Wynn-Davies). *Midwives* **9** (6), 231.

Sidgewick, C. (2006) Everybody's business: managing midwifery complaints. *British Journal of Midwifery* **14** (2), 70–71.

Symon, A. (2001) *Obstetric Litigation from A to Z*. Quay Books Division, Mark Allen Publishing Ltd, London.

Symon, A. (2006) Are we facing a complaints and litigation crisis in the health service? *British Journal of Midwifery* **14** (3), 164–5.

United Kingdom Central Council (UKCC) (1998) *Guidelines for Records and Record Keeping*, p. 56. UKCC, London.

Vincent, C., Young, M. & Phillpips, A. (1994) Why do people sue doctors? *NHS Litigation Authority Journal* **2**, 4.

Williams, B. & Arulkumaran, S. (2004) CTG and medicolegal issues. *Best Practice and Research* **18** (3), 457–66; reprinted in *MIDIRS* December 2004, 504–509.

23 Intrapartum blood tests

Julie Davis

Maternal blood tests

Maternal blood may be taken for a variety of reasons, routinely or in an emergency during pregnancy or labour. Normal reference ranges for blood results may vary slightly between different hospitals or laboratories and are normally based on population studies.

The word 'normal' may need qualification. A blood result may fall within the 'normal' accepted range, but it may be abnormal for a particular woman. Equally, a value may fall outside the 'normal' range but the woman is quite well and simply has a 'numerically non-standard' blood result.

This needs consideration particularly when allowing for the changes in haemodynamics in pregnancy. The increase in circulating plasma volume is 50% above non-pregnant values by the 34th week of gestation, lowering haemoglobin, haematocrit and red cell counts as well as placing an increased demand on maternal organs. This should be remembered when evaluating normal reference ranges for the pregnant women.

Taking blood

- Explain why you want to take blood and gain the woman's consent. She should subsequently be informed of the result and its significance: ensure she knows how and when this will be communicated to her.
- Always wear gloves for protection.
- Select a site: the antecubital fossa is usually best, as the cephalic, median, cubital and basilic veins are easily accessible near the skin surface (Coates, 1998).
- Collect blood into the correct bottles (there is no national colour coding for blood bottles at present), store appropriately with a completed request form and send to the laboratory as soon as possible. Record bloods taken in the mother's notes.

Biochemical tests

Electrolytes

Lithium heparin blood bottles

- Sodium (Na) is indirectly related to body water volume.
- Potassium (K) is important for normal cardiac electrical activity, and very high or low concentrations are associated with cardiac electrical abnormality (such as ventricular fibrillation or asystole) (Table 23.1).

Table 23.1 Electrolytes.

Constituent	Normal range
Na	135–145 mmol/l
K	3.4–5.2 mmol/l

Renal function tests

Lithium heparin blood bottles

- Creatinine is a nitrogenous end product of muscle metabolism. Creatinine is filtered by the glomeruli in the kidney, so the renal clearance rate provides an approximate measurement of the glomerular filtration rate. As the concentration of creatinine can be readily measured in the plasma, it is a useful indicator of renal function, particularly when sequential observations are made (Walton *et al.*, 1994).
- Uric acid is the end product of protein metabolism. Elevated uric acid levels may reflect decreased renal blood flow caused by vasoconstriction.
- Urea is a waste product of metabolism which is excreted via the kidneys (Table 23.2).

Table 23.2 Renal function tests.

Constituent	Normal range
Creatinine	60–120 mmol/l
Uric acid	0.2–0.4 mmol/l
Urea	2.5–6.5 mmol/l

Liver function tests

Studies suggest that pregnancy liver enzymes are lower than the non-pregnant reference ranges often used and that, in the absence of altered hepatic blood flow, physiological haemodilution alone may result in lower values for alanine transaminase (ALT), aspartate transaminase (AST) and bilirubin levels (Girling *et al.*, 1997) (Table 23.3).

Table 23.3   Liver function tests.

Constituent	Normal range
ALT	6–40 U/l
AST	10–40 U/l
ALP	40–120 U/l (↑ ++ at term so of no diagnostic value)
Albumin	34 g/l
Bilirubin	5–17 µmol/l

Alanine transaminase and aspartate transaminase

Lithium heparin blood bottles

The activities of ALT and AST are widely used as a sensitive, although non-specific, index of acute damage to liver cells, irrespective of its cause (Gaw *et al.*, 1999). Levels remain unchanged in normal pregnancy.

Alkaline phosphatase

Lithium heparin blood bottles

While other liver enzymes remain unchanged in normal pregnancy, alkaline phosphatase (ALP) does not. It is produced by the placenta from the first trimester onwards: by the third trimester it is so greatly raised that it has virtually no diagnostic value.

Total albumin

Clotted blood sample

Plasma albumin is also synthesised in the liver and so indicates liver function. In normal pregnancy the decrease in albumin levels is caused by haemodilution and not as a result of liver insufficiency (McKay, 1999).

Total bilirubin

Lithium heparin blood bottles

This test is to screen the liver for damage and to investigate the causes of anaemia. Haemoglobin destruction results in the production of bilirubin, which is conjugated in the liver and excreted in the bile. Any overload or blockage of the system raises levels (Bratt-Wyton, 1998). During a normal pregnancy levels do not usually rise. However, in HELLP (haemolysis, elevated liver enzymes, low platelets) syndrome levels can sometimes increase.

Haematological tests

Full blood count

Ethylenediamine-tetra-acetic acid (EDTA) blood bottles

- **Haemoglobin** (Hb) is the pigment contained in the red blood cells and enables them to transport oxygen around the body. Anaemia may cause tiredness and loss of energy: it has little effect on labour itself but can potentiate the effect of any haemorrhage at birth. There are no definitive ranges for Hb as there is a lot of variance in the literature. National Institute for Clinical Excellence (NICE) (2003) recommends iron supplementation if <10.5 g/dl after 28 weeks, but an Hb of >9 g/dl in labour is unlikely to cause major problems. Low Hb is often due to haemodilution of pregnancy; women are often falsely diagnosed as anaemic and treated unnecessarily with iron supplements, without consideration of the full blood picture. Interpret the Hb in the light of the MCV, MCH and haematocrit. If the haematocrit is low, and the MCV and MCH are normal, anaemia is unlikely.
- **Platelets** are essential for normal haemostasis. Platelets may be reduced in preeclampsia and HELLP syndrome. The function of platelets is related to many factors in the body's coagulation system. A platelet count is important as thrombocytopaenia (deficiency of the platelets) frequency accompanies other disorders (Star & Peipert, 1996).
- **White blood cells** (WBC). This test calculates the total number of all the different white cells. It indicates bone marrow health and if the immune system is being stimulated for any reason (Frye, 1998).
- **Haematocrit or packed cell volume** (PCV). This shows the concentration of red cells in the plasma. As with Hb, in normal pregnancy the haematocrit level will decrease during the second trimester. If the haematocrit is low, this means the blood is dilute and the Hb is likely to be low as well, as Hb is measured relative to the plasma volume.
- **Mean corpuscular volume** (MCV) is the average volume of a single red cell. It has been regarded as the most sensitive red cell index for the identification of iron deficiency. Values below 70 fl occur only with iron deficiency anaemia or thalassaemia minor (Kirkpatrick & Alexander, 1996).
- **Mean corpuscular haemoglobin** (MCH) measures the amount and volume of haemoglobin inside the red blood cell. A woman with a low Hb and normal MCH and MCV levels will probably not be anaemic (Table 23.4).

Table 23.4 Full blood count.

Constituent	Normal range
Hb	8–14 g/dl
Platelets	150–350 × 10^9/l
WBC	6–18 × 10^9/l
PCV	36–48%
MCV	80–96 fl

Serum ferritin

Ferritin is a protein inside the cell that stores iron for future use. Serum ferritin levels demonstrate how much iron the body has stored, and are therefore a more accurate (but more expensive) test for anaemia than haemoglobin estimation, which is affected by haemodilution. Normal levels range from 15 to 250 ng/ml.

Clotting screening

Sodium citrate blood bottles
  Samples must be tested as soon as possible on the day of collection.

- Activated partial thromboplastin time (APTT). This test measures the clotting time of plasma and indicates the overall efficiency of the intrinsic coagulation pathway.
- Prothrombin time (PT). This test measures the clotting time of plasma and indicates the efficiency of the extrinsic pathway.
- Fibrinogen is a protein formed in the liver. During tissue injury it is activated by thrombin to form fibrin, arresting haemorrhage (Tiran, 1997) (Table 23.5).

Table 23.5 Clotting tests.

Constituent	Normal range
Platelets	$150–350 \times 10^9/l$
APTT	29–37 s
PT	11–15 s
Fibrinogen	20–40 g/l

Other tests

Kleihauer test

Maternal blood 6 ml sample in EDTA bottle. Umbilical cord blood 1 ml sample in EDTA bottle. This test is offered to rhesus negative women to detect if any fetal cells have crossed over into the maternal circulation. Blood is taken from the mother's vein and from the baby's umbilical cord following birth. If the baby is found to be rhesus positive, an anti-immunoglobulin D injection can be offered to the mother. This directs any fetal cells away from stimulating the mother's immune system.

Group and save

EDTA blood bottles

This determines blood group and rhesus status. The serum is saved for 5–7 days. Antibody screening is also carried out. This may be done prior to caesarean section, or if a woman presents with an antepartum haemorrhage, placenta praevia, intrauterine death or any other medical or obstetric problem that may necessitate a blood transfusion.

Cross-matching

EDTA bottles

The donor's red blood cells and white cells are placed in the recipient's serum to confirm if the donated blood will be compatible with the potential recipient.

C-reactive protein

Clotted blood sample

The C-reactive protein is present in low concentration in plasma, but increases during an acute response phase, indicating a non-specific systemic response to inflammation or infection. Normal levels are <10 mg/l.

The D-dimer test

Sodium citrate bottles

This detects fibrin derivatives. The presence of a cross-linked D-dimer is diagnostic for the breaking down of a fibrin clot and is useful for detecting pulmonary, deep vein thrombosis and disseminated intravascular coagulation. Normal values are <0.5 ng/ml.

Blood tests for specific conditions and blood pictures

Pre-eclampsia

Bloods to take:

- Full blood count (FBC)
- Electrolytes
- Renal function tests (including uric acid)
- Liver function tests
- Clotting studies

Pre-eclampsia is a syndrome that affects all maternal organ systems. Pathophysiological changes suggest reduced organ perfusion of the kidneys, liver and brain (Roberts & Redman, 1993). The vascular system is subjected to raised peripheral resistance, reduced plasma volume, reduced cardiac output and sometimes haemolysis. The renal system has a reduced uric acid clearance, renal blood flow and glomerular filtration rate. As the liver is put under stress, liver enzymes become raised and the clotting system has a tendency towards coagulation in severe cases (Table 23.6).

Table 23.6 Blood picture for pre-eclampsia.

Sample	Level
Electrolytes	Unchanged
Hb	May increase
PCV	May increase
Platelets	May decrease
Clotting time	May be normal or prolonged in severe stages
Creatinine	May increase
Uric acid	Increased
Urea	May increase
Liver enzymes	Increased except for bilirubin (unchanged unless HELLP syndrome)

HELLP syndrome

Bloods to take:

- FBC
- Electrolytes
- Clotting
- Liver function tests
- Renal function tests (Table 23.7)

Table 23.7   Blood picture for HELLP syndrome.

Sample	Level
Hb	May decrease
MCV	Decreased
Platelets	Decreased
PT/APTT	Unchanged
Fibrinogen	Increased
Creatinine	Increased
Uric acid	Increased
Urea	Increased
Liver enzymes	Increased

Adapted from Poole (1988).

HELLP syndrome is characterised by haemolysis, elevated liver enzymes and low platelets, and is a serious, potentially fatal complication of pregnancy. It is most frequently found in conjunction with severe pre-eclampsia: the pathophysiological changes result in injury to the vascular system with hypoxic changes in the liver (Nutt, 1997). Arterial vasospasms damage small blood vessels forming lesions. These allow platelet aggregation and formation of a fibrin network. As red cells are forced through the network under pressure, haemolysis results. As the haemolytic process continues, the haematocrit levels fall and bilirubin levels rise (Poole, 1988). Diagnosis is aided by laboratory findings, and early diagnosis is essential to prevent further complications of disseminated intravascular coagulation, hepatic and renal failure (see HELLP in Chapter 19).

Disseminated intravascular coagulation

Disseminated intravascular coagulation (DIC) is not a disease; it is more of an underlying disorder secondary to another syndrome. It is a contradictory process involving coagulation and anticoagulation, and thrombosis can be overshadowed by haemorrhage. DIC is characterised by widespread activation of blood coagulation, resulting in the intravascular formation of fibrin, which may lead to thrombotic occlusion of small- and mid-sized vessels (Levi *et al.*, 2000). Acute DIC can occur after obstetric emergencies such as placental abruption, intrauterine death, amniotic fluid embolism, postpartum haemorrhage and infection, but is more commonly linked with eclampsia and HELLP syndrome.

Blood tests will both confirm DIC and help plan medication. They should include FBC with platelets, PT, APTT, fibrinogen, fibrin degradation products and the D-dimer test. Research suggests that the D-dimer test and fibrin degradation products are the best tests for the diagnosis of DIC, and that PT, APTT and platelet count, although sensitive are non-specific tests when examining DIC (Yu *et al.*, 2000) (Table 23.8).

Table 23.8 Blood picture for DIC.

Sample	Level
Platelets	Decreased
PT	Increased
APTT	Increased
Fibrinogen	Decreased in acute DIC
	May be normal in chronic DIC
D-dimer	Increased

Stillbirth

Local practice may vary, but usual bloods taken are the following:

- Full blood count
- Group and save
- Liver function tests
- Clotting studies
- Infection screen/TORCH/parvovirus
- Autoimmune antibodies (e.g. lupus, anticardiolipin)
- Kleihauer

If the cause of fetal death is known and a maternal disorder has contributed, then any bloods relating to this will obviously need to be taken. Genetic testing of both parents may also be indicated, but this will require further counselling and is unlikely to be performed in the immediate postnatal period.

If the baby has been dead for some time there is a small increased risk of DIC.

Fetal blood tests

Fetal pH measurements

Fetal blood pH is an important diagnostic and prognostic test measured during pregnancy, labour or in the cord after birth. Severe fetal acidaemia is associated with increased perinatal mortality and increased risk for later impaired neurodevelopment (Huch *et al.*, 1994).

Respiratory acidosis

This occurs due to the accumulation of carbon dioxide in the fetal blood as a result of interference in the exchange of gases between mother and baby. The PO_2 blood level will decrease and the pCO_2 level will increase. It can be caused by compression of the umbilical cord or uterine hyperstimulation. The baby will suffer no serious effects as long as there is sufficient oxygen to maintain aerobic metabolism.

Metabolic acidosis

If oxygen levels continue to decrease fetal metabolism changes from aerobic to anaerobic. During this time of reduced oxygen levels the baby's body begins to metabolise glucose resulting in lactic acid as a waste product. In the absence of oxygen, lactic acid cannot be broken down and its accumulation causes retention of hydrogen ions and therefore acidosis. The hydrogen ions are absorbed by a buffer base, but as more lactic acid builds up further buffer bases have to be used. The base deficit will be higher in a metabolic acidosis where more buffering capacity has been needed. By measuring the base deficit it is possible to see if acidaemia was respiratory or metabolic.

Fetal blood sampling

Electronic fetal heart monitoring (EFM) during labour has been associated with increased caesarean section rates and instrumental deliveries for assumed fetal distress. The fetal blood sampling (FBS) technique developed by Saling in 1967 allows capillary blood to be taken from the baby during labour to assess pH values and to give a complete acid-base status, therefore giving a clearer picture of the baby's condition (Table 23.9). The mother needs to fully understand and consent to the procedure, and she should be aware of the possible implications of an abnormal result. It is uncomfortable and can take 10 minutes or longer. The mother needs lots of support and can use entonox if required.

Table 23.9 Fetal blood pH and action to be taken.

Fetal blood pH	Recommended action
≥7.25	No action at present: repeat FBS in 1 h if FHR concern persists If later FBS stable and FHR unchanged, defer further FBS unless further FHR abnormalities develop
7.21–7.24	Repeat FBS in 30 min if FHR concern persists If later FBS stable and FHR unchanged, defer further FBS unless further FHR abnormalities develop
<7.20	Urgent birth is indicated

If a third FBS is contemplated or after an abnormal FBS result, consultant obstetric opinion should be sought.

Adapted from NICE (2007).

Contraindications to FBS

- Maternal HIV, hepatitis or *active* herpes.
- The woman does not give consent.
- Prematurity <34 weeks.
- Fetal bleeding disorders, e.g. haemophilia.

- If during the second stage of labour the EFM trace is ominous and there is clear evidence suggestive of acute fetal compromise (NICE, 2007). Instrumental or operative delivery is indicated at this point.

FBS procedure

For the sampling to be performed:
- The cervix must be adequately dilated to gain access to the presenting part, and membranes ruptured.
- The woman should be in the left lateral position to prevent aortocaval compression.
- An amnioscope is passed into the vagina and, once visualised, the presenting part cleaned and dried.
- Ethyl chloride may be sprayed on.
- A thin layer of liquid paraffin is usually applied to help give a good blood droplet.
- A small incision is made and the blood collected in a dry heparin-coated glass capillary tube for analysis.

Cord blood sampling

Cord blood analysis is useful to aid neonatal management, for medical audits and for litigation and legal purposes. There is no evidence to suggest that routine cord blood analysis should be the norm after all births and NICE (2007) advises against it.

Practices may vary between units. Selective reasons may be as follows:

- Abnormal fetal heart rate (FHR) in labour.
- Instrumental delivery or emergency caesarean section.
- Low Apgar score.
- Preterm birth.
- Any other situation where suspected fetal compromise has occurred.

Umbilical arteries carry blood away from the baby. Arterial blood reflects fetal wellbeing and acid-base levels. The umbilical vein carries blood to the baby from the placenta. Venous blood reflects placental status and placental tissue acid-base levels (Wallman, 1997). When carrying out umbilical cord samples after delivery, both the artery and the vein should be sampled (Tables 23.10 and 23.11). Firstly, this will ensure that the umbilical artery value can be recognised (the artery has a lower O_2 tension and saturation, a lower pH, a greater base deficit and a higher CO_2 tension). Secondly, as the umbilical artery represents fetal circulation and the umbilical vein blood shows the influence of the placenta, the balance between fetal acid production and placental oxygen can only be assessed by comparing both samples (Huch *et al.*, 1994).

The pH is a measure of the acid-base balance of the blood. The acid is the hydrogen ion donor and the base is the hydrogen ion receptor, and so by measuring pH values, hydrogen levels in the blood are determined. The base excess represents the deficit of bicarbonate in the blood.

There is some limited evidence that cord pH is a predictor for neonatal death and intrapartum-related hypoxic ischaemic encephalopathy (NICE, 2007). Whilst it does

Table 23.10   Umbilical venous blood analysis.

Venous blood	Normal range	Median
pH	7.17–7.48	7.35
pCO_2	3.5–7.9 kPa	5.3
Base deficit	−1.0 to 8.9 mmol/l	2.4 mmol/l

Adapted from Westgate *et al.* (1994).

Table 23.11   Umbilical arterial blood analysis.

Arterial blood	Normal range	Median
pH	7.05–7.38	7.26
pCO_2	4.9–10.7 kPa	7.3
Base deficit	−2.5 to 9.7 mmol/l	2.4 mmol/l

Adapted from Westgate *et al.* (1994).

not have a strong positive predictive value, it is believed that its highly negative predictive value for cerebral palsy means that its use is justified in cases of suspected fetal compromise.

References

Bratt-Wyton, R. (1998) Interpretation of routine blood tests. *Nursing Standard* **13** (12), 42–6.

Coates, T. (1998) Venepuncture and intravenous cannulation. *The Practising Midwife* **1** (1), 28–31.

Frye, A. (1998) *Holistic Midwifery*, Vol. 1. Labrys Press, Portland, Oregon.

Gaw, A., Cowan, R.A., O'Reilly, D.S.J., Stewart, M.J. & Shephard, J. (1999) *Clinical Biochemistry*, 2nd edn. Churchill Livingstone, Edinburgh.

Girling, J.C., Dow, E. & Smith, J.H. (1997) Liver function tests in pre-eclampsia – importance of comparison with a reference range derived for normal pregnancy. *British Journal of Obstetrics and Gynaecology* **104**, 246–50.

Huch, A., Huch, R. & Rooth, G. (1994) Guidelines for blood sampling and measurement of pH and blood gas values in obstetrics. *European Journal of Obstetrics and Gynaecology and Reproductive Biology* **54**, 165–75.

Kirkpatrick, C. & Alexander, S. (1996) Antepartum and postpartum assessment of haemoglobin, haematocrit and serum ferritin. In *When to Screen in Obstetrics and Gynaecology* (Wildschut, H., Weiner, C.P. & Peters, T.J., eds), pp. 180–95. WB Saunders, London.

Levi, M., de Jong, E., Van Der Poll, T. & Cate, H. (2000) Novel approaches to the management of DIC. *Critical Care Medicine* **28** (9), 520–24.

McKay, K. (1999) Biochemical and blood tests in midwifery practice. (1) Pre-eclampsia. *The Practising Midwife* **2** (8), 28–31.

National Institute for Clinical Excellence (NICE) (2003) *Antenatal Care: Routine Care for the Healthy Pregnant Woman – Clinical Guideline 6*. National Institute for Clinical Excellence, London.

National Institute for Clinical Excellence (NICE) (2007) *Clinical Guideline 55: Intrapartum Care*. National Institute for Clinical Excellence, London. Available at: www.nice.org (accessed March 2008).

Nutt, J. (1997) HELLP syndrome. *British Journal of Midwifery* **5** (1), 8–11.

Poole, J.H. (1988) Getting a perspective on HELLP syndrome. *American Journal of Maternal and Child Health* **13**, 432–7.

Roberts, J.M. & Redman, C.W.G. (1993) Pre-eclampsia: more than pregnancy induced hypertension. *The Lancet* **341**, 1447–53.

Star, J. & Peipert, J.F. (1996) Intrapartum coagulation studies. In *When to Screen in Obstetrics and Gynaecology* (Wildschut, H., Weiner, C.P. & Peters, T.J., eds), pp. 219–27.

Tiran, D. (1997) *Bailliere's Midwives Dictionary*, 9th edn. Bailliere Tindall, London.

Wallman, C.M. (1997) Interpretation of fetal cord blood gases. *Neonatal Network* **16** (1), 72–4.

Walton, J., Barondess, J.A. & Lock, S. (1994) *The Oxford Medical Companion*. Oxford University Press, Oxford.

Westgate, J., Garibaldi, J.M. & Greene, K.R. (1994) Umbilical cord blood gas analysis at delivery. *British Journal of Obstetrics and Gynaecology* **101**, 1054–63.

Yu, M., Nardella, A. & Pechet, L. (2000) Screening tests of DIC. Guidelines for rapid and specific laboratory diagnosis. *Critical Care Medicine* **28** (6), 1777–80.

24 Medicines and the midwife

Vicky Chapman and Sheila Miskelly

Introduction

'A practising midwife shall only supply and administer those medicines, including analgesics, in respect of which she has received the appropriate training as to use, dosage and methods of administration' (Rule 7: Administration of medicines, Nursing and Midwifery Council (NMC), 2004).

This chapter discusses the midwife's position regarding the supply and administration of medicines. It includes a pharmacopoeia listing some of the commonest drugs used during the intrapartum period. While every care has been taken to ensure this information is correct and up to date at the time of publication, it is intended as a guide only and midwives are advised to confirm information by referring to the NMC, local protocols and the British National Formulary (BNF) or MIMS which are updated as new evidence emerges.

Facts

- Most medicines the midwife supplies or administers are covered under *midwife exemptions*.
- Midwifery practice is subject to medicines legislation: the Medicines Act 1968, the Misuse of Drugs Act 1971, the Midwives Rules and Standards (NMC, 2004) and the NMC (2007) Standards for Medicines Management.
- Midwives should expect their supervisor of Midwives (SOM) to audit their drug administration records periodically (NMC, 2004).
- A woman has the right to use homeopathic and herbal medicines. However, if the midwife believes that using the medicines might be counterproductive she should discuss this with the woman (NMC, 2004).
- Midwives practising outside their employing authority, or outside the NHS, should seek advice from their SOM regarding any matters related to the supply, administration, storage, surrender and destruction of controlled drugs and other medicines (NMC, 2004).

- A woman who has not used a controlled drug, which has been prescribed by her general practitioner, can return the drug to the pharmacist from where it was obtained. Midwives must not do this for her. Alternatively, the woman can choose to destroy it – ideally with the midwife as a witness (NMC, 2004).

Drugs are classified as:

- **General sales list (GSL):** obtainable from retail outlets, e.g. supermarkets.
- **Pharmacy (P):** no prescription required but can only be bought from a pharmacy.
- **Prescription only medicines (POM):** may only be sold or supplied with a prescription.

Midwives and the supply and administration of medicines

Midwives exemptions

Provided it is in the course of their practice, registered midwives can *supply* and *administer*, on their own initiative, any medicines specified under midwives exemptions.
    Under these exemptions midwives may supply/administer:

- Without the need for a prescription or patient-specific written direction from a medical practitioner.
- Without the need for a patient group direction (PGD).

What medicines are covered by **midwives exemptions?**

All 'General sales list' medicines
All 'Pharmacy' medicines

- Examples of P and GSL medicines that midwives commonly use in their practice are paracetamol (GSL/P), oral iron preparations (P), oral laxatives (GSL/P) and entonox (P) (Royal College of Midwives (RCM), 2006).
  Certain 'Prescription Only medicines' are also covered
- Midwives can supply/administer specific POM in the course of their practice. These POMs are listed by the NMC (2004) and the RCM (2006).
- Examples of POMs the midwife can administer under the exemptions include diamorphine (heroin), lignocaine, oxytocins, pethidine hydrochloride and phytomenadione (vitamin K).
- Intravenous fluids are not covered under midwives exemptions.
- Any medicine covered under the midwife exemptions that appears in the pharmacopoeia below has been highlighted with*.

Standing orders

Many midwives work in units that provide standing orders. Standing orders may be helpful simply because they give written guidance on the route of administration, dosage and specific circumstances where midwives may supply and administer medicines.
    However, standing orders are not required in law under the current legislation and the actual term 'standing order' does not exist in any medicines legislation (NMC, 2005).

The NMC states that there is no legal requirement to replace standing orders with patient group directions if the administration and supply of medicines on standing orders is covered under the midwives exemptions.

Patient group directions

Patient group directions (PGDs) provide a local framework for the supply and administration of medicines by certain health professionals without a prescription. These medicines are approved for supply/administration by local doctors and pharmacists for patients in pre-identified clinical situations.

This is a complex topic and there is much confusion about whether midwives should be involved in PGDs. Part of the confusion is due to the fact that PGDs are intended for all health professionals, not just midwives.

- Most POMs the midwife uses are covered under midwives exemptions. If this is not the case, the midwife will require either a prescription or a PGD.
- None of the midwives exemptions has been replaced by the legislation concerning PGDs and there is, therefore, no legal requirement to move all existing locally agreed policies into PGDs.
- PGDs are not a form of prescribing, and while midwives should ideally be involved in drawing up and signing off PGDs, a PGD *must* be signed off by a doctor and pharmacist involved in the PGD development (NMC, 2007).
- PGDs can only be administered by midwives named in each PGD document: PGD administration cannot be delegated.

See also PGD guidance under 'Useful contacts'.

Documentation, record keeping and drug errors

Midwives are required to keep accurate, detailed records of the supply/administration of all medicines. Below are the guidelines for best practice adapted from the NMC.

Safety and good practice

- Correctly identify the woman or baby to whom the medicine is to be administered.
- Check that the woman is not allergic to the medicine before administration.
- Consider the dosage, method of administration, route and timing in the context of the woman's condition and any co-existing therapies.
- Check that the prescription, or the label on the medicine dispensed by a pharmacist, is clearly written and unambiguous.
- Check the expiry date.

Documentation

- Document immediately all medicines administered; avoid abbreviations.
- Ensure that all written entries are clear and legible, accurately dated, timed and signed with the signature printed alongside the first entry.
- Clearly countersign the signature of any student who is being supervised in the administration of medicines.

Errors in drug administration

- If a midwife makes or identifies an error in the administration of a drug, it should be reported immediately to the prescriber and the line manager/employer. A practising midwife should also inform their named SOM (RCM, 2006; NMC, 2007). Any error or near miss should be reported to the local risk management team.

To avoid errors in drug administration the NMC recommends that:

- A second *registered professional* checks any complex drug calculation.
- It is unacceptable to prepare substances for injection in advance of their immediate use. A practitioner does not administer medication drawn up by another practitioner when not in their presence (NMC, 2007).

The NMC supports the use of critical incident procedures for clinical errors but urges managers, when considering disciplinary action in relation to the administration of medicines to distinguish between:

'those cases where the error was the result of reckless or incompetent practice or was concealed, and those that resulted from other causes, such as serious pressure of work, and where there was immediate, honest disclosure in the patient's interest' (NMC, 2007).

Common abbreviations

The Joint Formulary Committee (2007) states that prescriptions should be in English without abbreviation; however, they do acknowledge that some abbreviations are used. Because of this, midwives should be able to use or interpret the abbreviations and their meaning (see Tables 24.1–24.3).

Table 24.1   Route of administration.

Abbreviation	Route of administration
IM	Intramuscular
IV	Intravenous
sc	Subcutaneous
po *per oram*	Oral
pr *per rectum*	Rectal
pv *per vaginum*	Vaginal

Drug calculations

Formula for liquids:

$$\frac{\text{What you want}}{\text{What you have}} \times \text{volume} = \text{dose to be administered}$$

100 mg of penicillin is prescribed; it comes as a preparation of 125 mg of penicillin in 5 ml solution

Example:

$$\frac{100 \text{ mg}}{125 \text{ mg}} \times 5 \text{ ml} = 4 \text{ ml}$$

Table 24.2   Frequency of drug administration.

Abbreviation	Frequency
stat	Immediately
od *omni die*	Once a day
bd *bis die*	Twice a day
tds *ter die sumendus*	Three times a day
qds *quatre die sumendus*	Four times a day
nocte	At night
prn *pro re nata*	As needed
hrly	Hourly

Table 24.3   Units of measurement.

Abbreviation	Unit
μg or mcg	Microgram
ng	Manogram
mg	Milligram
g	Gram
kg	Kilogram
ml or mL	Millilitre
l or L	Litre
IU	International units
mU	Milliunits

Pharmacopoeia of intrapartum drugs

Listed in *alphabetical order* below are some of the commonest drugs used in the intrapartum period. Drugs used in resuscitation are not listed here; please refer to Chapter 17 for more information.

Substances covered under midwife exemptions that appear in the list below have been highlighted with *.

IV fluids are not covered under midwives exemptions, so for example if it is planned to administer any drugs covered by midwife exemptions (e.g. syntocinon) in IV fluids, a prescription or PGD would be required.

Drug: Atosiban (Tractocile®)
(POM)
Action: Myometrial relaxant.
Dosage and frequency: **IV injection**:
- 6.75 mg over 1 min
- Followed by IV infusion 18 mg/hr for 3 hours - then 6 mg/hr

Maximum treatment duration 48 hours.

Indications: To delay uncomplicated preterm delivery 24–33 weeks gestation: allowing administration of corticosteroid therapy or transfer to specialist unit, following which there is no benefit in continuing the infusion (Royal College of Obstetricians and Gynaecologists (RCOG), 2002).

Route: IV bolus/infusion.

Contraindications: Severe pre-eclampsia or eclampsia, active bleeding/placenta praevia (as betamimetics relax the uterus); fetal death, preterm rupture of membranes >30 weeks and/or infection (where there is probably no benefit to stop labour) (Keirse, 2000; RCOG, 2002).

Side effects: Tachycardia, nausea, vomiting, hypotension, headache, dizziness, hot flushes, hyperglycaemia, less commonly rash, fever, pruritus.

Cautions: Intrauterine growth restriction; hepatic and renal impairment. Monitor postnatal blood loss.

Note: RCOG (2002) suggests 'it is reasonable not to use tocolytic drugs, as there is no clear evidence that they improve perinatal outcome' although as stated they may gain time if necessary, e.g. intrapartum transfer to a specialist centre. Tocolytic drugs have serious side effects; nifedipine (not licenced for this use in the UK) or atosiban is more effective and has fewer adverse effects than ritodrine (RCOG, 2002).

Drug: Betamethasone/dexamethasone (POM)

Action: Anti-inflammatory.

Dosage and frequency:
- 12 mg first dose.
- 12 mg second dose 12 hours later.

Indications: Prophylactic treatment administered to the mother at risk of preterm birth to promote surfactant production encouraging fetal lung maturation.

Route: Oral, IM.

Contraindications: Systemic infection (unless responding to appropriate treatment). Refer to JFC (2008).

Side effects: Side effects from steriods can be numerous, although these are often associated with longer-term steroid use and are listed extensively in the British National Formulary of drugs (BNF) (JFC, 2008).

Repeated prenatal exposure may suppress adrenal function in the baby but is rarely clinically significant (JFC, 2008); ongoing research is exploring possible more serious endocrine defects.

Cautions: Diabetes in the mother.

Note: See BNF for other uses of corticosteroids. Their use described here relates solely to prophylactic administration in threatened preterm labour. Every effort should be made to administer a prophylactic corticosteroid regime when clinical features indicate a possible preterm delivery (Confidential Enquiry into Stillbirths and Deaths in Infancy (CESDI), 2003; Roberts & Dalziel, 2007).

Drug: Bupivacaine/ropivacaine hydrochloride (Naropin®)
(POM)

Action: Local anaesthetic.

Dosage: Adjusted by the anaesthetist according to the woman's physical status and weight.
  Initial labour lumbar block:
  • *Bupivacaine:* 3–6 ml depending on concentration,
  • *Ropivacaine:* 10–20 ml 2 mg/ml solution.
  Continuous epidural infusion in labour (once block established):
  • *Bupivacaine:* 10–15 mg/h of 0.1% (1 mg/ml) or 0.125% (1.25 mg/ml) solution.
  • *Ropivacaine:* 6–14 ml/h of 0.2% (2 mg/ml) solution.

Indications: Regional local anaesthetic for labour pain, caesarean section, post-delivery procedures (e.g. suturing, manual removal of placenta).

Route: Lumbar epidural/spinal.

Contraindications: Hypovolaemia, hypotension, maternal infection, coagulation disorder or ongoing coagulation treatment, cardiac/respiratory impairment, epilepsy, complete heart block (JFC, 2008).

Side effects: Central nervous system effects: respiratory depression, convulsions, hypotension and bradycardia, also pyrexia and leg weakness. Ropivacaine may reduce risk of cardiac symptoms.

Note: Epidural/spinal anaesthesia can have secondary effects, i.e. poor mobility and less upright position leading to prolonged labour, increased fetal malposition, increased oxytocin augmentation and perineal trauma due to increased instrumental delivery (Leighton & Halpern, 2002; Lieberman & O'Donaghue, 2002; Howell, 2004). There may also be more subtle effects on natural mothering behaviour: maternal endorphin levels appear lower with epidurals (Abboud *et al.*, 1983).

Drug: Codeine, dihydrocodeine and paracetamol preparations* (including
(POM/P)   Co-codamol®, Co-dydramol®)

Action: Analgesic.

Dosage and frequency: 1–2 tablets 4–6 hourly; maximum dose 8 tablets in 24 h.

Indications:	Moderate postnatal pain (not recommended for pregnancy use).
Route:	Oral.
Contraindications:	Hepatic or renal disease, alcohol dependence, acute respiratory depression.
Side effects:	Commonly constipation, less commonly weakness, dizziness, sedation, nausea and vomiting, abdominal pain, rash, headache, euphoria, dysphoria hallucinations and minor visual disturbances. Rarely blood disorders. Overdose causes liver damage (EMC, 2006).
Note:	Different preparations have different ratios of opioid component combined with paracetamol. Co-codamol comes in 8 mg or (usually) 30 mg opioid component combined with 500 mg paracetamol; co-dydramol 10/500 ratio.

**Drug: Diclofenac sodium (Voltarol®)
(POM)**

Action:	Non-steroidal anti-inflammatory (NSAID).
Dosage and frequency:	50–150 mg doses; may be divided into 2–3 smaller doses; maximum 150 mg in 24 h (JFC, 2008).
Indications:	Pain and inflammation, usually for postnatal or post-operative analgesia. Not suitable for pregnancy use.
Route:	Oral (preferably after food), PR or IM.
Contraindications:	Pregnancy, hypersensitivity to aspirin or other NSAID drugs (JFC, 2008).
Side effects:	Gastric irritability, nausea, diarrhoea, ulceration, coagulation disorders leading to haemorrhage, headache, dizziness and vertigo. Suppositories may cause localised rectal irritation (JFC, 2008).
Cautions:	Asthma. Can also interact with other drugs, including analgesics, beta-blockers and hypertensives *causing increased hypertensive effects*, and in beta-blockers antagonism of hypertensive effects (JFC, 2008).
Note:	Diclofenac 100 mg suppository PR post-suturing is the drug of choice for postnatal perineal pain: it is an effective method of pain relief lasting around 24 hours (Dodd *et al.*, 2004).

**Drug: Entonox®/Equanox® (nitrous oxide and oxygen)*
(P)**

Action:	Analgesic.
Dosage and frequency:	Self-administered as required.
Indications:	Pain in labour.
Route:	Inhaled via a mask or mouthpiece.
Contraindications:	None.

Side effects:	Drowsiness, dry mouth, occasionally nausea and vomiting (Bannister, 2004). Suggested long-term high exposure risks for staff include miscarriage, myeloneuropathy and infertility for women (Rowland *et al.*, 1992; Ahlborg *et al.*, 1996a, b) and reduced fertility in men (Blair *et al.*, 1968).

Drug: Ergometrine maleate[*]
(POM)

Action:	Uterotonic oxytocic.
Dosage and frequency:	250–500 µg; maximum of two doses (as either Syntometrine or ergometrine).
Indications:	Postpartum haemorrhage (PPH) from uterine atony.
Route:	IM, or IV for quicker action.
Contraindications:	See Syntometrine.
Side effects:	Nausea, vomiting, hypertension, headaches, bradycardia, palpitations, dyspnoea, severe afterpains and rarely stroke and myocardial infarction (JFC, 2008).
Cautions:	Do not exceed two doses of ergometrine. Preferably placenta delivered prior to administration. Cardiac disease, hypertension, hepatic/renal impairment (JFC, 2008).
Note:	See also Syntometrine.

Drug: Hemabate® (Carboprost) (stored in fridge)
(POM)

Action:	Uterotonic prostaglandin.
Dosage and frequency:	• 250 µg (1 ml) deep IM injection • Repeat at 90 min intervals; • In severe cases the interval can be reduced – but no closer than 15 min apart **Maximum dose 2 mg (8 doses)** (JFC, 2008).
Indications:	Severe PPH unresponsive to oxytocin or ergometrine.
Route:	IM (give deep into the muscle).
Contraindications:	Cardiopulmonary hepatic or renal disease, untreated pelvic infection. Exercise caution in clients with a history of asthma, glaucoma, hypertension, hypotension, anemia, jaundice, diabetes or epilepsy.
Side effects:	Nausea, vomiting, flushing, headache, hyperthermia, diarrhoea hypertension, wheezing, asthma, hypertension and, very rarely, cardiovascular collapse. This drug will probably make the woman feel nauseated and very unwell. Common transient side effects usually pass when therapy ends (Pharmacia & Upjohn, 2002).
Note:	Risks, contraindications and side effects may be of secondary importance as this drug is only used in extreme circumstances; such concerns may be secondary to the immediate problem of catastrophic haemorrhage.

Drug: **Hydralazine hydrochloride**
(POM)

Action:	Antihypertensive.
Dosage and frequency:	Oral: 25–50 mg bd (maximum 50 mg bd).

IV usually titrated against the woman's blood pressure in labour.

By slow IV injection:

- 5–10 mg diluted with 10 ml sodium chloride 0.9%.
- 5 mg IV may be repeated after 20 min.
- Maximum cumulative dose 20 mg, i.e. 4 doses of 5 mg IV over 80 min (DoH, 2001).

By IV infusion:

- 200–300 µg/min initially, maintenance usually 50–150 µg/min.

Indications:	Moderate to severe hypertension.
Route:	Oral, IV injection or IV infusion.
Contraindications:	Idiopathic systemic lupus erythematosus, severe tachycardia, high output heart failure, myocardial insufficiency due to mechanical obstruction.
Side effects:	Tachycardia, palpitations, flushing, hypotension, fluid retention, gastrointestinal disturbances, headache, dizziness.
Cautions:	Consider colloid bolus of up to 500 ml (but no more) before treatment is initiated to maintain uteroplacental circulation. Anaesthetics enhance the drug's hypotensive effects (Bannister, 2004).

Drug: **Labetalol**
(POM)

Action:	Antihypertensive (beta-blocker).
Dosage and frequency:	**Oral:** 100 mg bd with food, increased at intervals of 14 days to usual dose of 200 mg bd; maximum daily dose 2.4 g.

IV injection: 50 mg over at least 1 min. Repeat after 5 min (maximum IV dose 200 mg).

IV infusion: 2 mg/min until satisfactory response then discontinue; usual total dose 50–200 mg.

Indications:	Hypertension in pregnancy, acute hypertension in labour.
Route:	Oral, IV.
Contraindications:	Asthma, bronchospasm.
Side effects:	Postural hypotension, tiredness, weakness, headache, rashes, scalp tingling, difficult micturation.
Cautions:	Avoid abrupt withdrawal (JFC, 2008).

Drug: **Lignocaine hydrochloride or lidocaine hydrochloride***
(POM)

Action:	Local anaesthetic

Dosage:	5–20 ml, depending on concentration and effectiveness 0.5% (5 mg/ml), 1% (10 mg/ml), 2% (20 mg/ml). Maximum dose 200 mg.
Indications:	Prior to performing an episiotomy or for suturing. (This drug is also used to treat specific cardiac problems including ventricular arrhythmias; see BNF.)
Route:	Tissue infiltration by injection.
Contraindications:	Cardiac problems including bradycardia, sinoatrial disorders and complete heart block.
Side effects:	Dizziness, paraesthesia, drowsiness, hypovolaemia, hypotension, bradycardia, rarely anaphylaxis, respiratory depression, convulsions; may lead to cardiac arrest (JFC, 2008).
Cautions:	Epilepsy, hepatic or respiratory or cardiac impairment, bradycardia.
Note:	Take care to avoid IV injection during perineal repair; this can lead to central nervous system excitory response including drowsiness, convulsions and respiratory arrest (Bannister, 2004).

Drug: Magnesium sulphate (POM)

Action:	Prevention of recurrent seizures in eclampsia.
Dosage and frequency:	Regimes vary between hospitals.

Loading dose:
- 4 g slowly by IV infusion pump over 5–15 min.
- 1 g/hour for at least 24 hours after last seizure or 24 hours after delivery.

Subsequent seizures should be treated:
- Further 2 g bolus (4 g if body weight ≥70 kg).
- Increase of infusion rate to 1.5 g or 2 g/hour.

Indications:	Severe pre-eclampsia, where there is a real and imminent risk of fitting (unlicenced), or following an actual eclamptic fit (licenced). Diazepam and phenytoin should *no longer* be used as first-line drugs following a fit: magnesium sulphate is the therapy of choice (Collaborative Eclampsia Trial, 1995; RCOG, 2006a).
Route:	IV
Contraindications:	–
Side effects:	Generally associated with hypermagnesaemia: nausea, vomiting, thirst, skin flushing, hypotension, arrhythmias, coma, respiratory depression, drowsiness, confusion, loss of tendon reflexes, muscle weakness.
Cautions:	Monitor for overdose, i.e. blood pressure, respiratory rate, urinary output and observe for signs of toxicity, e.g. confusion, slurred speech and loss of reflexes (see Chapter 19 for more detail). *Calcium gluconate injection* is used for the management of magnesium toxicity (JFC, 2008).

Drug: Naloxone hydrochloride
(POM)

Action:	Opioid antagonist (reversal of opioid-induced respiratory depression).
Dosage and frequency:	Given by weight either as a single IM dose: 200 µg (60 µg/kg) or 10 µg/kg repeated every 2–3 min
Indications:	Its use at birth is only for newborns *failing to respond to active resuscitation* and who have *received opiates* transplacentally in labour (see Chapter 17 on p. 246).
Route:	IM, SC, or IV.
Contradictions:	Maternal physical dependence on opioids (precipitates withdrawal) (JFC, 2008).
Side effects:	Nausea, vomiting, tachycardia, and fibrillation (JFC, 2008).
Cautions:	Has short duration of action (repeated doses or infusion may be necessary to reverse the effects of opioids with longer duration of action). The baby must be observed and monitored following administration.
Notes:	Gill and Colvin (2007) found many practitioners give naloxone inappropriately and often fail to monitor the baby following its administration. Their review highlights the potentially adverse effects of naloxone, scant evidence to support its use and questions whether it should be available on labour ward resuscitaires (Gill & Colvin, 2007).

Drug: Oxytocin (Syntocinon®) (stored in fridge)*
(POM)

Action:	Stimulates uterine contractions
Dosage:	Labour induction/augmentation (based on National Institute for Health and Clinical Excellence (NICE) 2001 guidelines): To reduce error, a standard dilution should always be used.

Suggested standardised dilutions and dose regimens include:

IV infusion:

30 IU in 500 ml normal saline; hence 1 ml/hour = 1 mU/min. Increase by 1 ml/hour at 30 min intervals until contracting 3–4:10 min (NICE, 2001).

Or

- 10 IU in 500 ml sodium chloride 0.9%; hence 3 ml/hour = 1 mU/min. Increase by 3 ml/hour at 30 min intervals until contracting 3–4:10 min (NICE, 2001).
- Most women should have adequate contractions at 12 mU/min; 20 mU/min is the maximum licenced dose.

Postpartum

- 10 IU IM (unlicenced route); this is the recommended choice of oxytocic as it reduces retained placenta (NICE, 2007).

- Can be given by slow IV bolus for faster action; but may cause transient hypotension if administered too rapidly (JFC, 2008).
- 10 IU IM (unlicenced route) instead of Syntometrine in hypertension (JFC, 2008).

Postpartum haemorrhage

- Oxytocin 10–30 IU in 500 ml infusion fluid given by IV infusion pump or device at a rate that controls uterine atony. Crafter (2002) notes that in practice sometimes ≥40 units used.

Do not confuse intrapartum and postpartum drug regimes, as large or bolus doses would be very dangerous if accidentally administered during labour.

Indications:	• Induction/augmentation of labour.
	• Active management for delivery of the placenta.
	• Retained placenta (see notes below).
	• Postpartum haemorrhage from uterine atony.
	• Use instead of Syntometrine or ergometrine in women with hypertension.
Route:	IV intrapartum, IM/IV postpartum.
Contraindications:	Hypertonic uterine contractions, fetal distress, severe pre-eclampsia and cardiovascular disease (Bannister, 2004).
Side effects:	**Maternal**: uterine hyperstimulation, hypotension, arrhythmias, nausea, vomiting, rash and anaphylaxis, placental abruption, amniotic fluid embolism, uterine spasm even at low dose. **Fetal**: heart rate abnormalities, asphyxia, intrauterine death.
Caution:	High doses and large volume infusion can cause water intoxication (JFC, 2008). Interactions can cause severe hypotension and arrhythmias when administered during anaesthetic (DoH, 2001). It can potentiate the effects of prostaglandins (Bannister, 2004).
Note:	In retained placenta: Syntocinon® may be administered into the maternal end of the umbilical cord to improve the chance of delivery (Carroli & Bergel, 2002); see Chapter 15 for more information.

Drug: Paracetamol* (GSL/P)

Action:	Analgesic.
Dosage and frequency:	500 mg to 1 g 4–6 hourly; maximum 4 g in 24 h.
Indications:	Mild to moderate pain, pyrexia.
Route:	Oral, PR.
Contraindications:	Hepatic or renal disease, alcohol dependence.
Side effects:	Rarely blood disorders, rashes; overdose causes liver damage.

Drug: **Pethidine hydrochloride***
(POM)

Action:	Opioid analgesic,
Dosage and frequency:	50–100 mg (maximum 400 mg in 24 h).
	50–100 mg 1–3 hourly depending on dosage. Maximum 400 mg in 24 hours. Smaller doses can be administered more frequently, including via patient-controlled analgesia (PCA); see BNF for more information.
Indications:	Short acting analgesia for moderate pain, also has a strong sedative effect. Not suitable for severe pain (JFC, 2008).
Route:	Usually administered IM, but occasionally oral, SC or via PCA.
Contraindications:	A compromised fetus, renal impairment, existing respiratory depression (Bannister, 2004; JFC, 2008).
Side effects:	**Maternal**: nausea, vomiting, drowsiness, respiratory depression, bradycardia, gastric stasis.
	Fetal/neonatal: crosses the placental barrier so can cause fetal bradycardia. It is only slowly excreted by the neonatal liver (Bannister, 2004), so may cause respiratory depression, drowsiness and depressed newborn reflexes including poor sucking (JFC, 2008).
Note:	Antiemetics should be given prophylactically with opioids (NICE, 2007).

Drug: **Prostaglandin PGE_2/dinoprostone (Prostin $E_2^{®}$)**
(POM)

Action:	Stimulates contractions.
Dosage:	Varies according to cervical favourability/maternal parity: Further dose after 6 hours depending on progress and parity.
	Gel
	• 1 mg or 2 mg
	• maximum gel dose: primigravida 4 mg, multigravida 3 mg.
	Vaginal tablets
	• 3 mg
	• maximum vaginal tablet dose: 6 mg for all women.
Indications:	Induction of labour.
Route:	Posterior fornix of vagina.
Contraindications:	Active cardiac, pulmonary, renal or hepatic disease, placenta praevia, unexplained vaginal bleeding during pregnancy, ruptured membranes, history of CS or major uterine surgery (JFC, 2008).
Side effects:	Nausea, vomiting, diarrhoea, uterine hypertonus, severe uterine contractions (many more: see BNF).
Cautions:	History of asthma, glaucoma/raised intra-ocular pressure, hepatic/renal impairment, hypertension, epilepsy (JFC, 2008).

Drug: **Ranitidine (Zantac®)***
(POM/P)

Action:	H₂ antagonist receptor.
Dosage and frequency:	150 mg at onset of labour then 6-hourly orally.
Indications:	Used for women at risk of CS as prophylaxis to reduce risk of acid aspiration/Mendelssohn's syndrome sometimes caused by general anaesthesia.
Route:	Oral (in labour), IV (pre-anaesthesia).
Contraindications:	Use with caution in pregnancy, breastfeeding, hepatic or renal impairment (JFC, 2008).
Side effects:	Gastrointestinal disturbance, headache, dizziness, rash and tiredness. Rarely bradycardia, AV block, confusion, agitation (JFC, 2008).

Drug: **Ritodrine hydrochloride (Yutopar®)**
(POM)

Action:	Myometrial relaxant.
Dosage and frequency:	Regimes vary. Commonly commenced at 50 µg/min, increased by 50 µg/min every 10 min until contractions stop or are <1:15 or maternal pulse 140 bpm. Stabilising dose is usually 150–350 µg/min. Maximum dose 350 µg/min (JFC, 2008).
Indications:	To delay uncomplicated preterm delivery (see also atosiban).
Route:	Oral, IV infusion.
Contraindications:	Cardiac disease, severe pre-eclampsia or eclampsia, active bleeding (as betamimetics relax the uterus) fetal death (JFC, 2008), preterm rupture of membranes and/or infection (in which there is probably no benefit to stopping labour) (Keirse, 2000).
Side effects:	Palpitations, tachycardia, chest pain, arrhythmias, tremor, nausea, vomiting, headache, thirst, hypokalaemia, restlessness and agitation, and, although rare, maternal death may result (JFC, 2008).
Cautions:	Avoided in diabetes (affects carbohydrate metabolism); hyperthyroidism, heart disease due to cardiovascular side effects, mild to moderate pre-eclampsia, hypertension, hypokalaemia (JFC, 2008). Stop the infusion if maternal HR >140 bpm or any chest pain or breathlessness (JFC, 2008).
Note:	See under notes for Atosiban. If hypotensive or abnormal fetal heart rate use left lateral position. Maintain fluid chart, as fluid overload may cause pulmonary oedema (RCOG, 2006b). Test maternal blood sugar and serum urea and electrolytes 6–12 hourly; auscultate chest 4–8 hourly for signs of oedema.

Drug: Syntometrine®*(oxytocin 5 IU and ergometrine maleate 500 µg)
(POM)   (stored in fridge)

Action:	Stimulates uterine contractions.
Dosage:	1 ml ampoule contains 5 IU Syntocinon oxytocin® and 0.5 mg ergometrine maleate. *Maximum dose* 1 mg ergometrine in either form, i.e. Syntometrine or ergometrine.
Indications:	For prevention or treatment of uterine haemorrhage.
Route:	IM only (JFC, 2008); takes >2 min to act (Crafter, 2002). Syntometrine lasts for several hours, as opposed to oxytocin alone which lasts for 30–60 min (Medsafe website).
Contraindications:	Labour, hypertension, pre-eclampsia/eclampsia, severe asthma, sepsis, renal impairment, hepatic/cardiac/pulmonary disease and some medical disorders (JFC, 2008).
Side effects:	Increased risk of retained placenta (NICE, 2007), nausea, vomiting, hypertension, headache, bradycardia, tinnitus, palpitations, chest pain, dyspnoea, severe afterpains and rarely stroke and myocardial infarction (JFC, 2008).
Caution:	Do not exceed 1 mg dose of ergometrine.
Note:	Avoid in retained placenta, as ergometrine maleate can close the cervical os, therefore Syntocinon® (oxytocin) is preferable (Crafter, 2002).

Drug: Vitamin K (phytomenadione)*/Konakion® MM paediatric
(POM)

Action:	Benefits manufacture of clotting agents.
Dosage and frequency:	In healthy neonates >36 weeks IM regime: • 1 mg/0.1 ml. Oral regime: • Oral 2 mg dose at birth. • Second 2 mg dose within first week. • Third 2 mg dose at 1 month – usually only in breastfed babies (JFC, 2008).
Indications:	NICE (2006) recommends all parents are offered IM vitamin K for their baby, and if this is declined should be offered an oral preparation as a 'second-line option'. Babies who receive vitamin K regime have a reduced risk of early onset haemorrhagic disease of the newborn (HDN).
Route:	IM (single dose); oral (2–3 dose regime).
Contraindications:	–
Side effects:	With IM administration in babies <36 weeks or small infants <2.5 kg, there is an increased risk of kernicterus and dose should be adjusted/reduced according to weight (Electronic Medicines Compendium, 2006).
Note:	In the UK >97% of babies receive vitamin K after birth (Ansell *et al.*, 2001). There is some debate about the routine use of Vitamin K (see Chapter 5).

Useful contacts

BNF (The British National Formulary)   A joint publication of the British Medical Association and the Royal Pharmaceutical Society of Great Britain aiming to give healthcare professionals up-to-date information about the use of medicines in the UK. It is published twice a year. Website: www.bnf.org

Electronic Medicines Compendium   Website: http://emc.medicines.org.uk

For PGD guidance   Website: www.portal.nelm.nhs.uk at www.nes.scot.nhs.uk/PGDs/ or 'maintaining competency in patient group directions' at www.npc.co.uk/

MIMS   Directory of prescription drugs and prescription medicine guidelines. Website: http://www.healthcarerepublic.com

NMC (The Nursing and Midwifery Council)   Information, guidelines, standards and rules on all aspects of midwifery practice including the supply and administration of drugs. Tel: 020 7637 7181. Website: www.nmc-uk.org.

References

Abboud, T., Sarkis, F., Hung, T., Khoo, S.S., Varakian, L., Henrickson, K., Noueihed, R. & Goebelsmann, L. (1983) Effects of epidural anaesthesia during labour on maternal plasma beta-endorphin levels. *Anaesthesiology* **59**, 1–5.

Ahlborg, G., Axelsson, G. & Bodin, L. (1996a) Shift work, nitrous oxide exposure and subfertility among Swedish midwives. *International Journal of Epidemiology* **25** (4), 783–90.

Ahlborg, G., Axelsson, G. & Bodin, L. (1996b) Shift work, nitrous oxide exposure and spontaneous abortion among Swedish midwives. *British Journal of Anaesthesia* **58** (12), 1348–56.

Ansell, P., Roman, E., Fear, N.T. & Renfrew, M.J. (2001) Vitamin K policies and midwives practice: questionnaire survey. *British Medical Journal* **322**, 150–52.

Bannister, C. (2004) *The Midwife's Pocket Formulary*, 2nd edn. Books for Midwives Press, Hale, Cheshire.

Blair, J., Steams, H. & Simpson, G. (1968) Vitamin B12 and fertility. *Lancet* **1** (7532), 49–50.

Carroli, G. & Bergel, E. (2002) Umbilical vein injection for management of retained placenta (Cochrane review). *Cochrane Database of Systematic Reviews*, Issue 4. Update Software, Oxford.

Collaborative Eclampsia Trial (1995) Which anticonvulsant for women with eclampsia? Evidence from the collaborative eclampsia trial. *Lancet* **345** (8963), 1455–63; erratum in *Lancet* 1995; **346**, 258.

Confidential Enquiry into Stillbirths and Deaths in Infancy (CESDI) (2003) *Project 27/28: An Enquiry into Quality and Care and Its Effects on Survival of Babies Born at 27/28 Weeks.* HMSO, London.

Crafter, H. (2002) Intrapartum and primary postpartum haemorrhage. In *Emergencies Around Childbirth – A Handbook for Midwives* (Boyle, M., ed.), pp. 113–26. Radcliffe Medical Press, Oxford.

Department of Health (DoH) (2001) *Why Mothers Die, 1997–1999. The Fifth Report of the Confidential Enquiries into Maternal Deaths in the United Kingdom.* Department of Health, RCOG Press, London.

Dodd, J.M., Hedayati, H., Pearce, E., Hotham, M. & Crowther, C.A. (2004) Rectal analgesia for the relief of pain after childbirth: a randomised controlled trial of diclofenac suppositories. *British Journal of Obstetrics and Gynaecology* **111** (10), 1059–64.

Electronic Medicines Compendium (2006) *Konakion MM Paediatric. Electronic Medicines Compendium.* Available at: http://emc.medicines.org.uk (accessed March 2008).

Gill, A. & Colvin, J. (2007) Use of naloxone during neonatal resuscitation in Australia: Compliance with published guidelines. *Journal of Paediatrics and Child Health* **43** (12), 795–8.

Howell, C. (2004) Epidural versus non-epidural analgesia for pain relief in labour (Cochrane Review). *Cochrane Library of Systematic Reviews*, Issue 1. Update Software, Oxford.

JFC Joint Formulary Committee (2008) *British National Formulary*, 55th edn. British Medical Association and Royal Pharmaceutical Society of Great Britain, London.

Keirse, M.J.N.C. (2000) Preterm birth. In *A Guide to Effective Care in Pregnancy and Childbirth*, 3rd edn (Enkin, M., Keirse, M.J.N.C., Neilson, J., Crowther, C., Duley L., Hodnett, E. & Hofmeyr, J., eds), pp. 214–23, 352. Oxford University Press, Oxford.

Leighton, B. & Halpern, S. (2002) The effects of epidural analgesia on labor, maternal and neonatal outcomes: a systematic review. *American Journal of Obstetrics and Gynecology* **186**, 69–77.

Lieberman, E. & O'Donaghue, C. (2002) Unintended effects of epidural analgesia in labor: a systematic review. *American Journal of Obstetrics and Gynecology* **186**, 531–68.

Medsafe data sheet: Available at: www.medsafe.gov.nz (accessed December 2007).

National Institute for Health and Clinical Excellence (NICE) (2001) *Clinical Guideline D – Induction of Labour*. National Institute for Health and Clinical Excellence, London.

National Institute for Health and Clinical Excellence (NICE) (2006) *Routine Postnatal Care of Women and Their Babies*. National Institute for Health and Clinical Evidence, London.

National Institute for Health and Clinical Excellence (NICE) (2007) *Clinical Guideline 55: Intrapartum Care*. National Institute for Clinical Excellence, London.

Nursing and Midwifery Council (NMC) (2004) *Midwives Rules and Standards*. Nursing and Midwifery Council, London.

Nursing and Midwifery Council (NMC) (2005) *Medicines Legislation: What It Means for Midwives*. Nursing and Midwifery Council, London.

Nursing and Midwifery Council (NMC) (2007) *Standards for Medicines Management*. Nursing and Midwifery Council, London.

Pharmacia & Upjohn (2002) *Hemabate Sterile Solution (Carboprost Tromethamine) Drug Company Literature for Physicians and Patients*. Pharmacia & Upjohn, a subsidiary of Pharmacia Corporation, Kalamazoo, MI, USA.

Roberts, D. & Dalziel, S. (2007) Antenatal corticosteroids for accelerating fetal lung maturation for women at risk of preterm birth (Cochrane Review). *Cochrane Database of Systemic Reviews*, Issue 4. Update Software, Oxford.

Rowland, A., Baird, D., Weinberg C., Shore, D., Shy, C. & Wilcox, A. (1992) Reduced fertility among women employed as dental nurses exposed to high levels of nitrous oxide. *New England Journal of Medicine* **327** (14), 993–7.

Royal College of Midwives (RCM) (2006) *Midwifery and Medicines Legislation: An Information Paper*. Royal College of Midwives, London. Available at: http://www.rcm.org.uk/info/pages/recentDocs.php (accessed December 2007).

Royal College of Obstetricians and Gynaecologists (RCOG) (2002) *Tocolytic Drugs for Women in Preterm Labour. RCOG Clinical Guideline No. 1(b)*. Royal College of Obstetricians and Gynaecologists, London.

Royal College of Obstetricians and Gynaecologists (RCOG) (2006a) *Management of Severe Pre-Eclampsia/Eclampsia. RCOG Clinical Guideline No 10a*. Royal College of Obstetricians and Gynaecologists, London.

Royal College of Obstetricians and Gynaecologists (RCOG) (2006b) *Preterm Prelabour Rupture of Membranes. RCOG Green-top Guideline No 44*. Royal College of Obstetricians and Gynaecologists, London.

Index

Boldface page numbers refer to key citations.